30ᵗʰ EDITION

MW00986397

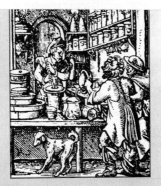

"Desire to take medicines ... distinguishes man from animals."
— Sir William Osler

Editor-in-Chief
Richard J. Hamilton, MD, FAAEM, FACMT, FACEP
Professor and Chair, Department of Emergency Medicine
Drexel University College of Medicine
Philadelphia, PA

JONES & BARTLETT
LEARNING

World Headquarters
Jones & Bartlett Learning
5 Wall Street
Burlington, MA 01803
978-443-5000
info@jblearning.com
www.jblearning.com

Jones & Bartlett Learning books and products are available through most bookstores and online booksellers. To contact Jones & Bartlett Learning directly, call 800-832-0034, fax 978-443-8000, or visit our website www.jblearning.com.

Substantial discounts on bulk quantities of Jones & Bartlett Learning publications are available to corporations, professional associations, and other qualified organizations. For details and specific discount information, contact the special sales department at Jones & Bartlett Learning via the above contact information or send an email to specialsales@jblearning.com.

The information in the *Pocket Pharmacopoeia* is compiled from sources believed to be reliable, and exhaustive efforts have been put forth to make the book as accurate as possible. The *Pocket Pharmacopoeia* is edited by a panel of drug information experts with extensive peer review and input from more than 50 practicing clinicians of multiple specialties. Our goal is to provide health professionals focused, core-prescribing information in a convenient, organized, and concise fashion. We include FDA-approved dosing indications and those off-label uses that have a reasonable basis to support their use. *However, the accuracy and completeness of this work cannot be guaranteed.* Despite our best efforts, this book may contain typographical errors and omissions. The *Pocket Pharmacopoeia* is intended as a quick and convenient reminder of information you have already learned elsewhere. The contents are to be used as a guide only, and healthcare professionals should use sound clinical judgment and individualize therapy to each specific patient care situation. This book is not meant to be a replacement for training, experience, continuing medical education, or studying the latest drug prescribing literature. This book is sold without warranties of any kind, expressed or implied, and the publisher and editors disclaim any liability, loss, or damage caused by the contents. Although drug companies purchase and distribute our books as promotional items, the Tarascon editorial staff alone determines all book content.

ISSN: 1945-9076

ISBN: 978-1-284-09529-6

6048

Printed in the United States of America

19 18 17 16 15 10 9 8 7 6 5 4 3 2 1

Production Credits

Chief Executive Officer: Ty Field
President: James Homer
V.P., Design and Production: Rebecca Goldthwaite
V.P., Manufacturing and Inventory Control: Therese Connell
Manufacturing and Inventory Control Supervisor: Amy Bacus
Executive Editor: Nancy Anastasi Duffy

Production Editor: Daniel Stone
Rights and Media Specialist: Wes DeShano
Digital Marketing Manager: Jennifer Sharp
Composition: Cenveo
Text and Cover Design: Anne Spencer/Kristin E. Parker
Printing and Binding: Cenveo
Cover Printing: Cenveo

If you obtained your *Pocket Pharmacopoeia* from a bookstore, please send your address to info@tarascon.com. This allows you to be the first to hear of updates! (We don't sell or distribute our mailing lists, by the way.)

The cover woodcut is *The Apothecary* by Jost Amman, Frankfurt, 1574.

Last year we asked about making calendars from numbered cubes. Popular desk calendars represent the 12 months of the year and the 31 days of the month using four cubes—for example 1,0,1,1 would be October 11th. What are the digits necessary on the six sides of each cube to represent every day of the year? The trick was to distribute the numbers this way: Cube one: 0,1,2,3,4,5; Cube two: 0,1,2,6,7,8; Cube three: 0,1,2,6,7,8; Cube four: 0,1,3,4,5,6; but you also need to know to flip the 6 to make a 9!

This year is much more pharmaco-logic. A patient is on an experimental regiment that requires of two very expensive medications: pill X and pill Y. Every day at the same time, the patient must take one X pill and one Y pill. One morning, while putting his medication into a pill cup, the patient accidentally puts in one X pill and two Y pills. Unfortunately, X and Y are both the same exact size and weight and are white, scored, uncoated tablets with no markings. They are indistinguishable from each other. The pills are expensive so he cannot just throw them out and start over and they MUST be taken together at the exact dose. What can the patient do to make sure that he only takes one X pill and one Y pill from these three pills?

CONTENTS

ANALGESICS......................1
Muscle Relaxants...............1
Non-Opioid Analgesic
  Combinations....................2
Non-Steroidal Anti-
  Inflammatories.................3
Opioid Agonist-
  Antagonists......................6
Opioid Agonists..................6
Opioid Analgesic
  Combinations....................9
Opioid Antagonists............11
Other Analgesics...............11
ANESTHESIA..................13
Anesthetics and
  Sedatives.........................13
Local Anesthetics.............13
Neuromuscular Blockade...14
Neuromuscular Blockers....14
ANTIMICROBIALS..........15
Aminoglycosides...............29
Antifungal Agents.............29
Antimalarials.....................31
Antimycobacterial Agents..32
Antiparasitics....................33
Antiviral Agents................35
Carbapenems....................48
Cephalosporins.................49
Glycopeptides...................51
Macrolides........................51
Penicillins.........................52
Quinolones........................54
Sulfonamides....................55
Tetracyclines....................56
Other Antimicrobials.........59
CARDIOVASCULAR........59
ACE Inhibitors..................65
Aldosterone Antagonists...66
Angiotensin Receptor
  Blockers (ARBs)..............66
Antiadrenergic
  Agents.............................67
Anti-Dysrhythmics/
  Cardiac Arrest................68
Antihypertensives............72
Antihyperlipidemic
  Agents.............................75
Antiplatelet Drugs.............79
Beta-Blockers...................81
Calcium Channel
  Blockers (CCBs)..............84

Diuretics...........................85
Nitrates............................87
Pressors/Inotropes...........88
Pulmonary Arterial
  Hypertension...................88
Thrombolytics...................90
Volume Expanders............91
Other................................91
CONTRAST MEDIA........93
MRI Contrast....................93
Radiography Contrast.......93
DERMATOLOGY............95
Acne Preparations............95
Actinic Keratosis
  Preparations....................98
Antibacterials (Topical)....98
Antifungals (Topical).........99
Antiparasitics (Topical)...100
Antipsoriatics.................101
Antivirals (Topical).........102
Atopic Dermatitis
  Preparations..................102
Corticosteroid/Antimicrobial
  Combinations.................103
Hemorrhoid Care.............103
Other Dermatologic
  Agents...........................103
**ENDOCRINE AND
  METABOLIC**.............107
Androgens/Anabolic
  Steroids.........................110
Bisphosphonates.............111
Corticosteroids...............112
Diabetes-Related............113
Diagnostic Agents...........120
Minerals.........................120
Nutritionals....................123
Phosphate Binders..........123
Thyroid Agents...............124
Vitamins.........................124
Other..............................127
ENT............................129
Antihistamines................130
Antitussives /
  Expectorants.................132
Combination Products.....132
Decongestants...............132
Ear Preparations.............133
Mouth and Lip
  Preparations..................134
Nasal Preparations.........134

GASTROENTEROLOGY.....137
Antidiarrheals.................137
Antiemetics.....................138
Antiulcer.........................140
Laxatives........................143
Ulcerative Colitis............146
Other GI Agents..............146
**HEMATOLOGY/
  ANTICOAGULANTS**......149
Anticoagulants................149
Colony-Stimulating
  Factors...........................155
Other Hematological
  Agents...........................155
**HERBAL AND ALTERNATIVE
  THERAPIES**.................157
IMMUNOLOGY..............163
Immunizations.................163
Immunoglobulins.............167
Immunosuppression.........167
Other..............................168
NEUROLOGY................169
Alzheimer's Disease........169
Anticonvulsants..............170
Migraine Therapy............175
Multiple Sclerosis...........176
Myasthenia Gravis..........177
Parkinsonian Agents........177
Other Agents...................179
OB/GYN.......................181
Contraceptives................184
Estrogens........................186
GnRH Agents...................187
Hormone Combinations....187
Labor Induction /
  Cervical Ripening...........188
Ovulation Stimulants.......188
Progestins.......................189
Selective Estrogen
  Receptor Modulators......189
Uterotonics.....................189
Vaginitis Preparations.....189
Other OB/GYN Agents.....190
ONCOLOGY...................191
OPHTHALMOLOGY.........193
Antiallergy......................193
Antibacterials.................194
Antiviral Agents..............195
Corticosteroid &
  Antibacterial
  Combinations.................195

Corticosteroids 196
Glaucoma Agents 197
Mydriatics & Cycloplegics..199
Non-Steroidal
  Anti-Inflammatories ..199
Other Ophthalmologic
  Agents.......................200
PSYCHIATRY.................201
Antidepressants 201
Antimanic (Bipolar)
  Agents......................205
Antipsychotics 207
Anxiolytics/Hypnotics......210

Combination Drugs 212
Drug Dependence Therapy.212
Stimulants/ADHD/
  Anorexiants................213
PULMONARY.................217
Beta Agonists 219
Combinations.................220
Inhaled Steroids 221
Leukotriene Inhibitors......222
Other Pulmonary
  Medications...............222
RHEUMATOLOGY...........225
Biologic Response
  Modifiers....................225

Disease-Modifying
  Antirheumatic Drugs ...228
Gout-Related..................230
Other 230
TOXICOLOGY.................231
UROLOGY......................233
Benign Prostatic
  Hyperplasia 233
Bladder Agents..............233
Erectile Dysfunction 234
Nephrolithiasis 235
INDEX..........................237
APPENDIX....................271

PAGE INDEX FOR TABLES

GENERAL
Abbreviations ix
Therapeutic drug levels.....x
Pediatric drugs...............xi
Pediatric vital signs and
  IV drugs.....................xii
Conversions.....................xii
P450 isozymes.................xiii
Inhibitors, inducers,
  and substrates of
  P-Glycoprotein xvi
Drug therapy reference
  websites xvii
Adult emergency drugs ...271
Cardiac dysrhythmia
  protocols..................272

ANALGESICS
Opioid equivalency 1
NSAIDs 4
Fentanyl transdermal.........7

ANTIMICROBIALS
Prophylaxis for bacterial
  endocarditis................15
Overview of bacterial
  pathogens...................15
Acute bacterial sinusitis in
  adults and children.......18
Anthrax: CDC and AAP
  Preferred Regimens 19
C. difficile infection
  in adults.....................21
Acute otitis media in
  children......................22
STDs/vaginitis.................24
Antiviral drugs for
  influenza.....................46

Cephalosporins.................49
Penicillins......................52
Quinolones......................54

CARDIOVASCULAR
ACE inhibitors.................59
Cardiac parameters.........59
Lipid change by class/
  agent..........................60
Cholesterol treatment
  recommendations.........61
HTN therapy....................62
QT interval drugs.............63
High- and moderate-intensity
  statin doses................64
Thrombolytic therapy for
  STEMI.........................64
Antihypertensive
  Combinations...............72

DERMATOLOGY
Topical steroids..............95

ENDOCRINE
A1C reduction in type 2
  diabetes....................107
IV solutions...................107
Corticosteroids 108
Diabetes numbers...........108
Injectable insulins 116
Fluoride
  supplementation..........121
Potassium (oral forms).....123

ENT
ENT combinations 129

GASTROENTEROLOGY
H. pylori treatment 137

HEMATOLOGY
Enoxaparin adult dosing...151

Heparin dosing for ACS...151
Heparin dosing for
  DVT/PE......................152
Warfarin—Selected Drug
  Interactions 153
Therapeutic goals for
  anticoagulation...........154

IMMUNOLOGY
Adult Immunizations 163
Childhood
  Immunizations............164
Tetanus 165

NEUROLOGY
Dermatomes..................169
Glasgow coma scale.... ..169

OB/GYN
Emergency
  contraception...............181
Oral contraceptives........181
Drugs in pregnancy........184

PSYCHIATRY
Body mass index 201
Antipsychotics 206

PULMONARY
Inhaler colors................217
Inhaled steroids 218
Peak flow......................219

RHEUMATOLOGY
Initial treatment of
  RA.............................225
Colchicine dosage
  reductions..................229

TOXICOLOGY
Antidotes......................231

*Affiliations are given for information purposes only, and no affiliation sponsorship is claimed.

PREFACE TO THE TARASCON POCKET PHARMACOPOEIA®

The *Tarascon Pocket Pharmacopoeia®* arranges drugs by clinical class with a comprehensive index in the back. Trade names are italicized and capitalized. Drug doses shown in mg/kg are generally intended for children, while fixed doses represent typical adult recommendations. Brackets indicate currently available formulations, although not all pharmacies stock all formulations. The availability of generic, over-the-counter, and scored formulations is mentioned. We have set the disease or indication in red for the pharmaceutical agent. It is meant to function as an aid to find information quickly. Codes are as follows:

▶ **METABOLISM & EXCRETION:** **L** = primarily liver, **K** = primarily kidney, **LK** = both, but liver > kidney, **KL** = both, but kidney > liver.

♀ **SAFETY IN PREGNANCY:** **A** = Safety established using human studies, **B** = Presumed safety based on animal studies, **C** = Uncertain safety; no human studies and animal studies show an adverse effect, **D** = Unsafe - evidence of risk that may in certain clinical circumstances be justifiable, **X** = Highly unsafe - risk of use outweighs any possible benefit. For drugs that have not been assigned a category: **+** = Generally accepted as safe, **?** Safety unknown or controversial, **−** Generally regarded as unsafe. **NOTE:** As of June 2015, the FDA no longer uses letter categories to describe pregnancy risk.

▶ **SAFETY IN LACTATION:** **+** = Generally accepted as safe, **?** Safety unknown or controversial, **−** Generally regarded as unsafe. Many of our "+" listings are from the AAP policy "The Transfer of Drugs and Other Chemicals Into Human Milk" (see www.aap.org) and may differ from those recommended by the manufacturer.

© **DEA CONTROLLED SUBSTANCES:** **I** = High abuse potential, no accepted use (e.g., heroin, marijuana), **II** = High abuse potential and severe dependence liability (e.g., morphine, codeine, hydromorphone, cocaine, amphetamines, methylphenidate, secobarbital). Some states require triplicates. **III** = Moderate dependence liability (e.g., *Tylenol #3, Vicodin*), **IV** = Limited dependence liability (benzodiazepines, propoxyphene, phentermine), **V** = Limited abuse potential (e.g., *Lomotil*).

$ **RELATIVE COST:** Cost codes used are "per month" of maintenance therapy (e.g., antihypertensives) or "per course" of short-term therapy (e.g., antibiotics). Codes are calculated using average wholesale prices (at press time in US dollars) for the most common indication and route of each drug at a typical adult dosage. For maintenance therapy, costs are calculated based upon a 30-day supply or the quantity that might typically be used in a given month. For short-term therapy (i.e., 10 days or less), costs are calculated on a single treatment course. When multiple forms are available

Code	Cost
$	< $25
$$	$25 to $49
$$$	$50 to $99
$$$$	$100 to $199
$$$$$	≥ $200

(e.g., generics), these codes reflect the least expensive generally available product. When drugs don't neatly fit into the classification scheme above, we have assigned codes based upon the relative cost of other similar drugs. *These codes should be used as a rough guide only*, as (1) they reflect cost, not charges, (2) pricing often varies substantially from location to location and time to time, and (3) HMOs, Medicaid, and buying groups often negotiate quite different pricing. Check with your local pharmacy if you have any questions.

🍁 **CANADIAN TRADE NAMES:** Unique common Canadian trade names not used in the US are listed after a maple leaf symbol. Trade names used in both nations or only in the US are displayed without such notation.

■ **BLACK BOX WARNINGS:** This icon indicates that there is a black box warning associated with this drug. Note that the warning itself is not listed.

ABBREVIATIONS IN TEXT

AAP	American Academy of Pediatrics	h	hour
ACCP	American College of Chest Physicians	HAART	highly active antiretroviral therapy
ACR	American College of Rheumatology	Hb	hemoglobin
ACT	activated clotting time	HBV	hepatitis B virus
ADHD	attention deficit hyperactivity disorder	HCTZ	hydrochlorothiazide
AHA	American Heart Association	HCV	hepatitis C virus
Al	aluminum	HIT	heparin-induced thrombocytopenia
ANC	absolute neutrophil count	HPV	human papillomavirus
ASA	aspirin	HSV	herpes simplex virus
BP	blood pressure	HTN	hypertension
BPH	benign prostatic hyperplasia	IM	intramuscular
BUN	blood urea nitrogen	INR	international normalized ratio
Ca	calcium	IU	international units
CAD	coronary artery disease	IV	intravenous
cap	capsule	JIA	juvenile idiopathic arthritis
cm	centimeter	kg	kilogram
CMV	cytomegalovirus	lb	pound
CNS	central nervous system	LFT	liver function test
COPD	chronic obstructive pulmonary disease	LV	left ventricular
CrCl	creatinine clearance	LVEF	left ventricular ejection fraction
CVA	stroke	m^2	square meters
CYP	cytochrome P450	MAOI	monoamine oxidase inhibitor
D5W	5% dextrose	mcg	microgram
dL	deciliter	MDI	metered dose inhaler
DM	diabetes mellitus	mEq	milliequivalent
DMARD	disease-modifying drug	mg	milligram
DPI	dry powder inhaler	Mg	magnesium
DRESS	drug rash eosinophilia and systemic symptoms	MI	myocardial infarction
ECG	electrocardiogram	min	minute
EPS	extrapyramidal symptoms	mL	milliliter
ET	endotracheal	mo	months old
g	gram	MRSA	methicillin-resistant *Staphylococcus aureus*
GERD	gastroesophageal reflux disease	ng	nanogram
gtts	drops	NHLBI	National Heart, Lung, and Blood Institute
GU	genitourinary	NPH	neutral protamine hagedorn

ABBREVIATIONS IN TEXT (continued)

NS	normal saline	sec	second
N/V	nausea/vomiting	soln	solution
NYHA	New York Heart Association	supp	suppository
OA	osteoarthritis	susp	suspension
oz	ounce	tab	tablet
pc	after meals	TB	tuberculosis
PO	by mouth	TCA	tricyclic antidepressant
PR	by rectum	TNF	tumor necrosis factor
prn	as needed	TPN	total parenteral nutrition
PTT	partial thromboplastin time	UTI	urinary tract infection
q	every	wt	weight
RA	rheumatoid arthritis	y	year
RSV	respiratory syncytial virus	yo	years old
SC	subcutaneous		

THERAPEUTIC DRUG LEVELS

Drug	Level	Optimal Timing
amikacin peak	20–35 mcg/mL	30 minutes after infusion
amikacin trough	<5 mcg/mL	Just prior to next dose
carbamazepine trough	4–12 mcg/mL	Just prior to next dose
cyclosporine trough	50–300 ng/mL	Just prior to next dose
digoxin	0.8–2.0 ng/mL	Just prior to next dose
ethosuximide trough	40–100 mcg/mL	Just prior to next dose
gentamicin peak	5–10 mcg/mL	30 minutes after infusion
gentamicin trough	<2 mcg/mL	Just prior to next dose
lidocaine	1.5–5 mcg/mL	12–24 hours after start of infusion
lithium trough	0.6–1.2 meq/L	Just prior to first morning dose
NAPA	10–30 mcg/mL	Just prior to next procainamide dose
phenobarbital trough	15–40 mcg/mL	Just prior to next dose
phenytoin trough	10–20 mcg/mL	Just prior to next dose
primidone trough	5–12 mcg/mL	Just prior to next dose
procainamide	4–10 mcg/mL	Just prior to next dose
quinidine	2–5 mcg/mL	Just prior to next dose
theophylline	5–15 mcg/mL	8–12 hours after once daily dose
tobramycin peak	5–10 mcg/mL	30 minutes after infusion
tobramycin trough	<2 mcg/mL	Just prior to next dose
valproate trough (epilepsy)	50–100 mcg/mL	Just prior to next dose
valproate trough (mania)	45–125 mcg/mL	Just prior to next dose
vancomycin trough[1]	10–20 mg/L	Just prior to next dose
zonisamide[2]	10–40 mcg/mL	Just prior to dose

[1]Maintain trough >10 mg/L to avoid resistance; optimal trough for complicated infections is 15–20 mg/L
[2]Ranges not firmly established but supported by clinical trial results

OUTPATIENT PEDIATRIC DRUGS		Age	2mo	4mo	6mo	9mo	12mo	15mo	2yo	3yo	5yo
		Kg	5	6½	8	9	10	11	13	15	19
		lbs	11	15	17	20	22	24	28	33	42
med	**strength**	**freq**	**teaspoons of liquid per dose** (1 tsp = 5 mL)								
Tylenol (mg)		q4h	80	80	120	120	160	160	200	240	280
Tylenol (tsp)	160/t	q4h	½	½	¾	¾	1	1	1¼	1½	1¾
ibuprofen (mg)		q6h	--	--	75†	75†	100	100	125	150	175
ibuprofen (tsp)	100/t	q6h	--	--	¾t	¾t	1	1	1¼	1½	1¾
amoxicillin or	125/t	bid	1	1¼	1½	1¾	1¾	2	2¼	2¾	3½
Augmentin	200/t	bid	½	¾	1	1	1¼	1¼	1½	1¾	2¼
(not otitis media)	250/t	bid	½	½	¾	¾	1	1	1¼	1¼	1¾
	400/t	bid	¼	½	½	½	¾	¾	¾	1	1
amoxicillin,	200/t	bid	1	1¼	1¾	2	2	2¼	2¾	3	4
(otitis media)‡	250/t	bid	¾	1¼	1½	1½	1¾	1¾	2¼	2½	3¼
	400/t	bid	½	¾	¾	1	1	1¼	1½	1½	2
Auamentin ES‡	600/t	bid	?	½	½	¾	¾	¾	1	1¼	1½
azithromycin*§	100/t	qd	¼†	½†	½	½	½	½	¾	¾	1
(5-day Rx)	200/t	qd	--	¼†	¼	¼	¼	¼	½	½	½
Bactrim/Septra	---	bid	½	¾	1	1	1	1¼	1½	1½	2
cefaclor*	125/t	bid	1	1	1¼	1½	1½	1¾	2	2½	3
"	250/t	bid	½	½	¾	¾	¾	1	1	1¼	1½
cefadroxil	125/t	bid	½	¾	1	1	1¼	1¼	1½	1¾	2¼
"	250/t	bid	¼	½	½	½	¾	¾	¾	1	1
cefdinir	125/t	qd	--	¾†	1	1	1	1¼	1½	1¾	2
cefixime	100/t	qd	½	½	¾	¾	¾	1	1	1¼	1½
cefprozil*	125/t	bid	--	¾†	1	1	1¼	1½	1½	2	2¼
"	250/t	bid	--	½†	½	½	¾	¾	¾	1	1¼
cefuroxime	125/t	bid	--	¾	¾	1	1	1	1½	1¾	2¼
cephalexin	125/t	qid	--	½	¾	¾	1	1	1¼	1½	1¾
"	250/t	qid	--	¼	¼	½	½	½	¾	¾	1
clarithromycin	125/t	bid	½†	½	½	½	¾	¾	¾	1	1¼
"	250/t	bid	--	--	--	¼	½	½	½	½	¾
dicloxacillin	62½/t	qid	½	¾	1	1	1¼	1¼	1½	1¾	2
nitrofurantoin	25/t	qid	¼	½	½	½	½	¾	¾	¾	1
penicillin V**	250/t	bid-tid	--	1	1	1	1	1	1	1	1
cetirizine	5/t	qd	--	--	½	½	½	½	½	½	½
Benadryl	12.5/t	q6h	½	½	¾	¾	1	1	1¼	1½	2
prednisolone	15/t	qd	¼	½	½	¾	¾	¾	1	1	1¼
prednisone	5/t	qd	1	1¼	1½	1¾	2	2¼	2½	3	3¾
Robitussin	---	q4h	--	--	¼†	¼†	½	½	¾	¾	1
Tylenol w/ codeine		q4h	--	--	--	--	--	--	--	1	1

* Dose shown is for otitis media only; see dosing in text for alternative indications.

† Dosing at this age/weight not recommended by manufacturer.

‡ AAP now recommends high dose (80-90 mg/kg/d) for all otitis media in children; with Augmentin used as ES only.

§ Give a double dose of azithromycin the first day.

**AHA dosing for streptococcal pharyngitis. Treat for 10 days.

tsp/t = teaspoon; q = every; h = hour; kg = kilogram; Lbs = pounds; ml = mililiter; bid = two times per day; qd = every day; qid = four times per day; tid = three times per day

PEDIATRIC VITAL SIGNS AND INTRAVENOUS DRUGS

Age		Pre-matr	New-born	2m	4m	6m	9m	12m	15m	2y	3y	5y
Weight	(kg)	2	3½	5	6½	8	9	10	11	13	15	19
	(lbs)	4¼	7½	11	15	17	20	22	24	28	33	42
Maint fluids	(mL/h)	8	14	20	26	32	36	40	42	46	50	58
ET tube	(mm)	2½	3/3½	3½	3½	3½	4	4	4½	4½	4½	5
Defib	(Joules)	4	7	10	13	16	18	20	22	26	30	38
Systolic BP	(high)	70	80	85	90	95	100	103	104	106	109	114
	(low)	40	60	70	70	70	70	70	70	75	75	80
Pulse rate	(high)	145	145	180	180	180	160	160	160	150	150	135
	(low)	100	100	110	110	110	100	100	100	90	90	65
Resp rate	(high)	60	60	50	50	50	46	46	30	30	25	25
	(low)	35	30	30	30	24	24	20	20	20	20	20
adenosine	(mg)	0.2	0.3	0.5	0.6	0.8	0.9	1	1.1	1.3	1.5	1.9
atropine	(mg)	0.1	0.1	0.1	0.13	0.16	0.18	0.2	0.22	0.26	0.30	0.38
Benadryl	(mg)	-	-	5	6½	8	9	10	11	13	15	19
bicarbonate	(meq)	2	3½	5	6½	8	9	10	11	13	15	19
dextrose	(g)	1	2	5	6½	8	9	10	11	13	15	19
epinephrine	(mg)	.02	.04	.05	.07	.08	.09	0.1	0.11	0.13	0.15	0.19
lidocaine	(mg)	2	3½	5	6½	8	9	10	11	13	15	19
morphine	(mg)	0.2	0.3	0.5	0.6	0.8	0.9	1	1.1	1.3	1.5	1.9
mannitol	(g)	2	3½	5	6½	8	9	10	11	13	15	19
naloxone	(mg)	.02	.04	.05	.07	.08	.09	0.1	0.11	0.13	0.15	0.19
diazepam	(mg)	0.6	1	1.5	2	2.5	2.7	3	3.3	3.9	4.5	5
fosphenytoin*	(PE)	40	70	100	130	160	180	200	220	260	300	380
lorazepam	(mg)		0.1	0.2	0.3	0.35	0.4	0.5	0.6	0.7	0.8	1.0
phenobarb	(mg)	30	60	75	100	125	125	150	175	200	225	275
phenytoin*	(mg)	40	70	100	130	160	180	200	220	260	300	380
ampicillin	(mg)	100	175	250	325	400	450	500	550	650	750	1000
ceftriaxone	(mg)	-	-	250	325	400	450	500	550	650	750	1000
cefotaxime	(mg)	100	175	250	325	400	450	500	550	650	750	1000
gentamicin	(mg)	5	8	12	16	20	22	25	27	32	37	47

*Loading doses; fosphenytoin dosed in "phenytoin equivalents."

CONVERSIONS	Liquid:	Weight:
Temperature:	1 fluid ounce = 30 mL	1 kilogram = 2.2 lbs
F = (1.8) C + 32	1 teaspoon = 5 mL	1 ounce = 30 g
C = (F − 32)/1.8	1 tablespoon = 15 mL	1 grain = 65 mg

INHIBITORS, INDUCERS, AND SUBSTRATES OF CYTOCHROME P450 ISOZYMES

INHIBITORS, INDUCERS, AND SUBSTRATES OF CYTOCHROME P450 ISOZYMES

The cytochrome P450 (CYP) inhibitors and inducers below do not necessarily cause clinically important interactions with substrates listed. We exclude in vitro data which can be inaccurate. Refer to other resources for more information if an interaction is suspected based on this chart. A drug that inhibits CYP subfamily activity can block the metabolism of substrates by that enzyme, which can lead to substrate accumulation and toxicity. CYP inhibitors are classified by how much they increase the area-under-the-curve (AUC) of a substrate: weak (1.25- to 2-fold), moderate (2- to 5-fold), or strong (≥5-fold). A drug that induces CYP subfamily activity increases substrate metabolism, which can lead to reduced substrate efficacy. CYP inducers are classified by how much they decrease the AUC of a substrate: weak (20 to 50%), moderate (50 to 80%) and strong (>80%). A drug is considered a sensitive substrate if a CYP inhibitor increases the AUC of that drug by ≥ 5-fold. While AUC increases of >50% often do not affect patient response, smaller increases can be important if the drug has a narrow therapeutic range (eg, theophylline, warfarin, cyclosporine). This table may be incomplete since new evidence about drug metabolism is continually being identified.

CYP1A2

Inhibitors. *Strong:* ciprofloxacin, fluvoxamine. ***Moderate:*** methoxalan, mexiletine, oral contraceptives, vemurafenib, zileuton. ***Weak:*** acyclovir, allopurinol, caffeine, cimetidine, deferasirox, disulfiram, echinacea, famotidine, propafenone, propranolol, simeprevir, terbinafine, verapamil. ***Unclassified:*** amiodarone, atazanavir, citalopram, clarithromycin, estradiol, isoniazid, peginterferon alfa-2a and 2b.

Inducers. *Moderate:* montelukast, phenytoin, smoking. ***Weak:*** omeprazole, phenobarbital. ***Unclassified:*** carbamazepine, charcoal-broiled foods, rifampin, ritonavir, tipranavir-ritonavir.

Substrates. *Sensitive:* caffeine, duloxetine, melatonin, ramelteon, tizanidine. ***Unclassified:*** acetaminophen, amitriptyline, asenapine, bendamustine, cinacalcet, clomipramine, clozapine, cyclobenzaprine, erlotinib, estradiol, fluvoxamine, haloperidol, imipramine, loxapine, mexiletine, mirtazapine, naproxen, olanzapine, ondansetron, pomalidomide, propranolol, rasagiline, riluzole, roflumilast, ropinirole, ropivacaine, R-warfarin, tasimelteon, theophylline, zileuton, zolmitriptan.

CYP2B6

Inhibitors. *Weak:* clopidogrel, prasugrel.

Inducers. *Moderate:* efavirenz, rifampin. ***Weak:*** isavuconazole, nevirapine, artemether (in ***Unclassified:*** baicalin (in Limbrel), ritonavir.

Substrates. *Sensitive:* bupropion, efavirenz. ***Unclassified:*** cyclophosphamide, ketamine, meperidine, methadone, nevirapine, prasugrel, propofol.

CYP2C8

Inhibitors. *Strong:* clopidogrel, gemfibrozil. ***Moderate:*** deferasirox. ***Weak:*** atazanavir, fluvoxamine, ketoconazole, pazopanib, trimethoprim.

Inducers. *Moderate:* rifampin. ***Unclassified:*** barbiturates, carbamazepine, rifabutin, ritonavir.

Substrates. *Sensitive:* repaglinide. ***Unclassified:*** amiodarone, carbamazepine, dabrafenib, ibuprofen, imatinib, isotretinoin, loperamide, montelukast, paclitaxel, pioglitazone, rosiglitazone, treprostinil.

(continues)

CYP2C9

Inhibitors. *Moderate:* amiodarone, fluconazole, miconazole, oxandrolone. *Weak:* capecitabine, cotrimoxazole, etravirine, fluvastatin, fluvoxamine, metronidazole, oritavancin, tigecycline, voriconazole, zafirlukast. *Unclassified:* cimetidine, fenofibrate, fenofibric acid, fluorouracil, imatinib, isoniazid, leflunomide, ritonavir.

Inducers. *Moderate:* carbamazepine, rifampin. *Weak:* aprepitant, bosentan, elvitegravir, phenobarbital, St John's wort. *Unclassified:* dabrafenib, rifapentine, ritonavir.

Substrates. *Sensitive:* celecoxib. *Unclassified:* azilsartan, bosentan, chlorpropamide, diclofenac, etravirine, fluoxetine, flurbiprofen, fluvastatin, formoterol, glimepiride, glipizide, glyburide, ibuprofen, irbesartan, losartan, mefenamic acid, meloxicam, montelukast, naproxen, nateglinide, ospemifene, phenytoin, piroxicam, ramelteon, ruxolitinib, sildenafil, tolbutamide, torsemide, vardenafil, voriconazole, S-warfarin, zafirlukast, zileuton.

CYP2C19

Inhibitors. *Strong:* fluconazole, fluvoxamine. *Moderate:* esomeprazole, fluoxetine, moclobemide, omeprazole, voriconazole. *Weak:* armodafinil, carbamazepine, cimetidine, etravirine, felbamate, human growth hormone, ketoconazole, oral contraceptives, oritavancin. *Unclassified:* chloramphenicol, eslicarbazepine, isoniazid, modafinil, oxcarbazepine.

Inducers. *Moderate:* rifampin. *Unclassified:* efavirenz, ritonavir, St John's wort, tipranavir.

Substrates. *Sensitive:* lansoprazole, omeprazole. *Unclassified:* amitriptyline, bortezomib, carisoprodol, cilostazol, citalopram, clobazam, clomipramine, clopidogrel, clozapine, cyclophosphamide, desipramine, dexlansoprazole, diazepam, escitalopram, esomeprazole, etravirine, flibanserin formoterol, imipramine, lacosamide, methadone, moclobamide, nelfinavir pantoprazole, phenytoin, progesterone, proguanil, propranolol, rabeprazole, sertraline, tofacitinib, voriconazole, R-warfarin.

CYP2D6

Inhibitors. *Strong:* bupropion, fluoxetine, paroxetine, quinidine. *Moderate:* cinacalcet, dronedarone, duloxetine, mirabegron, rolapitant, terbinafine. *Weak:* amiodarone, asenapine, celecoxib, cimetidine, desvenlafaxine, diltiazem, diphenhydramine, echinacea, escitalopram, febuxostat, gefitinib, hydralazine, hydroxychloroquine, imitinib, methadone, oral contraceptives, pazopanib, propafenone, ranitidine, ritonavir, sertraline, telithromycin, venlafaxine, vemurafenib, verapamil. *Unclassified:* abiraterone, chloroquine, clobazam, clomipramine, cobicistat, darunavir-ritonavir, fluphenazine, haloperidol, lorcaserin, lumefantrine (in *Coartem*), metoclopramide, moclobamide, panobinostat, peginterferon alfa-2b, perphenazine, quinine, ranolazine, thioridazine, tipranavir-ritonavir.

Inducers. None known.

Substrates. *Sensitive:* atomoxetine, desipramine, dextromethorphan, metoprolol, nebivolol, perphenazine, tolterodine, venlafaxine. *Unclassified:* amitriptyline, aripiprazole, brexpiprazole, carvedilol, cevimeline, chlorpheniramine, chlorpromazine, clozapine, cinacalcet, clomipramine, codeine*, darifenacin, dihydrocodeine, dolasetron, donepezil, doxepin, duloxetine, fesoterodine, flecainide, fluoxetine, formoterol, galantamine, haloperidol, hydrocodone, iloperidone, imipramine, loratadine, loxapine, maprotiline, meclizine, methadone, methamphetamine, metoclopramide, mexiletine, mirtazapine, morphine, nortriptyline, ondansetron, paroxetine, pimozide, primaquine, promethazine, propafenone, propranolol, quetiapine, risperidone, ritonavir, tamoxifen, tamsulosin, tetrabenazine, thioridazine, timolol, tramadol*, trazodone, trimipramine, vortioxetine.

* Metabolism by CYP2D6 required to convert to active analgesic metabolite; analgesia may be impaired by CYP2D6 inhibitors.

(continues)

CYP3A4

Inhibitors. *Strong:* clarithromycin, cobicistat, conivaptan, indinavir, itraconazole, ketoconazole, lopinavir-ritonavir, nefazodone, nelfinavir, posaconazole, ritonavir, saquinavir, telithromycin, voriconazole. *Moderate:* aprepitant, atazanavir, ciprofloxacin, crizotinib, darunavir-ritonavir, diltiazem, dronedarone, erythromycin, fluconazole, fosamprenavir, grapefruit juice (variable), imatinib, isavuconazole, netupitant (in Akynzeo), verapamil. *Weak:* alprazolam, amiodarone, amlodipine, atorvastatin, bicalutamide, cilostazol, cimetidine, cyclosporine, everolimus, fluoxetine, fluvoxamine, ginko, goldenseal, isoniazid, ivacaftor, lapatinib, lomitapide, nilotinib, oral contraceptives, pazopanib, ranitidine, ranolazine, simeprevir, ticagrelor, tipranavir-ritonavir, zileuton. *Unclassified:* danazol, miconazole, palbociclib, quinine, quinupristin-dalfopristin, sertraline.

Inducers. *Strong:* carbamazepine, mitotane, phenytoin, rifampin, rifapentine, St Johns wort. *Moderate:* bosentan, efavirenz, etravirine, modafinil, nafcillin. *Weak:* aprepitant, armodafinil, clobazam, echinacea, fosamprenavir, oritavancin, pioglitazone, rufinamide. *Unclassified:* artemether (in Coartem), barbiturates, bexarotene, dabrafenib, dexamethasone, eslicarbazepine, ethosuximide, griseofulvin, nevirapine, oxcarbazepine, primidone, rifabutin, ritonavir, tocilizumab, vemurafenib.

Substrates. *Sensitive:* alfentanil, aprepitant, budesonide, buspirone, conivaptan, darifenacin, darunavir, dasatinib, dronedarone, eletriptan, eplerenone, everolimus, felodipine, fluticasone, ibrutinib, indinavir, isavuconazole, ivacaftor, lomitapide, lopinavir (in Kaletra), lovastatin, lurasidone, maraviroc, midazolam, nisoldipine, quetiapine, saquinavir, sildenafil, simvastatin, sirolimus, tipranavir, tolvaptan, triazolam, vardenafil. *Unclassified:* alfuzosin, aliskiren, almotriptan, alprazolam, amiodarone, amlodipine, apixaban, apremilast, aripiprazole, armodafinil, artemether (in Coartem), atazanavir, atorvastatin, avanafil, axitinib, bedaquiline, bortezomib, bosentan, bosutinib, brentuximab, brexpiprazole, bromocriptine, buprenorphine, cabazitaxel, cabozantinib, carbamazepine, cariprazine, ceritinib, cevimeline, cilostazol, cinacalcet, cisapride, citalopram, clarithromycin, clobazam, clomipramine, clonazepam, clopidogrel, clozapine, cobicistat, colchicine, corticosteroids, crizotinib, cyclophosphamide, cyclosporine, dabrafenib, daclatasivr, dapsone, desogestrel, desvenlafaxine, dexamethasone, dexlansoprazole, diazepam, dihydroergotamine, diltiazem, disopyramide, docetaxel, dofetilide, dolasetron, domperidone, donepezil, doxorubicin, dutasteride, efavirenz, elvitegravir, ergotamine, erlotinib, erythromycin, escitalopram, esomeprazole, eszopiclone, ethinyl estradiol, etoposide, etravirine, fentanyl, fesoterodine, finasteride, flibanserin, fosamprenavir, fosaprepitant, galantamine, gefitinib, guanfacine, haloperidol, hydrocodone, ivabradine, ifosfamide, iloperidone, imatinib, imipramine, irinotecan, isradipine, itraconazole, ixabepilone, ketamine, ketoconazole, lansoprazole, lapatinib, letrozole, levonorgestrel, lidocaine, loratadine, loxapine, lumefantrine (in Coartem), macitentan, methylergonovine, mifepristone, mirtazapine, modafinil, mometasone, naloxegol, nateglinide, nefazodone, nelfinavir, netupitant (in Akynzeo), nevirapine, nicardipine, nifedipine, nilotinib, nimodipine, nintedanib (minor), olaparib, ondansetron, ospemifene, oxybutynin, oxycodone, paclitaxel, panobinostat, pantoprazole, paritaprevir (in Viekira Pak), palbociclib, pazopanib, pimozide, pioglitazone, pomalidomide, ponatinib, prasugrel, praziquantel, quinidine, quinine, rabeprazole, rameltreon, ranolazine, regorafenib, repaglinide, rifabutin, rifampin, ritonavir, rivaroxaban, roflumilast, romidepsin, ruxolitinib, saxagliptin, sertraline, silodosin, solifenacin, sonidegib, sufentanil, sunitinib, tacrolimus, tadalafil, tamoxifen, tamsulosin, tasimelteon, telithromycin, temsirolimus, testosterone, tiagabine, ticagrelor, tinidazole, tofacitinib, tolterodine, tramadol, trazodone, verapamil, vilazodone, vinblastine, vincristine, vinorelbine, vorapaxar, voriconazole, R-warfarin, zaleplon, ziprasidone, zolpidem, zonisamide.

INHIBITORS, INDUCERS, AND SUBSTRATES OF P-GLYCOPROTEIN

INHIBITORS, INDUCERS, AND SUBSTRATES OF P-GLYCOPROTEIN

The p-glycoprotein (P-gp) inhibitors and inducers listed below do not necessarily cause clinically important interactions with P-gp substrates. We attempt to exclude in vitro data which can be inaccurate. Refer to other resources for more information if an interaction is suspected based on this chart. P-gp is an efflux transporter that pumps drugs out of cells. In the gut, P-gp reduces drug absorption by pumping drugs into the gut lumen. In the kidney, it increases drug excretion by pumping drugs into urine. P-gp inhibitors can increase exposure to P-gp substrates, potentially increasing their risk of toxicity. P-gp inducers can reduce exposure to P-gp substrates, potentially increasing the risk of treatment failure. Some drugs are dual inhibitors of P-gp and CYP3A4 (e.g., clarithromycin, dronedarone, erythromycin, itraconazole, ketoconazole, verapamil), while others are dual inducers of P-gp and CYP3A4 (e.g., carbamazepine, phenytoin, rifampin, St John's wort). Potent P-gp inhibitors are defined here as drugs that increase the area-under-the-curve (AUC) of a P-gp substrate (digoxin or fexofenadine) by ≥1.5-fold. This table may be incomplete since new evidence about drug interactions is continually being identified.

Inhibitors. *Potent:* amiodarone, clarithromycin, cyclosporine, dronedarone, flibanserin, itraconazole, lapatinib, lopinavir-ritonavir, ranolazine, ritonavir, verapamil. ***Unclassified:*** atorvastatin, azithromycin, captopril, carvedilol, cobicistat, conivaptan, daclatasvir, darunavir-ritonavir, diltiazem, dipyridamole, erythromycin, etravirine, everolimus, felodipine, indinavir, isavuconazole, isradipine, ketoconazole, ledipasvir, lomitapide, naproxen, nifedipine, nilotinib, posaconazole, quinidine, rolapitant saquinavir-ritonavir, simeprevir, telmisartan, ticagrelor.

Inducers: carbamazepine, fosamprenavir, phenytoin, rifampin, St John's wort, tipranavir-ritonavir*.
*Tipranavir induces CYP3A4 and P-gp, while ritonavir inhibits both pathways. This makes it difficult to predict the effect of ritonavir-boosted tipranavir on substrates of P-gp.

Substrates: afatinib, aliskiren, ambrisentan, apixaban, ceritinib, clobazam, clopidogrel, colchicine, cyclosporine, dabigatran, dasabuvir (in *Viekira Pak*), digoxin, diltiazem, docetaxel, dolutegravir, edoxaban, etoposide, everolimus, fexofenadine, fosamprenavir, imatinib, indinavir, lapatinib, ledipasvir (in *Harvoni*), linagliptin, loperamide, lovastatin, maraviroc, morphine, nadolol, nilotinib, nintedanib, ombitasvir (in *Viekira Pak*), paclitaxel, paliperidone, paritaprevir (in *Viekira Pak*), pomalidomide, posaconazole, pravastatin, propranolol, quinidine, ranolazine, rifaximin, ritonavir, rivaroxaban, romidepsin, saquinavir, saxagliptin, silodosin, simeprevir, sirolimus, sitagliptin, sofosbuvir, tacrolimus, tenofovir, tolvaptan, topotecan, vinblastine, vincristine.

DRUG THERAPY REFERENCE WEBSITES (selected)

Professional societies or governmental agencies with drug therapy guidelines

AAP	American Academy of Pediatrics	www.aap.org
ACC	American College of Cardiology	www.acc.org
ACCP	American College of Chest Physicians	www.chestnet.org
ACCP	American College of Clinical Pharmacy	www.accp.com
ACR	American College of Rheumatology	www.rheumatology.org
ADA	American Diabetes Association	www.diabetes.org
AHA	American Heart Association	www.heart.org
AHRQ	Agency for Healthcare Research and Quality	www.ahcpr.gov
AIDSinfo	HIV Treatment, Prevention, and Research	www.aidsinfo.nih.gov
AMA	American Medical Association	www.ama-assn.org
APA	American Psychiatric Association	www.psych.org
APA	American Psychological Association	www.apa.org
ASHP	Amer. Society Health-Systems Pharmacists Drug Shortages Resource Center	www.ashp.org/shortages
ATS	American Thoracic Society	www.thoracic.org
CDC	Centers for Disease Control and Prevention	www.cdc.gov
CDC	CDC bioterrorism and radiation exposures	www.bt.cdc.gov
IDSA	Infectious Diseases Society of America	www.idsociety.org
MHA	Malignant Hyperthermia Association	www.mhaus.org

Other therapy reference sites

Cochrane library	www.cochrane.org
Emergency Contraception Website	www.not-2-late.com
Immunization Action Coalition	www.immunize.org
QTDrug lists	www.crediblemeds.org
Managing Contraception	www.managingcontraception.com

ANALGESICS

OPIOID EQUIVALENCY[*]

Opioid	PO	IV/SC/IM	Opioid	PO	IV/SC/IM
buprenorphine	n/a	0.3–0.4 mg	meperidine	300 mg	75 mg
butorphanol	n/a	2 mg	methadone	5–15 mg	2.5–10 mg
codeine	130 mg	75 mg	morphine	30 mg	10 mg
fentanyl	?	0.1 mg	nalbuphine	n/a	10 mg
hydrocodone	20 mg	n/a	oxycodone	20 mg	n/a
hydromorphone	7.5 mg	1.5 mg	oxymorphone	10 mg	1 mg
levorphanol	4 mg	2 mg	pentazocine	50 mg	30 mg

[*]Approximate equianalgesic doses as adapted from the 2003 American Pain Society (www.ampainsoc.org) guidelines and the 1992 AHCPR guidelines. Not available = "n/a." See drug entries themselves for starting doses. Many recommend initially using lower than equivalent doses when switching between different opiods. IV doses should be titrated slowly with appropriate monitoring. All PO dosing is with immediate-release preparations. Individualize all dosing, especially in the elderly, children, and in those with chronic pain, opioid naïve, or hepatic/renal insufficiency.

Muscle Relaxants

BACLOFEN (✦Lioresal, Lioresal D.S.) Spasticity related to MS or spinal cord disease/injury: Start 5 mg PO three times per day, then increase by 5 mg/dose q 3 days until 20 mg PO three times per day. Max dose 20 mg four times per day. [Generic only: Tabs 10, 20 mg.] ▶K ♀C ▶+ $

CARISOPRODOL (Soma) Acute musculoskeletal pain: 350 mg PO three to four times per day. Abuse potential. [Generic/Trade: Tabs 250, 350 mg.] ▶LK ♀? ▶–⊚IV $

CHLORZOXAZONE (Parafon Forte DSC, Lorzone, Remular-S) Musculoskeletal pain: 500 to 750 mg PO three to four times per day to start. Decrease to 250 mg three to four times per day. [Generic/Trade: Tabs 500 mg (Parafon Forte DSC 500 mg tabs, scored). Trade only: Tabs 250 mg (Remular-S), Tabs 375 , 750 mg (Lorzone).] ▶LK ♀C ▶? $

CYCLOBENZAPRINE (Amrix, Flexeril, Fexmid) Musculoskeletal pain: Start 5 to 10 mg PO three times per day, max 30 mg/day or 15 to 30 mg (extended-release) PO daily. Not recommended in elderly. [Generic/Trade: Tab 5, 7.5, 10 mg. Extended-release caps 15, 30 mg ($$$$).] ▶LK ♀B ▶? $

DANTROLENE (Dantrium, Revonto, Ryanodex) Chronic spasticity related to spinal cord injury, CVA, cerebral palsy, MS: 25 mg PO daily to start, up to max of 100 mg

(cont.)

two to four times per day if necessary. Malignant hyperthermia: 2.5 mg/kg rapid IV push q 5 to 10 min continuing until symptoms subside or to a max total dose of 10 mg/kg (Dantrium, Revonto). Minimum of 1 mg/kg IV push with additional doses administered if necessary up to a total max dose of 10 mg/kg (Ryanodex). Prevention of malignant hyperthermia in patients at high risk: 2.5 mg/kg over a period of at least 1 min approximately 75 minutes before surgery (Ryanodex). Additiional doses may be given if surgery is prolonged. [Generic/Trade: Caps 25, 50, 100 mg. Trade only: Vials 20 mg (Dantrium, Revonto), 250 mg (Ryanodex).] ▶LK ♀C ▶? –$$$$ ■

METAXALONE (*Skelaxin*) Musculoskeletal pain: 800 mg PO three to four times per day. [Generic/Trade: Tabs 800 mg, scored. Generic only: Tabs 400 mg.] ▶LK ♀? ▶? $$$$

METHOCARBAMOL (*Robaxin, Robaxin-750*) Acute musculoskeletal pain: 1500 mg PO four times per day or 1000 mg IM/IV three times per day for 48 to 72 h. Maintenance: 1000 mg PO four times per day, 750 mg PO q 4 h, or 1500 mg PO three times per day. Tetanus: Specialized dosing. [Generic/Trade: Tabs 500, 750 mg. OTC in Canada.] ▶LK ♀C ▶? $

ORPHENADRINE (*Norflex*) Musculoskeletal pain: 100 mg PO two times per day. 60 mg IV/IM two times per day. [Generic only: 100 mg extended-release. OTC in Canada.] ▶LK ♀C ▶? $$

TIZANIDINE (*Zanaflex*) Muscle spasticity due to MS or spinal cord injury: 4 to 8 mg PO q 6 to 8 h prn, max 36 mg/day. [Generic/Trade: Tabs 4 mg, scored. Caps 2, 4, 6 mg. Generic only: Tabs 2 mg.] ▶ L ♀C ▶? $$$$

Non-Opioid Analgesic Combinations

ASCRIPTIN (acetylsalicylic acid + aluminum hydroxide + magnesium hydroxide + calcium carbonate) Multiple strengths. 1 to 2 tabs PO q 4 h. [OTC Trade only: Tabs 325 mg aspirin/50 mg magnesium hydroxide/50 mg Al hydroxide/50 mg Ca carbonate (Ascriptin and Aspir-Mox). 500 mg aspirin/33 mg magnesium hydroxide/33 mg Al hydroxide/ 237 mg Ca carbonate (Ascriptin Maximum Strength).] ▶ ♀D ▶? $

BUFFERIN (acetylsalicylic acid + calcium carbonate + magnesium oxide + magnesium carbonate) 1 to 2 tabs/caps PO q 4 h. Max 12 tabs/caps in 24 h. [OTC Trade only: Tabs/caps 325 mg aspirin/158 mg Ca carbonate/63 mg of magnesium oxide/34 mg of magnesium carbonate. Bufferin ES: 500 mg aspirin/222.3 mg Ca carbonate/88.9 mg of magnesium oxide/55.6 mg of Mg carbonate.] ▶K ♀D ▶? $

ESGIC (acetaminophen + butalbital + caffeine) 1 to 2 tabs or caps PO q 4 h. Max 6 in 24 h. [Generic only: Tabs/caps, 325 mg acetaminophen/50 mg butalbital/40 mg caffeine. Oral soln 325/50/40 per 15 mL. Generic/Trade: Tabs, Esgic Plus is 500/50/40 mg.] ▶LK ♀C ▶? $

EXCEDRIN MIGRAINE (acetaminophen + acetylsalicylic acid + caffeine) 2 tabs/caps/geltabs PO q 6 h while symptoms persist. Max 8 tabs/caps/geltabs in 24 h. [OTC Generic/Trade: Tabs/caps/geltabs 250 mg acetaminophen/250 mg aspirin/65 mg caffeine.] ▶LK ♀D ▶? $

FIORICET (acetaminophen + butalbital + caffeine) 1 to 2 caps PO q 4 h. Max 6 caps in 24 h. [Generic/Trade: Tabs 325 mg acetaminophen/50 mg butalbital/40 mg caffeine.] ▶LK ♀C ▶? $

FIORINAL (acetylsalicylic acid + butalbital + caffeine, ✦Trianal) 1 to 2 tabs PO q 4 h. Max 6 tabs in 24 h. [Generic/Trade: Caps 325 mg aspirin/ 50 mg butalbital/40 mg caffeine.] ▶KL ♀D ▶─◉III $$

GOODY'S EXTRA STRENGTH HEADACHE POWDER (acetaminophen + acetylsalicylic acid + caffeine) 1 powder PO followed with liquid, or stir powder into a glass of water or other liquid. Repeat in 4 to 6 h prn. Max 4 powders in 24 h. [OTC trade only: 260 mg acetaminophen/520 mg aspirin/32.5 mg caffeine per powder paper.] ▶LK ♀D ▶? $

NORGESIC (orphenadrine + acetylsalicylic acid + caffeine) Multiple strengths; write specific product on Rx. Norgesic: 1 to 2 tabs PO three to four times per day. Norgesic Forte: 1 tab PO three to four times per day. [Generic only: Tabs 25 mg orphenadrine/385 mg aspirin/30 mg caffeine (Norgesic). Tabs 50/770/60 mg (Norgesic Forte).] ▶KL ♀D ▶? $$$

PHRENILIN (acetaminophen + butalbital) Tension or muscle contraction headache: 1 to 2 tabs PO q 4 h. Max 6 in 24 h. [Generic/Trade: Tabs, 325 mg acetaminophen/50 mg butalbital (Phrenilin). Caps, 650/50 mg (Phrenilin Forte).] ▶LK ♀C ▶? $$

SEDAPAP (acetaminophen + butalbital) 1 to 2 tabs PO q 4 h. Max 6 tabs in 24 h. [Generic only: Tabs 650 mg acetaminophen/50 mg butalbital.] ▶LK ♀C ▶? $

SOMA COMPOUND (carisoprodol + acetylsalicylic acid) 1 to 2 tabs PO four times per day. Abuse potential. [Generic only: Tabs 200 mg carisoprodol/325 mg aspirin.] ▶LK ♀D ▶─◉IV $$$

ULTRACET (tramadol + acetaminophen, ✦Tramacet) Acute pain: 2 tabs PO q 4 to 6 h prn (up to 8 tabs/day for no more than 5 days). Adjust dose in elderly and renal dysfunction. Avoid in opioid-dependent patients. Seizures may occur if concurrent antidepressants or seizure disorder. [Generic/Trade: Tabs 37.5 mg tramadol/325 mg acetaminophen.] ▶KL ♀C ▶─◉IV $$

Non-Steroidal Anti-Inflammatories—COX-2 Inhibitors

CELECOXIB (*Celebrex*) OA, ankylosing spondylitis: 200 mg PO daily or 100 mg PO two times per day. RA: 100 to 200 mg PO two times per day. Familial adenomatous polyposis: 400 mg PO two times per day with food. Acute pain, dysmenorrhea: 400 mg single dose, then 200 mg two times per day prn. An additional 200 mg dose may be given on day 1 if needed. JRA: Give 50 mg PO two times per day for age 2 to 17 yo and wt 10 to 25 kg, give 100 mg PO two times per day for wt greater than 25 kg. Contraindicated in sulfonamide allergy. [Generic/Trade: Caps 50, 100, 200, 400 mg.] ▶L ♀C (D in 3rd trimester) ▶? $$$$$ ■

Non-Steroidal Anti-Inflammatories—Salicylic Acid Derivatives

ACETYLSALICYLIC ACID (*Ecotrin, Empirin, Halfprin, Bayer, Anacin, Zorprin, aspirin,* ✦*Asaphen, Entrophen, Novasen*) Analgesia: 325 to 650 mg PO/PR q 4 to

(cont.)

6 h. Platelet aggregation inhibition: 81 to 325 mg PO daily. [Generic/Trade (OTC): Tabs, 325, 500 mg; chewable 81 mg; enteric-coated 81, 162 mg (Halfprin), 81, 325, 500 mg (Ecotrin), 650, 975 mg. Trade only: Tabs, controlled-release 650, 800 mg (ZORprin, Rx). Generic only (OTC): Supps 60, 120, 200, 300, 600 mg.] ▶K ♀D ▷? $

CHOLINE MAGNESIUM TRISALICYLATE (*Trilisate***)** RA/OA: 1500 mg PO two times per day. [Generic only: Tabs 500, 750, 1000 mg. Soln 500 mg/5 mL.] ▶K ♀C (D in 3rd trimester) ▷? $$

DIFLUNISAL (*Dolobid***)** Pain: 500 to 1000 mg initially, then 250 to 500 mg PO q 8 to 12 h. RA/OA: 500 mg to 1 g PO divided two times per day. [Generic only: Tabs 500 mg.] ▶K ♀C (D in 3rd trimester) ▶– $$$ ▪

SALSALATE (*Salflex, Disalcid, Amigesic***)** RA/OA: 3000 mg/day PO divided q 8 to 12 h. [Generic only: Tabs 500, 750 mg, scored.] ▶K ♀C (D in 3rd trimester) ▷? $$ ▪

ANALGESICS—NSAIDs

Salicylic acid derivatives	ASA, diflunisal, salsalate, Trilisate
Propionic acids	flurbiprofen, ibuprofen, ketoprofen, naproxen, oxaprozin
Acetic acids	diclofenac, etodolac, indomethacin, ketorolac, nabumetone, sulindac, tolmetin
Fenamates	meclofenamate
Oxicams	meloxicam, piroxicam
COX-2 inhibitors	celecoxib

Note: If one class fails, consider another.

Non-Steroidal Anti-Inflammatories—Other

ARTHROTEC (*diclofenac + misoprostol***)** OA: One 50/200 tab PO three times per day. RA: One 50/200 tab PO three to four times per day. If intolerant, may use 50/200 or 75/200 PO two times per day. Misoprostol is an abortifacient. [Generic/Trade: Tabs 50 mg/200 mcg, 75 mg/200 mcg, diclofenac/misoprostol.] ▶LK ♀X ▶– $$$$$ ▪

DICLOFENAC (*Voltaren, Voltaren XR, Cataflam, Flector, Zipsor, Cambia, Zorvolex, ✦Voltaren Rapide***)** Multiple strengths; write specific product on Rx. Immediate- or delayed-release: 50 mg PO two to three times per day or 75 mg PO two times per day. Extended-release (Voltaren XR): 100 to 200 mg PO daily. Patch (Flector): Apply 1 patch to painful area two times per day. Gel: 2 to 4 g to affected area four times per day. Acute migraine with or without aura: 50 mg single dose (Cambia). [Generic/Trade: Tabs, immediate-release (Cataflam) 50 mg, extended-release (Voltaren XR) 100 mg. Generic only: Tabs, delayed-release 25, 50, 75 mg. Trade only: Patch (Flector) 1.3% diclofenac epolamine. Topical gel (Voltaren) 1% 100 g tube. Trade only: Caps, liquid-filled (Zipsor) 25 mg. Caps (Zorvolex) 18, 35 mg. Trade only: Powder for oral soln (Cambia) 50 mg.] ▶L ♀B (D in 3rd trimester) ▶– $$$ ▪

ETODOLAC Multiple strengths; write specific product on Rx. Immediate-release: 200 to 400 mg PO two to three times per day. Extended-release: 400 to 1200 mg PO daily. [Generic only: Caps, immediate-release: 200, 300 mg. Tabs, immediate-release: 400, 500 mg. Tabs, extended-release: 400, 500, 600 mg.] ▶L ♀C (D in 3rd trimester) ▶– $ ■

FLURBIPROFEN (*Ansaid*) 200 to 300 mg/day PO divided two to four times per day. [Generic/Trade: Tabs, immediate-release 50, 100 mg.] ▶L ♀B (D in 3rd trimester) ▶+ $$$ ■

IBUPROFEN (*Motrin, Advil, Nuprin, Rufen, NeoProfen, Caldolor*) 200 to 800 mg PO three to four times per day. Peds older than 6 mo: 5 to 10 mg/kg PO q 6 to 8 h. GI perforation and necrotizing enterocolitis has been reported with NeoProfen. [OTC: Caps/Liqui-Gel Caps 200 mg. Tabs 100, 200 mg. Chewable tabs 100 mg. Susp (infant gtts) 50 mg/1.25 mL (with calibrated dropper), 100 mg/5 mL. Rx Generic/Trade: Tabs 400, 600, 800 mg.] ▶L ♀B (D in 3rd trimester) ▶+ $ ■

INDOMETHACIN (*Indocin, Indocin SR, Indocin IV*) Multiple strengths; write specific product on Rx. Immediate-release preparations: 25 to 50 mg cap PO three times per day. Sustained-release: 75 mg cap PO one to two times per day. [Generic only: Caps, immediate-release 25, 50 mg. Caps, sustained-release 75 mg. Trade only: Suppository 50 mg. Oral susp 25 mg/5 mL (237 mL).] ▶L ♀B (D in 3rd trimester) ▶+ $ ■

KETOPROFEN (*Orudis, Orudis KT, Actron, Oruvail*) Immediate-release: 25 to 75 mg PO three to four times per day. Extended-release: 100 to 200 mg cap PO daily. [Rx Generic only: Caps, extended-release 200 mg. Caps, immediate-release 50, 75 mg.] ▶L ♀C (D in 3rd trimester) ▶– $$$ ■

KETOROLAC (*Toradol*) Moderately severe acute pain: 15 to 30 mg IV/IM q 6 h or 10 mg PO q 4 to 6 h prn. Combined duration IV/IM and PO is not to exceed 5 days. Moderately severe, acute pain, single-dose treatment: 60 mg IM or 30 mg IV if patient younger than 65 yo, 30 mg IM or 15 mg IV if patient 65 yo or older, has renal impairment, or wt less than 50 kg. [Generic only: Tabs 10 mg.] ▶L ♀C (D in 3rd trimester) ▶+ $ ■

MECLOFENAMATE Mild to moderate pain: 50 mg PO q 4 to 6 h prn. Max dose 400 mg/day. Menorrhagia and primary dysmenorrhea: 100 mg PO three times per day for up to 6 days. RA/OA: 200 to 400 mg/day PO divided three to four times per day. [Generic only: Caps 50, 100 mg.] ▶L ♀B (D in 3rd trimester) ▶– $$$ ■

MEFENAMIC ACID (*Ponstel, +Ponstan*) Mild to moderate pain, primary dysmenorrhea: 500 mg PO initially, then 250 mg PO q 6 h prn for no more than 1 week. [Generic/Trade: Caps 250 mg.] ▶L ♀C (D in 3rd trimester) ▶– $$$$$ ■

MELOXICAM (*Mobic, +Mobicox*) RA/OA: 7.5 mg PO daily. JRA age 2 yo or older: 0.125 mg/kg PO daily. [Generic/Trade: Tabs 7.5, 15 mg. Susp 7.5 mg/5 mL (1.5 mg/mL).] ▶L ♀C (D in 3rd trimester) ▶? $ ■

NABUMETONE (*Relafen*) RA/OA: Initial: Two 500 mg tabs (1000 mg) PO daily. May increase to 1500 to 2000 mg PO daily or divided two times per day. [Generic only: Tabs 500, 750 mg.] ▶L ♀C (D in 3rd trimester) ▶– $$ ■

NAPROXEN (*Naprosyn, Aleve, Anaprox, EC-Naprosyn, Naprelan, Prevacid NapraPAC*) Immediate-release: 250 to 500 mg PO two times per day.

(cont.)

Delayed-release: 375 to 500 mg PO two times per day (do not crush or chew). Controlled-release: 750 to 1000 mg PO daily. JRA: Give 2.5 mL PO two times per day for wt 13 kg or less, give 5 mL PO two times per day for 14 to 25 kg, give 7.5 mL PO two times per day for 26 to 38 kg. 500 mg naproxen equivalent to 550 mg naproxen sodium. [OTC Generic/Trade (Aleve): Tabs, immediate-release 200 mg. OTC Trade only (Aleve): Caps, Gelcaps, immediate-release 200 mg. Rx Generic/Trade: Tabs, immediate-release (Naprosyn) 250, 375, 500 mg. (Anaprox) 275, 550 mg. Tabs, delayed-release enteric-coated (EC-Naprosyn) 375, 500 mg. Tabs, controlled-release (Naprelan) 375, 500, 750 mg. Susp (Naprosyn) 125 mg/5 mL. Prevacid NapraPAC: 7 lansoprazole 15 mg caps packaged with 14 naproxen tabs 375 mg or 500 mg.] ▶L ♀B (D in 3rd trimester) ▶+ $$$ ■

OXAPROZIN (*Daypro*) 1200 mg PO daily. [Generic/Trade: Tabs 600 mg, trade scored.] ▶L ♀C (D in 3rd trimester) ▶– $$$ ■

PIROXICAM (*Feldene, Fexicam*) 20 mg PO daily. [Generic/Trade: Caps 10, 20 mg.] ▶L ♀B (D in 3rd trimester) ▶+ $$$

SULINDAC (*Clinoril*) 150 to 200 mg PO two times per day. [Generic/Trade: Tabs 200 mg. Generic only: Tabs 150 mg.] ▶L ♀B (D in 3rd trimester) ▶– $ ■

TOLMETIN (*Tolectin*) 200 to 600 mg PO three times per day. [Generic only: Tabs 200 (scored), 600 mg. Caps 400 mg.] ▶L ♀C (D in 3rd trimester) ▶+ $$$ ■

Opioid Agonist-Antagonists

BUPRENORPHINE (*Buprenex, Butrans, Subutex*) Analgesia: 0.3 to 0.6 mg IV/IM q 6 h prn. Treatment of opioid dependence (must undergo special training and be registered to prescribe for this indication): Induction 8 mg SL on day 1, 16 mg SL on day 2. Maintenance: 16 mg SL daily. Can individualize to range of 4 to 24 mg SL daily. Moderate to severe chronic pain: 5 to 20 mcg/h patch changed q 7 days. [Generic only: SL Tabs 2, 8 mg. Trade only (Butrans): transdermal patches 5, 10, 20 mcg/h.] ▶L ♀C ▶– ⊙III $ IV, $$$$$ SL ■

BUTORPHANOL (*Stadol, Stadol NS*) 0.5 to 2 mg IV or 1 to 4 mg IM q 3 to 4 h prn. Nasal spray (Stadol NS): 1 spray (1 mg) in 1 nostril q 3 to 4 h. Abuse potential. [Generic only: Nasal spray 1 mg/spray, 2.5 mL bottle (14 to 15 doses/bottle).] ▶LK ♀C ▶+ ⊙IV $$$ ■

NALBUPHINE (*Nubain*) 10 to 20 mg IV/IM/SC q 3 to 6 h prn. ▶LK ♀? ▶? $

PENTAZOCINE (*Talwin NX*) 30 mg IV/IM q 3 to 4 h prn (Talwin). 1 tab PO q 3 to 4 h. (Talwin NX = 50 mg pentazocine/0.5 mg naloxone). [Generic/Trade: Tabs 50 mg with 0.5 mg naloxone, trade scored.] ▶LK ♀C ▶? ⊙IV $$$ ■

Opioid Agonists

CODEINE 0.5 to 1 mg/kg up to 15 to 60 mg PO/IM/IV/SC q 4 to 6 h. Do not use IV in children. [Generic only: Tabs 15, 30, 60 mg. Oral soln: 30 mg/5 mL.] ▶LK ♀C ▶– ⊙II $ ■

FENTANYL (*Duragesic, Actiq, Fentora, Sublimaze, Abstral, Subsys, Lazanda, Onsolis*) Transdermal (Duragesic): 1 patch q 72 h (some with chronic pain

(cont.)

ANALGESICS

FENTANYL TRANSDERMALDOSE (Dosing based on ongoing morphine requirement.)

Morphine* (IV/IM)	Morphine* (PO)	Transdermal fentanyl*
10–22 mg/d	60–134 mg/d	25 mcg/h
23–37 mg/d	135–224 mg/d	50 mcg/h
38–52 mg/d	225–314 mg/d	75 mcg/h
53–67 mg/d	315–404 mg/d	100 mcg/h

*For higher morphine doses, see product insert for transdermal fentanyl equivalencies.

may require q 48 h dosing). May wear more than 1 patch to achieve the correct analgesic effect. Transmucosal lozenge (Actiq) for breakthrough cancer pain: 200 to 1600 mcg, goal is 4 lozenges on a stick per day in conjunction with long-acting opioid. Buccal tab (Fentora) for breakthrough cancer pain: 100 to 800 mcg, titrated to pain relief. Buccal soluble film (Onsolis) for breakthrough cancer pain: 200 to 1200 mcg, titrated to pain relief. Sublingual tab (Abstral) for breakthrough cancer pain: 100 mcg, may repeat once after 30 minutes. Sublingual spray (Subsys) for breakthrough cancer pain: 100 mcg, may repeat once after 30 minutes. Nasal spray (Lazanda) for breakthrough cancer pain: 100 mcg. Adult analgesia/procedural sedation: 50 to 100 mcg slow IV over 1 to 2 min; carefully titrate to effect. Analgesia: 50 to 100 mcg IM q 1 to 2 h prn. [Generic/Trade: Transdermal patches 12, 25, 50, 75, 100 mcg/h. Actiq lozenges on a stick, berry flavored 200, 400, 600, 800, 1200, 1600 mcg. Trade only: (Fentora) buccal tab 100, 200, 400, 600, 800 mcg, packs of 4 or 28 tabs. Trade only: (Onsolis) buccal soluble film 200, 400, 600, 800, 1200 mcg in child-resistant, protective foil, packs of 30 films. Trade only: (Abstral) sublingual tab: 100, 200, 300, 400, 600, 800 mcg, packs of 4 or 32 tabs. Trade only: (Subsys) sublingual spray: 100, 200, 400, 600, 800, 1200, 1600 mcg blister packs in cartons of 10 and 30 (30 only for 1200 and 1600 mcg). Trade only: (Lazanda) nasal spray: 100, 400 mcg/spray, 8 sprays/bottle.] ▶L ♀C ▶+ ⊚ll $ - varies by therapy ■

HYDROMORPHONE (*Dilaudid, Exalgo, ✦Hydromorph Contin*) Adults: 2 to 4 mg PO q 4 to 6 h. 0.5 to 2 mg IM/SC or slow IV q 4 to 6 h. 3 mg PR q 6 to 8 h. Titrate dose as high as necessary to relieve cancer or nonmalignant pain where chronic opioids are necessary. Peds age 12 yo or younger: 0.03 to 0.08 mg/kg PO q 4 to 6 h prn or give 0.015 mg/kg/dose IV q 4 to 6 h prn. Controlled-release tabs: 8 to 64 mg daily. [Generic/Trade: Tabs 2, 4, 8 mg (8 mg trade scored). Oral soln 5 mg/5 mL. Controlled-release tabs (Exalgo): 8, 12, 16, 32 mg.] ▶L ♀C ▶? ⊚ll $$ ■

LEVORPHANOL (*Levo-Dromoran*) 2 mg PO q 6 to 8 h prn. [Generic only: Tabs 2 mg, scored.] ▶L ♀C ▶? ⊚ll $$$$

MEPERIDINE (*Demerol, pethidine*) 1 to 1.8 mg/kg up to 150 mg IM/SC/PO or slow IV q 3 to 4 h. 75 mg meperidine IV/IM/SC is equivalent to 300 mg meperidine PO. [Generic/Trade: Tabs 50 (trade scored), 100 mg. Generic only: Syrup 50 mg/5 mL.] ▶LK ♀C but + ▶+ ⊚ll $$

METHADONE (*Diskets, Dolophine, Methadose, ✦Metadol*) Severe pain in opioid-tolerant patients: Initial dose is 2.5 mg IM/SC/PO q 8 to 12 h prn. Titrate up by 2.5 mg per dose q 5 to 7 days as necessary to relieve cancer or nonmalignant pain where chronic opioids are necessary. May start as high as 10 mg per dose if opioid-dependent patient and dosing is managed by experienced practitioner using an opioid conversion formula. Opioid dependence: Typical dose to prevent withdrawal is 20 mg PO daily but must be managed by an experienced practitioner. Treatment longer than 3 weeks is maintenance and only permitted in approved treatment programs. Opioid-naive patients: Not recommended in opioid-naive patients as 1st-line treatment of acute pain, mild chronic pain, postoperative pain, or as a prn medication.   [Generic/Trade: Tabs 5, 10 mg. Dispersible tabs 40 mg (for opioid dependence only). Oral concentrate (Intensol): 10 mg/mL. Generic only: Oral soln 5, 10 mg/5 mL.] ▶L ♀C ▷? ⊙II $ ■

MORPHINE (*MS Contin, Kadian, Avinza, Roxanol, Oramorph SR, MSIR, DepoDur, ✦Statex, M.O.S., Doloral, M-Eslon*) Controlled-release tabs (MS Contin, Oramorph SR): Start at 30 mg PO q 8 to 12 h. Controlled-release caps (Kadian): 20 mg PO q 12 to 24 h. Extended-release caps (Avinza): Start at 30 mg PO daily. Do not break, chew, or crush MS Contin or Oramorph SR. Kadian and Avinza caps may be opened and sprinkled in applesauce for easier administration; however, the pellets should not be crushed or chewed. Give 0.1 to 0.2 mg/kg up to 15 mg IM/SC or slow IV q 4 h. Titrate dose as high as necessary to relieve cancer or nonmalignant pain where chronic opioids are necessary. [Generic only: Tabs, immediate-release 15, 30 mg ($). Oral soln: 10 mg/5 mL, 20 mg/5 mL, 20 mg/mL (concentrate). Rectal supps 5, 10, 20, 30 mg. Generic/Trade: Controlled-release tabs (MS Contin) 15, 30, 60, 100, 200 mg ($$$$). Controlled-release caps (Kadian) 10, 20, 30, 50, 60, 80, 100 mg ($$$$$). Extended-release caps (Avinza) 30, 45, 60, 75, 90, 120 mg. Trade only: Controlled-release caps (Kadian) 40, 200 mg.] ▶LK ♀C ▷+ ⊙II varies by therapy ■

OXYCODONE (*Roxicodone, OxyContin, Percolone, OxyIR, OxyFAST, Oxecta, ✦Endocodone, Supeudol, OxyNEO*) Immediate-release preparations: 5 mg PO q 4 to 6 h prn. Controlled-release (OxyContin): 10 to 40 mg PO q 12 h (no supporting data for shorter dosing intervals for controlled-release tabs). Titrate dose as high as necessary to relieve cancer or nonmalignant pain where chronic opioids are necessary. Do not break, chew, or crush controlled-release preparations or Oxecta. [Generic only: Immediate-release: Tabs 5, 10, 20 mg. Caps 5 mg. Oral soln 5 mg/5 mL. Generic/Trade: Tab 15, 30 mg. Oral concentrate 20 mg/mL. Trade only: Immediate-release abuse-deterrent tabs (Oxecta): 5, 7.5 mg. Controlled-release tabs: 10, 15, 20, 30, 40, 60, 80 mg ($$$$$).] ▶L ♀B ▷- ⊙II $ - varies by therapy ■

OXYMORPHONE (*Opana, Opana ER*) 10 to 20 mg PO q 4 to 6 h (immediate-release) or 5 mg q 12 h (extended-release) in opioid-naive patients, 1 h before or 2 h after meals. 1 to 1.5 mg IM/SC q 4 to 6 h prn. 0.5 mg IV q 4 to 6 h prn, increase dose until pain adequately controlled. [Generic/Trade: immediate-release (IR) tabs 5, 10 mg. Extended-release tabs (ER) 5, 7.5, 10, 15, 20, 30, 40 mg. Trade only: Injection 1 mg/mL.] ▶L ♀C ▷? ⊙II $$$$$ ■

Opioid Analgesic Combinations

NOTE: *Refer to individual components for further information. May cause drowsiness and/or sedation, which may be enhanced by alcohol and other CNS depressants. Opioids, carisoprodol, and butalbital may be habit forming. Avoid exceeding 4 g/day of acetaminophen in combination products. Caution people who drink 3 or more alcoholic drinks/day to limit acetaminophen use to 2.5 g/ day due to additive liver toxicity. Opioids commonly cause constipation; concurrent laxatives are recommended. All opioids are pregnancy class D if used for prolonged periods or in high doses at term.*

ANEXSIA (hydrocodone + acetaminophen) Multiple strengths; write specific product on Rx. 1 tab PO q 4 to 6 h prn. [Generic only: Tabs 5/325, 7.5/325, 10/325 mg hydrocodone/mg acetaminophen, scored.] ▶LK ♀C ▶– ⊙ll $

CAPITAL WITH CODEINE SUSPENSION (acetaminophen + codeine) 15 mL PO q 4 h prn. Give 5 mL q 4 to 6 h prn for age 3 to 6 yo, give 10 mL PO q 4 to 6 h prn for age 7 to 12 yo, use adult dose for age older than 12 yo. [Generic only: Soln 120 mg/5 mL, 12 mg/5 mL (APAP/Codeine). Trade only: Susp 120 mg/5 mL, 12 mg/5 mL (APAP/Codeine).] ▶LK ♀C ▶? ⊙V $

COMBUNOX (oxycodone + ibuprofen) 1 tab PO q 6 h prn for no more than 7 days. Max 4 tabs per day. [Generic only: Tabs 5 mg oxycodone/ 400 mg ibuprofen.] ▶L ♀C (D in 3rd trimester) ▶? ⊙ll $$$

EMPIRIN WITH CODEINE (acetylsalicylic acid + codeine, ✦292 tab) Multiple strengths; write specific product on Rx. 1 to 2 tabs PO q 4 h prn. [Generic/Trade: No US formulation available. Tabs 325/30, 325/60 mg aspirin/mg codeine] ▶LK ♀D ▶– ⊙ll $

FIORICET WITH CODEINE (acetaminophen + butalbital + caffeine + codeine) 1 to 2 caps PO q 4 h prn. Max 6 caps per day. [Generic/Trade: Caps 325 mg acetaminophen/50 mg butalbital/40 mg caffeine/ 30 mg codeine.] ▶LK ♀C ▶– ⊙lll $$$

FIORINAL WITH CODEINE (acetylsalicylic acid + butalbital + caffeine + codeine, ✦Fiorinal C-1/4, Fiorinal C-1/2, Trianal C-1/2, Trianal C-1/2) 1 to 2 caps PO q 4 h prn. Max 6 caps/24 h. [Generic/Trade: Caps 325 mg aspirin/50 mg butalbital/40 mg caffeine/30 mg codeine.] ▶LK ♀D ▶– ⊙lll $$$

IBUDONE, REPREXAIN (hydrocodone + ibuprofen) 1 tab PO q 4 to 6 h prn, max dose 5 tabs/day. [Generic/Trade: Tabs 2.5/200, 5/200, and 10/200 mg hydrocodone/ibuprofen.] ▶LK ♀– ▶? ⊙ll $$

LORCET (hydrocodone + acetaminophen) 1 to 2 caps (5/325) PO q 4 to 6 h prn, max dose 8 caps/day. 1 tab PO q 4 to 6 h prn (7.5/325 and 10/325), max dose 6 tabs/day. [Generic/Trade: Tabs 5/325, 7.5/325, 10/325 mg hydrocodone/ acetaminophen.] ▶LK ♀C ▶– ⊙ll $

LORTAB (hydrocodone + acetaminophen) 1 to 2 tabs (2.5/325 and 5/325) PO q 4 to 6 h prn, max dose 8 tabs/day. 1 tab (7.5/325 and 10/325 PO) q 4 to 6 h prn, max dose 5 tabs/day. [Generic/Trade: Lortab 5/325 (scored), Lortab 7.5/325 (trade scored), Lortab 10/325 mg hydrocodone/mg acetaminophen. Generic only: Tabs 2.5/325 mg.] ▶LK ♀C ▶– ⊙ll $

MERSYNDOL WITH CODEINE (acetaminophen + codeine + doxylamine) Canada only. 1 to 2 tabs PO q 4 to 6 h prn. Max 12 tabs per day. [Canada Trade only: OTC tab 325 mg acetaminophen/8 mg codeine phosphate/5 mg doxylamine.] ▶LK ♀C ▶? $

NORCO (hydrocodone + acetaminophen) 1 to 2 tabs PO q 4 to 6 h prn (5/325), max dose 12 tabs/day. 1 tab (7.5/325 and 10/325) PO q 4 to 6 h prn, max dose 8 and 6 tabs/day respectively. [Generic/Trade: Tabs 5/325, 7.5/325, 10/325 mg hydrocodone/acetaminophen, scored. Generic only: solution 7.5/325 mg per 15 mL.] ▶L ♀C ▶? ⊚ll $$

PERCOCET (oxycodone + acetaminophen, ✦Percocet-demi, Oxycocet, Endocet) Multiple strengths; write specific product on Rx. 1 to 2 tabs PO q 4 to 6 h prn (2.5/325 and 5/325 mg). 1 tab PO q 4 to 6 h prn (7.5/325 and 10/325 mg). [Generic/Trade: oxycodone/acetaminophen Tabs 2.5/325, 5/325, 7.5/325, 10/325 mg. Trade only: (Primlev) tabs 2.5/300, 5/300, 7.5/300, 10/300 mg. Generic only: 10/325 mg.] ▶L ♀C ▶– ⊚ll $

PERCODAN (oxycodone + acetylsalicylic acid, ✦Oxycodan) 1 tab PO q 6 h prn. [Generic/Trade: Tabs 4.88/325 mg oxycodone/aspirin (trade scored).] ▶LK ♀D ▶– ⊚ll $$

ROXICET (oxycodone + acetaminophen) Multiple strengths; write specific product on Rx. 1 tab PO q 6 h prn. Soln: 5 mL PO q 6 h prn. [Generic/Trade: Tabs 5/325 mg. Caps/Caplets 5/325 mg. Soln 5/325 per 5 mL, mg oxycodone/acetaminophen.] ▶L ♀C ▶– ⊚ll $

SOMA COMPOUND WITH CODEINE (carisoprodol + acetylsalicylic acid + codeine) Moderate to severe musculoskeletal pain: 1 to 2 tabs PO four times per day prn. [Generic only: Tabs 200 mg carisoprodol/ 325 mg aspirin/16 mg codeine.] ▶L ♀D ▶– ⊚ll $$$$

SYNALGOS-DC (dihydrocodeine + acetylsalicylic acid + caffeine) 2 caps PO q 4 h prn. [Generic/Trade: Caps 16 mg dihydrocodeine/ 356.4 mg aspirin/30 mg caffeine.] ▶L ♀C ▶– ⊚lll $$$

TYLENOL WITH CODEINE (codeine + acetaminophen, ✦Tylenol #1, Tylenol #2, Tylenol #3, Tylenol #4, Atasol 8, Atasol 15, Atasol 30) Multiple strengths; write specific product on Rx. Give 1 to 2 tabs PO q 4 h prn. Elixir: give 5 mL q 4 to 6 h prn for age 3 to 6 yo; give 10 mL q 4 to 6 h prn for age 7 to 12 yo. [Generic only: Tabs Tylenol #2 (15/300). Tylenol with Codeine Elixir/Susp/Soln 12/120 per 5 mL, mg codeine/mg acetaminophen. Generic/Trade: Tabs Tylenol #3 (30/300), Tylenol #4 (60/300).] ▶LK ♀C ▶? ⊚lll $

TYLOX (oxycodone + acetaminophen) 1 cap PO q 6 h prn. [Trade only: Caps 5 mg oxycodone/325 mg acetaminophen.] ▶L ♀C ▶– ⊚ll $

VICODIN (hydrocodone + acetaminophen) 5/300 mg (max dose 8 tabs/day) and 7.5/300 mg (max dose of 6 tabs/day): 1 to 2 tabs PO q 4 to 6 h prn. 10/300 mg: 1 tab PO q 4 to 6 h prn (max of 6 tabs/day). [Generic/Trade: Tabs Vicodin (5/300), Vicodin ES (7.5/300), Vicodin HP (10/300), scored, mg hydrocodone/mg acetaminophen.] ▶LK ♀C ▶? ⊚lll $$$

VICOPROFEN (hydrocodone + ibuprofen) 1 tab PO q 4 to 6 h prn, max dose 5 tabs/day. [Generic/Trade: Tabs 7.5/200 mg hydrocodone/ibuprofen. Generic only: Tabs 2.5/200, 5/200, 10/200 mg.] ▶LK ♀– ▶? ⊚ll $$

XODOL (**hydrocodone + acetaminophen**) 1 tab PO q 4 to 6 h prn, max 6 doses/day. [Generic/Trade only: Tabs 5/300, 7.5/300, 10/300 mg hydrocodone/acetaminophen.] ▶LK ♀C ▶– ⊚II $$$

Opioid Antagonists

NALOXONE (*Narcan*) Adult opioid overdose: 0.4 to 2 mg q 2 to 3 min prn. Adult post-op reversal: 0.1 to 0.2 mg q 2 to 3 min prn. Peds opioid overdose: 0.01 mg/kg IV; may give 0.1 mg/kg if inadequate response. Peds post-op reversal: 0.005 to 0.01 mg q 2 to 3 min prn. May use IM/SC/ET if IV not available. ▶LK ♀B ▶? $

Other Analgesics

ACETAMINOPHEN (*Tylenol, Panadol, Tempra, Ofirmev, paracetamol, ✦Abenol, Atasol, Pediatrix*) 325 to 650 mg PO/PR q 4 to 6 h prn. Max dose 4 g/day, possibly changing to 3 g/day in near future. Adults and adolescents wt less than 50 kg, give 15 mg/kg IV q 6 h or 12.5 mg/kg IV q 4 h. Max dose 75 mg/kg/day. Adults and adolescents wt 50 kg or greater, give 1000 mg IV q 6 h or 650 mg IV q 4 h. Max dose 4 g/day. OA: 2 extended-release caplets (ie, 1300 mg) PO q 8 h around the clock. Peds: 10 to 15 mg/kg/dose PO/PR q 4 to 6 h prn. Children age 2 to 12 yo, give 15 mg/kg IV q 6 h or 12.5 mg/kg q 4 h. Max dose 75 mg/kg/day. [OTC: Tabs 325, 500, 650 mg. Chewable Tabs 80 mg. Oral disintegrating Tabs 80, 160 mg. Caps/Gelcaps 500 mg. Extended-release caplets 650 mg. Liquid 160 mg/5 mL, 500 mg/15 mL. Supps 80, 120, 325, 650 mg.] ▶LK ♀B ▶+ $

MIDOL TEEN FORMULA (**acetaminophen + pamabrom**) 2 caps PO q 4 to 6 h. [Generic/Trade OTC: Caps 325 mg acetaminophen/25 mg pamabrom (diuretic).] ▶LK ♀B ▶+ $

TAPENTADOL (*Nucynta, Nucynta ER*) Moderate to severe acute pain: Immediate-release: 50 to 100 mg PO q 4 to 6 h prn, max 600 mg/day. Moderate to severe chronic pain: Extended-release: 50 to 250 mg PO twice daily. Adjust dose in elderly, renal and hepatic dysfunction. Avoid in opioid-dependent patients. Seizures may occur with concurrent antidepressants or seizure disorder. [Trade only: Immediate-release ($$$$): Tabs 50, 75, 100 mg. Extended-release ($$$$$): Tabs 50, 100, 150, 200, 250 mg.] ▶LK ♀C ▶– ⊚II $$$$

TRAMADOL (*Ultram, Ultram ER, Ryzolt, ConZip, Rybix ODT, ✦Zytram XL, Tridural, Ralivia, Durela*) Moderate to moderately severe pain: 50 to 100 mg PO q 4 to 6 h prn, max 400 mg/day. Chronic pain, extended-release: 100 to 300 mg PO daily. Adjust dose in elderly, renal, and hepatic dysfunction. Avoid in opioid-dependent patients. Seizures may occur with concurrent serotonergic agents or seizure disorder. [Generic/Trade: Tabs, immediate-release 50 mg. Extended-release tabs 100, 200, 300 mg. Trade only: (ConZip) Extended-release caps 100, 150, 200, 300 mg. (Rybix) ODT 50 mg.] ▶KL ♀C ▶– ⊚IV $$$

ANESTHESIA

Anesthetics and Sedatives

DEXMEDETOMIDINE (*Precedex*) ICU sedation less than 24 h: Load 1 mcg/kg over 10 min followed by infusion 0.2 to 0.7 mcg/kg/h titrated to desired sedation endpoint. Beware of bradycardia and hypotension. ▶LK ♀C ▶? $$$$$

ETOMIDATE (*Amidate*) Induction: Give 0.3 mg/kg IV. ▶L ♀C ▶? $

KETAMINE (*Ketalar*) Dissociative sedation, induction: Adult: 1 to 2 mg/kg IV over 1 to 2 min (produces 5 to 10 min dissociative state) or 6.5 to 13 mg/kg IM (produces 10 to 20 min dissociative state). Consider concurrent administration of benzodiazepine and atropine (minimizes hypersalivation). Peds: Age older than 3 mo: 1 to 2 mg/kg IV over 1 to 2 min or 4 to 5 mg/kg IM. [Generic/Trade: 10 mg/mL, 50 mg/mL, 100 mg/mL.] ▶L ♀? ▶? ⊙III $ ■

METHOHEXITAL (*Brevital*) Anesthesia induction: 1 to 1.5 mg/kg IV, duration 5 min. ▶LK ♀D ▶? ⊙IV $$

MIDAZOLAM (*Versed*) Adult sedation/anxiolysis: 5 mg or 0.07 mg/kg IM; or 1 mg IV slowly q 2 to 3 min up to 5 mg. Peds: 0.25 to 1 mg/kg to max of 20 mg PO, or 0.1 to 0.15 mg/kg IM. IV route (6 mo to 5 yo): initial dose 0.05 to 0.1 mg/kg IV, then titrated to max 0.6 mg/kg. IV route (6 to 12 yo): initial dose 0.025 to 0.05 mg/kg IV, then titrated to max 0.4 mg/kg. Monitor for respiratory depression. [Generic only: Injection: 1 mg/mL, 5 mg/mL, Oral liquid 2 mg/mL.] ▶LK ♀D ▶– ⊙IV $

PROPOFOL (*Diprivan*) Induction: 40 mg IV q 10 sec until induction (2 to 2.5 mg/kg). ICU ventilator sedation: Infusion 5 to 50 mcg/kg/min. Deep sedation: 1 mg/kg IV over 20 to 30 seconds. Repeat 0.5 mg/kg IV prn. ▶L ♀B ▶– $

Local Anesthetics

NOTE: *Risk of chondrolysis in patients receiving intra-articular infusions of local anesthetics following arthroscopic and other surgical procedures.*

ARTICAINE (*Septocaine, Zorcaine*) 4% injection (includes epinephrine) up to 7 mg/kg total dose [4% (includes epinephrine 1:100,000).] ▶LK ♀C ▶? $

BUPIVACAINE (*Marcaine, Sensorcaine*) Up to 2.5 mg/kg without epinephrine and up 3.0 mg/kg with epinephrine [0.25%, 0.5%, 0.75%, all with or without epinephrine.] ▶LK ♀C ▶? $ ■

EMLA (prilocaine—topical + lidocaine—topical) Topical anesthesia: Apply 2.5 g cream or 1 disc to region at least 1 h before procedure. Cover with occlusive dressing. [Generic/Trade: Cream (2.5% lidocaine + 2.5% prilocaine) 5, 30 g.] ▶LK ♀B ▶? $$

LIDOCAINE—LOCAL ANESTHETIC (*Xylocaine*) Without epinephrine: Max dose 4.5 mg/kg not to exceed 300 mg. With epinephrine: Max dose 7 mg/kg not exceed 500 mg. Dose for regional block varies by region. [0.5, 1, 1.5, 2%. With epi: 0.5, 1, 1.5, 2%.] ▶LK ♀B ▶? $

MEPIVACAINE (*Carbocaine, Polocaine*) Onset 3 to 5 min, duration 45 to 90 min. Amide group. Max local dose 5 to 6 mg/kg. [1, 1.5, 2, 3%.] ▶LK ♀C ▶? $

PRILOCAINE (*Citanest*) Contraindicated if younger than 6 to 9 mo. If younger than 5 yo, maximum local dose is 3 to 4 mg/kg (with or without epinephrine). If 5 yo or older, maximum local dose is 5 mg/kg without epinephrine and 7 mg/kg with epinephrine. [4%, 4% with epinephrine] ▶LK ♀B ▶? $

Neuromuscular Blockade Reversal Agents

NEOSTIGMINE (*Bloxiverz*) 0.03 to 0.07 mg/kg slow IV (preceded by atropine or glycopyrrolate). Max 0.07 mg/kg or 5 mg, whichever is less. ▶L ♀C ▶? $$$$

Neuromuscular Blockers

CISATRACURIUM (*Nimbex*) Paralysis: 0.15 to 0.2 mg/kg IV. Peds: 0.1 mg/kg. Duration 30 to 60 min. ▶plasma ♀B ▶? $

ROCURONIUM (*Zemuron*) Paralysis: 0.6 mg/kg IV. Duration 30 min. Rapid-sequence intubation: 0.6 to 1.2 mg/kg IV. ▶L ♀B ▶? $$

SUCCINYLCHOLINE (*Anectine, Quelicin*) Paralysis: 0.6 to 1.1 mg/kg IV. Peds: 2 mg/kg IV. ▶plasma ♀C ▶? $

VECURONIUM (*Norcuron*) Paralysis: 0.08 to 0.1 mg/kg IV. Duration 15 to 30 min. ▶LK ♀C ▶? $

ANTIMICROBIALS

PROPHYLAXIS FOR BACTERIAL ENDOCARDITIS*

Limited to dental or respiratory tract procedures in patients at highest risk. All regimens are single dose administered 30–60 minutes prior to procedure.	
Standard regimen	Amoxicillin 2 g PO
Unable to take oral meds	Ampicillin 2 g IM/IV; or cefazolin† or ceftriaxone† 1 g IM/IV
Allergic to penicillin	Clindamycin 600 mg PO; or cephalexin† 2 g PO; or azithromycin or clarithromycin 500 mg PO
Allergic to penicillin and unable to take oral meds	Clindamycin 600 mg IM/IV; or cefazolin† or ceftriaxone† 1 g IM/IV
Pediatric drug doses	Pediatric dose should not exceed adult dose. Amoxicillin 50 mg/kg, ampicillin 50 mg/kg, azithromycin 15 mg/kg, cephalexin† 50 mg/kg, cefazolin† 50 mg/kg, ceftriaxone† 50 mg/kg, clarithromycin 15 mg/kg, clindamycin 20 mg/kg.

*For additional details of the 2007 AHA guidelines, see http://www.heart.org.
†Avoid cephalosporins if prior penicillin-associated anaphylaxis, angioedema, or urticaria.

OVERVIEW OF BACTERIAL PATHOGENS (Selected)

By bacterial class

Gram-positive aerobic cocci: Staphylococci: *S. epidermidis* (coagulase-negative), *S. aureus* (coagulase-positive); Streptococci: *S. pneumoniae* (*pneumococcus*), *S. pyogenes* (Group A), *S. agalactiae* (Group B), enterococcus
Gram-positive aerobic/facultatively anaerobic bacilli: Bacillus,Corynebacterium diphtheriae, Erysipelothrix rhusiopathiae, Listeria monocytogenes, Nocardia
Gram-negative aerobic diplococci: Moraxella catarrhalis, Neisseria gonorrhoeae, Neisseria meningitidis
Gram-negative aerobic coccobacilli: Haemophilus ducreyi, H. influenzae
Gram-negative aerobic bacilli: Acinetobacter, Bartonella species, Bordetella pertussis, Brucella, Burkholderia cepacia, Campylobacter, Francisella tularensis, Helicobacter pylori, Legionella pneumophila, Pseudomonas aeruginosa, Stenotrophomonas maltophilia, Vibrio cholerae, Yersinia
Gram-negative facultatively anaerobic bacilli: Aeromonas hydrophila, Eikenella corrodens, Pasteurella multocida; Enterobacteriaceae: E. coli, Citrobacter, Shigella, Salmonella, Klebsiella, Enterobacter, Hafnia, Serratia, Proteus, Providencia
Anaerobes: Actinomyces, Bacteroides fragilis, Clostridium botulinum, Clostridium difficile, Clostridium perfringens, Clostridium tetani, Fusobacterium, Lactobacillus, Peptostreptococcus

ANTIMICROBIALS

(cont.)

OVERVIEW OF BACTERIAL PATHOGENS (Selected) (*continued*)

By bacterial class (*continued*)
<u>**Defective Cell Wall Bacteria:**</u> *Chlamydia pneumoniae, Chlamydia psittaci, Chlamydia trachomatis, Coxiella burnetii, Mycoplasma pneumoniae, Rickettsia prowazekii, Rickettsia rickettsii, Rickettsia typhi, Ureaplasma urealyticum*   <u>**Spirochetes:**</u> *Borrelia burgdorferi, Leptospira, Treponema pallidum*   <u>**Mycobacteria:**</u> *M. avium* complex, *M. kansasii, M. leprae, M. tuberculosis*

By bacterial name
Acinetobacter **Gram-negative aerobic bacilli**
Actinomyces **Anaerobes**
Aeromonas hydrophila **Gram-negative facultatively anaerobic bacilli**
Bacillus **Gram-positive aerobic/facultatively anaerobic bacilli**
Bacteroides fragilis **Anaerobes**
Bartonella species **Gram-negative aerobic bacilli**
Bordetella pertussis **Gram-negative aerobic bacilli**
Borrelia burgdorferi **Spirochetes**
Brucella **Gram-negative aerobic bacilli**
Burkholderia cepacia **Gram-negative aerobic bacilli**
Campylobacter **Gram-negative aerobic bacilli**
Chlamydia pneumoniae **Defective cell wall bacteria**
Chlamydia psittaci **Defective cell wall bacteria**
Chlamydia trachomatis **Defective cell wall bacteria**
Citrobacter **Gram-negative facultatively anaerobic bacilli**
Clostridium botulinum **Anaerobes**
Clostridium difficile **Anaerobes**
Clostridium perfringens **Anaerobes**
Clostridium tetani **Anaerobes**
Corynebacterium diphtheriae **Gram-positive aerobic/facultatively anaerobic bacilli**
Coxiella burnetii **Defective cell wall bacteria**
E. coli **Gram-negative facultatively anaerobic bacilli**
Eikenella corrodens **Gram-negative facultatively anaerobic bacilli**
Enterobacter **Gram-negative facultatively anaerobic bacilli**
Enterobacteriaceae **Gram-negative facultatively anaerobic bacilli**
Enterococcus **Gram-positive aerobic cocci**
Erysipelothrix rhusiopathiae **Gram-positive aerobic/facultatively anaerobic bacilli**
Francisella tularensis **Gram-negative aerobic bacilli**
Fusobacterium **Anaerobes**
Haemophilus ducreyi **Gram-negative aerobic coccobacilli**
Haemophilus influenzae **Gram-negative aerobic coccobacilli**
Hafnia **Gram-negative facultatively anaerobic bacilli**
Helicobacter pylori **Gram-negative aerobic bacilli**
Klebsiella **Gram-negative facultatively anaerobic bacilli**

(cont.)

OVERVIEW OF BACTERIAL PATHOGENS (Selected) (*continued*)

By bacterial name (*continued*)

Lactobacillus **Anaerobes**
Legionella pneumophila **Gram-negative aerobic bacilli**
Leptospira **Spirochetes**
Listeria monocytogenes **Gram-positive aerobic/facultatively anaerobic bacilli**
M. avium complex **Mycobacteria**
M. kansasii **Mycobacteria**
M. leprae **Mycobacteria**
M. tuberculosis **Mycobacteria**
Moraxella catarrhalis **Gram-negative aerobic diplococci**
Myocoplasma pneumoniae **Defective cell wall bacteria**
Neisseria gonorrhoeae **Gram-negative aerobic diplococci**
Neisseria meningitidis **Gram-negative aerobic diplococci**
Nocardia **Gram-positiv eaerobic/facultatively anaerobic bacilli**
Pasteurella multocida **Gram-negative facultatively anaerobic bacilli**
Peptostreptococcus **Anaerobes**
Pneumococcus **Gram-positive aerobic cocci**
Proteus **Gram-negative facultatively anaerobic bacilli**
Providencia **Gram-negative facultatively anaerobic bacilli**
Pseudomonas aeruginosa **Gram-negative aerobic bacilli**
Rickettsia prowazekii **Defective cell wall bacteria**
Rickettsia rickettsii **Defective cell wall bacteria**
Rickettsia typhi **Defective cell wall bacteria**
Salmonella **Gram-negative facultatively anaerobic bacilli**
Serratia **Gram-negative facultatively anaerobic bacilli**
Shigella **Gram-negative facultatively anaerobic bacilli**
Staph aureus (coagulase positive) **Gram-positive aerobic cocci**
Staph epidermidis (coagulasenegative) **Gram-negative aerobic cocci**
Stenotrophomonas maltophilia **Gram-negative aerobic bacilli**
Strep agalactiae (Group B) **Gram-positive aerobic cocci**
Strep pneumoniae (pneumococcus) **Gram-positive aerobic cocci**
Strep pyogenes (GroupA) **Gram-positive aerobic cocci**
Streptococci **Gram-positive aerobic cocci**
Treponema pallidum **Spirochetes**
Ureaplasma urealyticum **Defective cell wall bacteria**
Vibrio cholerae **Gram-negative aerobic bacilli**
Yersinia **Gram-negative aerobic bacilli**

ACUTE BACTERIAL SINUSITIS IN ADULTS AND CHILDREN:[a] IDSA TREATMENT RECOMMENDATIONS

Initial therapy in patients with mild to moderate infection and no risk factors for resistance	
Adults: Treat for 5 to 7 days with: 1) Amoxicillin-clavulanate 500 mg/125 mg PO three times per day or 875/125 mg PO two times per day for 5 to 7 days 2) Doxycycline 100 mg PO two times per day or 200 mg PO once daily	Peds: Amoxicillin-clavulanate[a] 45 mg /kg/day PO two times per day for 10 to 14 days
Initial therapy in patients with severe infection, risk factors for resistance,[c] or high endemic rate of invasive penicillin-nonsusceptible *S. pneumoniae* (≥10%)	
Adults: Treat for 5 to 7 days with: 1) Amoxicillin-clavulanate[b] 2000 mg /125 mg PO two times per day 2) Doxycycline 100 mg PO two times per day or 200 mg PO once daily	Peds: Amoxicillin-clavulanate[b] 90 mg/kg/day PO two times per day for 10 to 14 days
Beta-lactam allergy	
Adults: Treat for 5 to 7 days with: 1) Doxycycline 100 mg PO two times per day or 200 mg PO once daily 2) Levofloxacin 500 mg PO once daily 3) Moxifloxacin 400 mg PO once daily	Peds, type 1 hypersensitivity: Levofloxacin 10 to 20 mg/kg/day PO q 12-24 h for 10 to 14 days Peds, not type 1 hypersensitivity: Clindamycin[d] 30 to 40 mg/kg/day PO three times per day plus cefixime 8 mg/kg/day PO two times per day or cefpodoxime 10 mg/kg/day PO two times per day for 10 to 14 days
Risk factors for antibiotic resistance[†] or failed first-line therapy	
Adults: Treat for 5 to 7 days with: 1) Amoxicillin-clavulanate[b] 2000 mg /125 mg PO two times per day 2) Levofloxacin 500 mg PO once daily 3) Moxifloxacin 400 mg PO once daily	Peds: Treat for 10 to 14 days with: 1) Amoxicillin-clavulanate[b] 90 mg/kg/day PO two times per day 2) Clindamycin[d] 30 to 40 mg/kg/day PO three times per day plus cefixime 8 mg/kg/day PO two times per day or cefpodoxime 10 mg/kg/day PO two times per day 3) Levofloxacin 10 to 20 mg/kg/day PO q 12 to 24 h
Severe infection requiring hospitalization	
Adults: 1) Ampicillin-sulbactam 1.5 to 3 g IV q 6 h 2) Levofloxacin 500 mg PO/IV once daily 3) Moxifloxacin 400 mg PO/IV once daily 4) Ceftriaxone 1 to 2 g IV q 12 to 24 h 5) Cefotaxime 2 g IV q 4 to 6 h	Peds: 1) Ampicillin-sulbactam 200 to 400 mg/kg/day IV q 6 h 2) Ceftriaxone 50 mg/kg/day IV q 12 h 3) Cefotaxime 100 to 200 mg/kg/day IV q 6 h 4) Levofloxacin 10 to 20 mg/kg/day IV q 12 to 24 h

(cont.)

ACUTE BACTERIAL SINUSITIS IN ADULTS AND CHILDREN:[a] IDSA TREATMENT RECOMMENDATIONS (*continued*)

Adapted from *Clin Infect Dis* 2012;54(8):e72-e112. Available online at: http://www.idsociety.org.

[a] AAP guideline for sinusitis in children (Pediatrics 2013;132:e262-e280; pediatrics.aappublications.org) recommends amoxicillin as first-line treatment of uncomplicated acute sinusitis when antimicrobial resistance is not suspected. It recommends amoxicillin 45 mg/kg/day divided two times per day for mild-moderate sinusitis in children 2 years old or older who do not attend daycare and have not received an antibiotic in the past month. It recommends amoxicillin 80 to 90 mg/kg/day divided two times daily (max 2 g/dose) in communities with a high prevalence of nonsusceptible *S. pneumoniae* (at least 10%). Amoxicillin-clavulanate 80 to 90 mg/kg/day divided two times per day (max 2 g/dose) is an option for moderate-severe sinusitis, and for children less than 2 years old, attending daycare, or who received an antibiotic in the past month.

[b] High-dose amoxicillin-clavulanate is recommended for geographic regions with high endemic rates (at least 10%) of invasive penicillin-nonsusceptible *S. pneumoniae*, severe infection (eg, evidence of systemic toxicity with fever of 39° C or higher, and threat of suppurative complications), or risk factors for antibiotic resistance. Use the 14:1 formulation that provides amoxicillin 90 mg/kg/day and clavulanate 6.4 mg/kg/day. In Canada, where the 14:1 formulation of amoxicillin-clavulanate is not available, use the 7:1 formulation with additional amoxicillin. Do not increase the dose of the 4:1 or 7:1 formulation in order to achieve a higher dose of amoxicillin; this results in an excessive clavulanate dose and increases the risk of diarrhea.

[c] Risk factors for antibiotic resistance include attendance at daycare, age younger than 2 yo or older than 65 yo, recent hospitalization, antibiotic use within the past month, or patients who are immunocompromised.

[d] Clindamycin resistance in *S. pneumoniae* is common in some areas of the United states.

Anthrax: CDC and AAP Preferred Regimens

Adults[a]	Children, 1 month of age and older[b]
Post-exposure prophylaxis.[c] Treat for 60 days with:	
Ciprofloxacin 500 mg PO q 12 h OR Doxycycline 100 mg PO q 12 h	Ciprofloxacin 30 mg/kg/day PO divided q 12 h (max 500 mg/dose) OR Doxycycline[g] 4.4 mg/kg/day PO divided q 12 h for wt <45 kg (max 100 mg/dose); 100 mg PO divided q 12 h for wt >45 kg
Cutaneous anthrax without systemic involvement.[c, d] Treat naturally-acquired disease for 7 to 10 days; treat bioterrorism-related disease for 60 days with:	
Ciprofloxacin 500 mg PO q 12 h OR Doxycycline 100 mg PO q 12 h OR Levofloxacin 750 mg PO q 24 h OR Moxifloxacin 400 mg PO q 24 h	Ciprofloxacin 30 mg/kg/day PO divided q 12 h (max 500 mg/dose)

ANTIMICROBIALS

Anthrax: CDC and AAP Preferred Regimens (*continued*)

Adults[a]	Children, 1 month of age and older[b]
Systemic anthrax[d] without meningitis. Treat for at least 2 weeks and until clinically stable with:[e]	
Ciprofloxacin 400 mg IV q 8 h[c] PLUS Clindamycin 900 mg IV q 8 h OR Linezolid 600 mg IV q 12 h[f]	Ciprofloxacin 30 mg/kg/day IV divided q 8 h (max 400 mg/dose)[c] PLUS Clindamycin 40 mg/kg/day IV divided q 8 h (max 900 mg/dose)
Systemic anthrax[d] with possible/confirmed meningitis. Treat for 2 to 3 weeks and until clinically stable with:[e]	
Ciprofloxacin 400 mg IV q 8 h PLUS Meropenem 2 g IV q 8 h[c] PLUS Linezolid 600 mg IV q 12 h[f]	Ciprofloxacin 30 mg/kg/day IV divided q 8 h (max 400 mg/dose) PLUS Meropenem 120 mg/kg/day divided q 8 h (max 2 g/dose)[e] PLUS Linezolid 30 mg/kg/day divided q 8 h for age less than 12 yo; divide q 12 h for age 12 yo and older (max 600 mg/dose)[f]

Adapted from Emerg Infect Dis [Internet]. 2014 Feb. http://dx.doi.org/10.3201/eid2002.130687 and Pediatrics 2014;133(5):e1411 at http://pediatrics.aappublications.org/content/early/2014/04/22/peds.2014-0563.

a For women who are pregnant or breastfeeding, refer to Emerg Infect Dis [Internet]. 2014 Feb. http://dx.doi.org/10.3201/eid2002.130611.

b Refer to AAP clinical report cited above for dosage regimens to treat infants less than 1 mo.

c Alternatives for penicillin-susceptible strains. Post-exposure prophylaxis or cutaneous anthrax. Adults: amoxicillin 1000 mg PO q 8 h OR Penicillin 500 mg PO q 6 h. Children: amoxicillin 75 mg/kg/day PO divided q 8 h (max 1 g/dose) OR penicillin 50 to 75 mg/kg/day divided q 6 to 8 h. Systemic anthrax. Adults: penicillin G 4 million units IV q 4 h OR ampicillin 3 g IV q 6 h. Children: penicillin G 400,000 units/kg/day IV divided q 4 h (max 4 million units/dose).

d Systemic anthrax is inhalation, injection, or GI anthrax; cutaneous anthrax with systemic involvement, extensive edema, or lesions of the head or neck; or meningitis. In addition to antimicrobials, patients with suspected systemic infection should receive anthrax immune globulin IV or raxibacumab.

e For patients exposed to aerosolized spores, provide prophylaxis to complete 60 days of treatment from the onset of illness.

f Linezolid can cause myelosuppression; monitor CBC weekly esp. in patients with myelosuppression and for courses longer than 2 weeks.

g In children younger than 8 yo, the benefit of preventing anthrax outweighs the risk of permanent tooth staining with doxycycline.

C. difficile Infection (CDI) in Adults: IDSA/SHEA and ACG Treatment Recommendations

Clinical signs	Treatment
Initial episode: mild to moderate	
IDSA: WBC ≤15,000 AND serum creatinine <1.5 times premorbid level ACG: Diarrhea with signs or symptoms not meeting severe or complicated criteria	Metronidazole 500 mg PO q 8 h for 10 to 14 days[a] ACG: If no response to metronidazole in 5 to 7 days, consider vancomycin. If unable to take metronidazole, use vancomycin 125 mg PO q 6 h for 10 days.
Initial episode: severe	
IDSA: WBC ≥15,000 OR serum creatinine ≥1.5 times premorbid level ACG: Serum albumin <3 g/dL plus either: • WBC ≥15,000 • Abdominal tenderness	Vancomycin 125 mg PO q 6 h for 10 to 14 days
Initial episode: severe and complicated	
IDSA: Hypotension or shock, ileus, megacolon ACG: Any of the following attributable to CDI: • ICU admission for CDI • Hypotension ± required use of vasopressors • Fever ≥38.5°C • Ileus or significant abdominal distention • Mental status changes • WBC ≥35,000 or <2000 • Serum lactate >2.2 mmol/L • End organ failure	Vancomycin 500 mg PO/NG q 6 h plus metronidazole 500 mg IV q 8 h IDSA: Consider adding vancomycin 500 mg/100 mL[c] normal saline retention enema q 6 h if complete ileus. ACG: Add vancomycin 500 mg/500 mL[c] normal saline enema q 6 h if complicated CDI with ileus or toxic colon and/or significant abdominal distention.
First recurrent episode	
	Same as initial episode, stratified by severity. IDSA: Use vancomycin if WBC ≥15,000 or serum creatinine is increasing.
Second recurrent episode	
	Vancomycin taper and/or pulsed regimen[d]

Adapted from: Infect Control Hosp Epidemiol 2010;31:431. Available online at: http://www.idsociety.org.
Am J Gastroenterol 2013;108:478–98. Available online at: http://gi.org.

(cont.)

C. difficile Infection (CDI) in Adults: IDSA/SHEA and ACG Treatment Recommendations (*continued*)

[a] ACG recommends 10 days of therapy because that is what clinical trials evaluated.

[b] IDSA: Consider colectomy for severe CDI. ACG: Consult surgeon for complicated CDI. Consider surgery for any of the following attributed to CDI: hypotension requiring vasopressors; clinical signs of sepsis and organ dysfunction; mental status changes; WBC ≥50,000; lactate ≥5 mmol/L; or failure to improve after 5 days on medical therapy.

[c] IDSA recommends diluting vancomycin in 100 mL for administration as enema. ACG recommends diluting vancomycin in a larger volume (500 mL) in order to ensure delivery to ascending and transverse colon.

[d] IDSA taper example: Vancomycin 125 mg PO QID for 10 to 14 days, then 125 mg two times per day for 7 days, then 125 mg once daily for 7 days, then 125 mg every 2 or 3 days for 2 to 8 weeks. ACG proposed pulse regimen: Vancomycin 125 mg PO q 6 h for 10 days, then 125 mg once every 3 days for 10 doses. Note: If there is a third recurrence after a pulsed vancomycin regimen, ACG recommends considering fecal microbiota transplant.

ACUTE OTITIS MEDIA (AOM) IN CHILDREN: AMERICAN ACADEMY OF PEDIATRICS

Initial Treatment (immediate or delayed[a])	
First-line	**Alternative for Penicillin Allergy[d]**
Amoxicillin 80 to 90 mg/kg/day PO divided 2 times per day[b] OR Amoxicillin-clavulanate[c] 90 mg/kg/day PO divided 2 times per day[b]	Cefdinir 14 mg/kg/day PO divided 1 or 2 times per day[b] OR Cefuroxime 30 mg/kg/day PO divided 2 times per day[b] OR Cefpodoxime 10 mg/kg/day PO divided 2 times per day[b] OR Ceftriaxone 50 mg IM/IV once daily for 1 or 3 days
Treatment After First Antibiotic Failure	
If initial treatment was amoxicillin, use amoxicillin-clavulanate[c] 90 mg/kg/day PO divided 2 times per day. If initial treatment was amoxicillin-clavulanate or oral 3rd generation cephalosporin, use ceftriaxone 50 mg IM/IV once daily for 3 days. Consider clindamycin 30 to 40 mg/kg/day PO divided 3 times per day ± 3rd generation cephalosporin if penicillin-resistant *S pneumoniae* suspected.[b]	

(cont.)

ACUTE OTITIS MEDIA (AOM) IN CHILDREN: AMERICAN ACADEMY OF PEDIATRICS *(continued)*

Treatment After Second Antibiotic Failure
Clindamycin 30 to 40 mg/kg/day PO divided 3 times per day + 3rd generation cephalosporin.[b] Consider tympanocentesis and consult infectious diseases specialist if multidrug-resistant bacteria detected.

Adapted from *Pediatrics* 2013;131:e964–e999. Available online at: http://pediatrics.aappublications.org.

[a] This guideline is for uncomplicated AOM in children age 6 mo to 12 yo. Immediate treatment is recommended for children with otorrhea or severe symptoms (moderate to severe pain, pain for ≥48 h, or temperature ≥39°C), and bilateral AOM in children age 6 to 23 mo. Observation for 48 to 72 h before antibiotic therapy is an option for children age 6 to 23 mo with unilateral AOM and mild symptoms (mild pain for <48 h and temperature <39°C), or children 2 yo and older with unilateral/bilateral AOM and mild symptoms. Observation must have mechanism for follow-up and initiation of antibiotic if child worsens or does not improve within 48 to 72 h of symptom onset. Do not use observation if follow-up is unsure.

[b] The duration of oral treatment is 10 days for age <2 yo and children of any age with severe symptoms, 7 days for age 2 to 5 yo with mild to moderate symptoms, and 5 to 7 days for age ≥6 yo with mild to moderate symptoms.

[c] Consider in patients who have received amoxicillin in the past 30 days or who have the otitis-conjunctivitis syndrome. Use the 14:1 formulation of amoxicillin-clavulanate that provides amoxicillin 90 mg/kg/day and clavulanate 6.4 mg/kg/day. In Canada, where the 14:1 formulation of amoxicillin-clavulanate is not available, give the 7:1 formulation with additional amoxicillin. Do not increase the dose of a 4:1 or 7:1 formulation in order to achieve a higher dose of amoxicillin; this provides an excessive clavulanate dose and increases the risk of diarrhea.

[d] Cefdinir, cefuroxime, cefpodoxime, and ceftriaxone are highly unlikely to cross-react with penicillin. Excluding patients with a history of a severe reaction, the reaction rate in patients who have not undergone penicillin skin testing is estimated at 0.1%. A drug allergy practice parameter (Ann Allergy Asthma Immunol 2010;105:259–73; available at http://www.allergyparameters.org) recommends that a cephalosporin can be given to patients who do not have a history of a severe and/or recent allergic reaction to penicillin. Options for patients with a history of an IgE-mediated reaction to penicillin include substitution of a non-beta-lactam antibiotic, or penicillin or cephalosporin skin testing to evaluate the risk of cephalosporin administration.

ANTIMICROBIALS

SEXUALLY TRANSMITTED DISEASES & VAGINITIS*

Bacterial vaginosis	(1) metronidazole 5 g of 0.75% gel intravaginally daily for 5 days OR 500 mg PO two times per day for 7 days; (2) clindamycin 5 g of 2% cream intravaginally at bedtime for 7 days. Alternative: (1) tinidazole 2 g PO once daily for 2 days OR 1 g PO once daily for 5 days; (2) clindamycin 300 mg PO two times per day for 7 days. Treat all symptomatic pregnant women.
Candidal vaginitis	(1) Intravaginal butoconazole, clotrimazole, miconazole, terconazole, or tioconazole; (2) fluconazole 150 mg PO single dose
Cervicitis	Treat based on NAAT results for chlamydia and gonorrhea. Presumptively treat at-risk women (age <25 yo; sex partner is new, has other partners, or has STD), esp if follow-up not ensured or NAAT not available. Presumptive regimen: (1) azithromycin 1 g PO single dose; (2) doxycycline 100 mg PO two times per day for 7 days. Presumptively treat for gonorrhea if at-risk or high community prevalence.
Chancroid	(1) azithromycin 1 g PO single dose; (2) ceftriaxone 250 mg IM single dose; (3) ciprofloxacin 500 mg PO two times per day for 3 days; (4) erythromycin base 500 mg PO three times per day for 7 days.
Chlamydia	(1) azithromycin 1 g PO single dose; (2) doxycycline 100 mg PO two times per day for 7 days. Alternative: (1) erythromycin base 500 mg PO four times per day for 7 days; (2) levofloxacin 500 mg PO once daily for 7 days. In pregnancy: azithromycin 1 g PO single dose. Alternative: (1) amoxicillin 500 mg PO three times per day for 7 days. (2) erythromycin base 500 mg PO four times per day for 7 days or 250 mg PO four times per day for 14 days. Repeat NAAT 3 to 4 weeks after treatment in pregnant women.
Lymphogranuloma venereum *(Chlamydia trachomatis)*	(1) doxycycline 100 mg PO two times per day for 21 days. Alternative: erythromycin base 500 mg PO four times per day for 21 days.
Epididymitis, acute	Chlamydia and gonorrhea likely: ceftriaxone 250 mg IM single dose + doxycycline 100 mg PO two times per day for 10 days. Chlamydia-gonorrhea and enteric organisms likely: ceftriaxone 250 mg IM single dose + levofloxacin 500 mg PO once daily for 10 days. Enteric organisms likely: levofloxacin 500 mg PO once daily for 10 days.

(cont.)

SEXUALLY TRANSMITTED DISEASES & VAGINITIS* (*continued*)

Genital herpes, first episode	(1) acyclovir 400 mg PO three times per day for 7 to 10 days; (2) famciclovir 250 mg PO three times per day for 7 to 10 days; (3) valacyclovir 1 g PO two times per day for 7 to 10 days.
Genital herpes, recurrent	(1) acyclovir 400 mg PO three times per day for 5 days; (2) acyclovir 800 mg PO three times per day for 2 days or two times per day for 5 days; (3) famciclovir 125 mg PO two times per day for 5 days; (4) famciclovir 1 g PO two times per day for 1 day; (5) famciclovir 500 mg PO 1st dose, then 250 mg PO two times per day for 2 days; (6) valacyclovir 500 mg PO two times per day for 3 days; (7) valacyclovir 1 g PO daily for 5 days.
Genital herpes, suppressive therapy	(1) acyclovir 400 mg PO two times per day; (2) famciclovir 250 mg PO two times per day; (3) valacyclovir 500 or 1000 mg PO daily. Valacyclovir 500 mg PO daily reduces transmission in patients with 9 or fewer recurrences per year, but other valacyclovir/acyclovir regimens may be more effective for suppression in patients who have 10 or more recurrences per year. Pregnant women with recurrent genital herpes: Start at 36 weeks gestation with (1) acyclovir 400 mg PO three times per day; (2) valacyclovir 500 mg PO two times per day.
Genital herpes, recurrent in HIV infection	(1) acyclovir 400 mg PO three times per day for 5 to 10 days; (2) famciclovir 500 mg PO two times per day for 5 to 10 days; (3) valacyclovir 1 g PO two times per day for 5 to 10 days.
Genital herpes, suppressive therapy in HIV infection	(1) acyclovir 400 to 800 mg PO two or three times per day; (2) famciclovir 500 mg PO two times per day; (3) valacyclovir 500 mg PO two times per day.
Genital warts	External anogenital, patient-applied: (1) imiquimod 3.75% or 5% cream; (2) podofilox 0.5% soln or gel; (3) sinecatechins 15% ointment. External anogenital, provider-administered: (1) cryotherapy with liquid nitrogen or cryoprobe; (2) surgical removal; (3) trichloroacetic or bichloroacetic acid 80% to 90% soln. Urethral meatus: (1) cryotherapy with liquid nitrogen; (2) surgical removal. Vaginal, cervical, or intra-anal: (1) cryotherapy with liquid nitrogen; (2) surgical removal; (3) trichloroacetic or bichloroacetic acid 80% to 90% soln.

ANTIMICROBIALS

(cont.)

SEXUALLY TRANSMITTED DISEASES & VAGINITIS* (continued)

Gonorrhea[a]	Ceftriaxone 250 mg IM single dose + azithromycin 1 g PO single dose. For cervix, urethra, and rectum if ceftriaxone is unavailable: cefixime 400 mg PO single dose + azithromycin 1 g PO single dose.[a] Ceftriaxone-allergic: consult infectious disease expert and consider (1) gemifloxacin 320 mg PO single dose + azithromycin 2 g PO single dose; (2) gentamicin 240 mg IM single dose + azithromycin 2 g PO single dose.
Gonorrhea, disseminated	Arthritis/arthritis-dermatitis syndrome: ceftriaxone 1 g IM/IV q 24 h + azithromycin 1 g PO single dose. After substantial improvement, can switch to PO drug based on antimicrobial susceptibility to complete at least 7 days of treatment. Alternative: cefotaxime 1 g IV q 8 h OR ceftizoxime 1 g IV q 8 h + azithromycin 1 g PO single dose. Meningitis, endocarditis: ceftriaxone 1 to 2 g IV q 12 to 24 h + azithromycin 1 g PO single dose. Treat IM/IV for at least 10 to 14 days for meningitis, and at least 4 weeks for endocarditis.
Granuloma inguinale	Azithromycin 1 g PO once weekly or 500 mg PO once daily for at least 3 weeks and until lesions completely healed. See STD guideline for alternative treatment regimens.
Non-gonococcal urethrits (NGU)	(1) azithromycin 1 g PO single dose; (2) doxycycline 100 mg PO two times per day for 7 days. Alternative: (1) erythromycin base 500 mg PO four times per day for 7 days; (2) levofloxacin 500 mg PO once per day for 7 days. Persistant/recurrent: (1) azithromycin 1 g PO single dose for men who initially received doxycycline; (2) moxifloxacin 400 mg PO once daily for 7 days if azithromycin failed; (3) metronidazole or tinidazole 2 g PO single dose for heterosexual men in areas of high *T vaginalis* prevalence.

[a] For suspected cephalosporin treatment failure, consult infectious disease specialist, an STD/HIV Prevention Training Center clinical expert (www.nnptc.org), or local/state health department STD program or CDC (phone 404-639-8659). Report suspected treatment failure to health department within 24 hours of diagnosis. When reinfection is likely, retreat with ceftriaxone 250 mg IM + azithromycin 1 g PO. For suspected treatment failure after cefixime-azithromycin regimen: Treat with ceftriaxone 250 mg IM single dose + azithromycin 2 g PO single dose. Obtain test-of-cure 7 to 14 days later, preferably with culture (and susceptibility testing of *N. gonorrhoeae* if isolated) and simultaneous NAAT.

(cont.)

SEXUALLY TRANSMITTED DISEASES & VAGINITIS* (*continued*)

Pelvic inflammatory disease (PID)	Parenteral: (1) cefotetan 2 g IV q 12 h + doxycycline 100 mg IV/PO q 12 h OR cefoxitin 2 g IV q 6 h + doxycycline 100 mg IV/PO q 12 h. After 24 to 48 h of improvement, switch to PO doxycycline to complete 14 days. (2) clindamycin 900 mg IV q 8 h + gentamicin IM/IV 2 mg/kg loading dose, then 1.5 mg/kg q 8 h (can substitute 3 to 5 mg/kg once-daily dosing). After 24 to 48 h of improvement, switch to clindamycin 450 mg PO four times per day or doxycycline 100 mg PO two times per day to complete 14 days. For tubo-ovarian abscess, add clindamycin 450 mg PO four times per day or metronidazole 500 mg PO two times per day to doxycycline to provide anaerobic activity. IM/oral regimen: ceftriaxone 250 mg IM single dose + doxycycline 100 mg PO two times per day ± metronidazole 500 mg PO two times per day for 14 days. Metronidazole is added to provide anaerobic coverage and treat bacterial vaginosis.
Proctitis	Ceftriaxone 250 mg IM single dose + doxycycline 100 mg PO two times per day for 7 days.
Pubic lice	(1) permethrin 1% cream rinse (2) pyrethrins with piperonyl butoxide. Apply to affected areas and wash off after 10 minutes. Alternatives: (1) malathion 0.5% lotion; apply to affected areas and wash off after 8 to 12 h (can be used if treatment failure may be due to resistance); (2) ivermectin 250 mcg/kg PO taken with food; repeat in 2 weeks.
Scabies	(1) permethrin 5% cream applied to body from neck down and washed off after 8 to 14 h; (2) ivermectin 200 mcg/kg PO taken with food; repeat in 2 weeks. Use permethrin for infants and children. Alternative: lindane 1% 1 oz of lotion or 30 g of cream applied to body from neck down and thoroughly washed off after 8 h; not for age less than 10 yo. Crusted scabies: 5% benzyl benzoate or 5% permethrin cream, full-body application daily for 7 days then twice weekly until discharge or cure + ivermectin 200 mcg/kg PO on days 1, 2, 8, 9, and 15. Consider additional doses on days 22 and 29 if severe.
Sexual assault prophylaxis	Ceftriaxone 250 mg IM single dose + metronidazole or tinidazole 2 g PO single dose + azithromycin 1 g PO single dose. Consider HBV and HPV vaccination and HIV prophylaxis when appropriate.

ANTIMICROBIALS

(cont.)

SEXUALLY TRANSMITTED DISEASES & VAGINITIS* (*continued*)

Syphilis, primary, secondary, or early latent, ie, duration less than 1 year	Benzathine penicillin 2.4 million units IM single dose. Penicillin-allergic: doxycycline 100 mg PO two times per day for 14 days if primary or secondary syphilis and 28 days if early latent syphilis. Use skin testing and penicillin desensitization protocol if medication compliance or follow-up cannot be ensured.
Syphilis, late latent or unknown duration	Benzathine penicillin 2.4 million units IM q week for 3 doses. Penicillin-allergic: doxycycline 100 mg PO two times per day for 4 weeks.
Syphilis, tertiary	Benzathine penicillin 2.4 million units IM q week for 3 doses. This regimen is for patients with normal CSF exam; use neurosyphilis regimen if CSF abnormalities. Consult infectious disease specialist for management of penicillin-allergic patients.
Syphilis, neuro and ocular	(1) penicillin G 18 to 24 million units/day continuous IV infusion or 3 to 4 million units IV q 4 h for 10 to 14 days; (2) if compliance can be ensured, consider procaine penicillin 2.4 million units IM daily + probenecid 500 mg PO four times per day, both for 10 to 14 days. Penicillin-allergic: (1) ceftriaxone 2 g IM/IV once daily for 10 to 14 days; (2) skin testing and penicillin desensitization protocol.
Syphilis in pregnancy	Treat with penicillin regimen for stage of syphilis as noted above. For primary, secondary, or early latent syphilis, consider a second dose of benzathine penicillin 2.4 million units IM one week after initial dose. Use skin-testing and penicillin-desensitization protocol if penicillin-allergic.
Trichomoniasis	Metronidazole or tinidazole 2 g PO single dose. Use metronidazole if pregnant. Persistent/recurrent: metronidazole 500 mg PO two times per day for 7 days. Treatment-failure: metronidazole or tinidazole 2 g PO two times per day for 7 days. HIV-infected women: metronidazole 500 mg PO two times per day for 7 days.

*MMWR 2015;64(No. RR-3): 1–137 or www.cdc.gov/std/tg2015/default.htm. Treat sexual partners for all except herpes, candida, and bacterial vaginosis. Refer to the STD guideline for additional alternative regimens.

NAAT = nucleic acid amplification test.

Aminoglycosides

NOTE: *See also Dermatology and Ophthalmology. Can cause nephrotoxicity, ototoxicity.*

AMIKACIN 15 mg/kg/day (up to 1500 mg/day) IM/IV divided q 8 to 12 h. Peak 20 to 35 mcg/mL, trough less than 5 mcg/mL. Alternative 15 mg/kg IV q 24 h. ▶K ♀D ▶? $$ ■

GENTAMICIN Adults: 3 to 5 mg/kg/day IM/IV divided q 8 h. Peak 5 to 10 mcg/mL, trough less than 2 mcg/mL. Alternative 5 to 7 mg/kg IV q 24 h. Peds: 2 to 2.5 mg/kg q 8 h. ▶K ♀D ▶+ $$ ■

STREPTOMYCIN Combo therapy for TB: 15 mg/kg (up to 1 g) IM daily. 10 mg/kg (up to 750 mg) for age 60 yo or older. Peds: 20 to 40 mg/kg (up to 1 g) IM daily. ▶K ♀D ▶+ $$$$$ ■

TOBRAMYCIN (*Bethkis, Kitabis Pak, Tobi*) Adults: 3 to 5 mg/kg/day IM/IV divided q 8 h. Peak 5 to 10 mcg/mL, trough less than 2 mcg/mL. Alternative 5 to 7 mg/kg IV q 24 h. Peds: 2 to 2.5 mg/kg q 8 h. Cystic fibrosis, age 6 yo to adult: 300 mg nebulized or 4 caps inhaled (Tobi Podhaler) two times per day 28 days on, then 28 days off. [Generic/Trade (Tobi): 300 mg/5 mL ampules for nebulizer ($$$$$). Trade only: Bethkis 300 mg/4 mL ampules for nebulizer ($$$$$). Tobi Podhaler 28 mg caps for inhalation ($$$$$). Kitabis Pak 300 mg/5 mL ampules copackaged with nebulizer ($$$$$).] ▶K ♀D ▶+ $$ ■

Antifungal Agents—Azoles

CLOTRIMAZOLE Oral troches five times per day for 14 days. [Generic only: Oral troches 10 mg.] ▶L ♀C ▶? $$$$

FLUCONAZOLE (*Diflucan, ★CanesOral*) Vaginal candidiasis: 150 mg PO single dose ($). All other dosing regimens IV/PO. Oropharyngeal candidiasis: 100 to 200 mg daily for 7 to 14 days. Esophageal candidiasis: 200 to 400 mg daily for 14 to 21 days. Candidemia: 800 mg on 1st day, then 400 mg daily. Cryptococcal meningitis (per IDSA guideline): Amphotericin B preferably in combo with flucytosine for at least 2 weeks (induction), followed by fluconazole 400 mg PO once daily for 8 weeks (consolidation), then chronic suppression with fluconazole 200 mg PO once daily until immune system reconstitution. Peds: Oropharyngeal candidiasis: 6 mg/kg on 1st day, then 3 mg/kg daily for 7 to 14 days. Esophageal candidiasis: 12 mg/kg on 1st day, then 6 mg/kg daily for 14 to 21 days. Systemic candidiasis; cryptococcal meningitis in AIDS: 12 mg/kg on 1st day, then 6 to 12 mg/kg daily. Many drug interactions. [Generic/Trade: Tabs 50, 100, 150, 200 mg. 150 mg tab in single-dose blister pack. Susp 10, 40 mg/mL (35 mL).] ▶K ♀C for single-dose treatment of vaginal candidiasis, D for all other indications ▶+ $$$$

ISAVUCONAZONIUM (*Cresemba*, isavuconazole) Invasive aspergillosis, mucormycosis: Loading dose of 372 mg isavuconazonium IV/PO q 8 h for 6 doses, then 372 mg IV/PO once daily starting 12 to 24 h after last loading dose. Infuse IV doses over at least 1 h with in-line filter. Isavuconazonium is prodrug of isavuconazole; 372 mg isavuconazonium = 200 mg isavuconazole. [Trade only: Caps 186 mg (100 mg isavuconazole).] ▶L glucuronidation ♀C ▶− $$$$$

ITRACONAZOLE (*Onmel, Sporanox*) Oral caps for onychomycosis "pulse dosing": 200 mg PO two times per day for 1st week of month for 2 months (fingernails) or 3 to 4 months (toenails). Standard regimen, toenail onychomycosis: 200 mg PO daily with full meal for 12 weeks. Fluconazole-refractory oropharyngeal or esophageal candidiasis: Oral soln 200 mg PO daily for 14 to 21 days. Strong CYP3A4 and P-glycoprotein inhibitor; contraindicated with many drugs due to risk of drug interactions. Negative inotrope; do not use for onychomycosis if ventricular dysfunction. [Trade only: Tabs 200 mg (Onmel). Oral soln 10 mg/mL (Sporanox-150 mL). Generic/Trade: Caps 100 mg.] ▶L ♀C ▶– $$$$$ ■

MICONAZOLE—BUCCAL (*Oravig*) Oropharyngeal candidiasis: Apply 50 mg buccal tab to gums once daily for 14 days. Increased INR with warfarin. [Trade only: Buccal tabs 50 mg.] ▶L ♀C ▶? $$$$$

POSACONAZOLE (*Noxafil, ✦Posanol*) Prevention of invasive *Aspergillus* or *Candida* infection, age 13 yo or older: 200 mg (5 mL) susp PO three times per day OR 300 mg delayed-release tabs PO two times per day on the 1st day, then 300 mg PO once daily OR 300 mg IV two times per day on 1st day, then 300 IV mg once daily. Oropharyngeal candidiasis, age 13 yo or older: 100 mg (2.5 mL) PO two times on day 1, then 100 mg PO once daily for 13 days. Oropharyngeal candidiasis resistant to itraconazole/fluconazole, age 13 yo or older: 400 mg (10 mL) PO two times per day. Take susp with full meal or liquid nutritional supplement. Take delayed-release tabs with food. Strong CYP3A4 inhibitor. IV posaconazole: Can give 1st dose by peripheral IV infusion over 30 minutes; infuse additional doses over 90 minutes by central venous line or peripherally inserted central catheter. [Trade only: Delayed-release tabs 100 mg. Oral susp 40 mg/mL (105 mL).] ▶Glucuronidation ♀C ▶– $$$$$

VORICONAZOLE (*Vfend*) Aspergillosis, systemic *Candida* infections: 6 mg/kg IV q 12 h for 2 doses, then 3 to 4 mg/kg IV q 12 h (use 4 mg/kg for aspergillosis). Esophageal candidiasis or maintenance therapy of aspergillosis/candidiasis: 200 mg PO two times per day. For wt less than 40 kg, reduce to 100 mg PO two times per day. Dosage adjustment for efavirenz: Voriconazole 400 mg PO two times per day with efavirenz 300 mg PO once daily (use caps). Peds younger than 12 yo: 7 mg/kg IV q 12 h. Infuse IV over 2 h. Take tabs or susp 1 h before or after meals. Strong CYP3A4 inhibitor. Many drug interactions. [Generic/Trade: Tabs 50, 200 mg (contains lactose). Susp 40 mg/mL (75 mL).] ▶L ♀D ▶? $$$$$

Antifungal Agents—Echinocandins

ANIDULAFUNGIN (*Eraxis*) Candidemia: 200 mg IV load on day 1, then 100 mg IV once daily. Esophageal candidiasis: 100 mg IV load on day 1, then 50 mg IV once daily. Max infusion rate of 1.1 mg/min to prevent histamine reactions. ▶Degraded chemically ♀C ▶? $$$$$

CASPOFUNGIN (*Cancidas*) Infuse IV over 1 h. Aspergillosis, candidemia, empiric therapy in febrile neutropenia: Give 70 mg IV loading dose on day 1, then 50 mg once daily. Esophageal candidiasis: 50 mg IV once daily. Peds, age 3 mo and older: 70 mg/m² IV loading dose on day 1, then 50 mg/m² once daily (max of 70 mg/day). ▶KL ♀C ▶? $$$$$

MICAFUNGIN (*Mycamine*) Esophageal candidiasis, age 4 mo and older: 3 mg/kg IV once daily for wt 30 kg or less; 2.5 mg/kg IV up to 150 mg once daily for wt greater than 30 kg. Candidemia, acute disseminated candidiasis, *Candida* peritonitis/abscess, age 4 mo and older: 2 mg/kg up to 100 mg IV once daily. Prevention of candidal infections in bone marrow transplant patients, age 4 mo and older: 1 mg/kg up to 50 mg IV once daily. Infuse over 1 h. Histamine-mediated reactions possible with more rapid infusion. For peds, infuse concentrations greater than 1.5 mg/mL by central catheter. Flush existing IV lines with NS before micafungin infusion. ▶L, feces ♀C ▶? $$$$$

Antifungal Agents—Polyenes

AMPHOTERICIN B DEOXYCHOLATE Test dose 0.1 mg/kg up to 1 mg slow IV. Wait 2 to 4 h, and if tolerated then begin 0.25 mg/kg IV daily and advance to 0.5 to 1.5 mg/kg/day depending on fungal type. Max dose 1.5 mg/kg/day. ▶Tissues ♀B ▶? $$$$$ ■

AMPHOTERICIN B LIPID FORMULATIONS (*Abelcet, AmBisome*) Abelcet: 5 mg/kg/day IV at 2.5 mg/kg/h. AmBisome: 3 to 5 mg/kg/day IV over 2 h. ▶? ♀B ▶? $$$$$

Antifungal Agents—Other

FLUCYTOSINE (*Ancobon*) 50 to 150 mg/kg/day PO divided four times per day. Myelosuppression. [Generic/Trade: Caps 250, 500 mg.] ▶K ♀C ▶– $$$$$ ■

GRISEOFULVIN (*Grifulvin V*) Tinea capitis: 500 mg PO daily in adults; 15 to 20 mg/kg (up to 1 g) PO daily in peds. Treat for 4 to 6 weeks, continuing for 2 weeks past symptom resolution. [Generic/Trade: Susp 125 mg/5 mL (120 mL). Tabs 500 mg. Generic only: Tabs 250 mg.] ▶Skin ♀C ▶? $$$$

NYSTATIN Thrush: 4 to 6 mL PO, swish and swallow four times per day. Infants: 2 mL/dose with 1 mL in each cheek four times per day. Non-esophageal mucus membrane gastrointestinal candidiasis: 1 to 2 tabs PO three times per day. [Generic only: Susp 100,000 units/mL (60, 480 mL). Film-coated tabs 500,000 units.] ▶Not absorbed ♀B ▶+ $

TERBINAFINE (*Lamisil*) Onychomycosis: 250 mg PO daily for 6 weeks to treat fingernails, for 12 weeks to treat toenails. Tinea capitis, age 4 yo or older: Give granules PO once daily with food for 6 weeks: 125 mg for wt less than 25 kg, 187.5 mg for wt 25 to 35 kg, 250 mg for wt more than 35 kg. [Generic/Trade: Tabs 250 mg. Trade only: Oral granules 125, 187.5 mg/packet.] ▶LK ♀B ▶– $$$$$

Antimalarials

NOTE: *For help treating malaria or getting antimalarials, see www.cdc.gov/malaria or call the "malaria hotline"; (770) 488-7788 Monday-Friday 9:00 am to 5:00 pm EST; after hours/weekend (770) 488-7100. Pediatric doses of antimalarials should never exceed adult doses.*

CHLOROQUINE (*Aralen*) Malaria prophylaxis, chloroquine-sensitive areas: 8 mg/kg up to 500 mg PO q week starting 1 to 2 weeks before exposure to 4 weeks after

(cont.)

ANTIMICROBIALS

exposure. Chloroquine resistance is widespread. Can prolong QT interval and cause torsades. [Generic only: Tabs 250 mg. Generic/Trade: Tabs 500 mg (500 mg phosphate equivalent to 300 mg base).] ▶KL ♀C but –▶+ $ ■

COARTEM (artemether + lumefantrine) Uncomplicated malaria: Take PO with food two times per day for 3 days. On day 1, give 2nd dose 8 h after 1st dose. Dose based on wt: 1 tab for 5 to 14 kg; 2 tabs for 15 to 24 kg; 3 tabs for 25 to 34 kg; 4 tabs for 35 kg or greater. Repeat dose if vomiting occurs within 1 to 2 h. Can prolong QT interval. [Trade only: Tabs, artemether 20 mg + lumefantrine 120 mg.] ▶L ♀C ▶? $$$$

MALARONE (atovaquone + proguanil) Prevention of malaria: Give the following dose PO once daily from 1 to 2 days before exposure until 7 days after. Dose based on wt: ½ ped tab for 5 to 8 kg; ¾ ped tab for 9 to 10 kg; 1 ped tab for 11 to 20 kg; 2 ped tabs for 21 to 30 kg; 3 ped tabs for 31 to 40 kg; 1 adult tab for all patients wt greater than 40 kg. Treatment of malaria: Give the following dose PO once daily for 3 days. Dose based on wt: 2 ped tabs for 5 to 8 kg; 3 ped tabs for 9 to 10 kg; 1 adult tab for 11 to 20 kg; 2 adult tabs for 21 to 30 kg; 3 adult tabs for 31 to 40 kg; 4 adult tabs for all patients wt greater than 40 kg. Take with food or milky drink. [Generic/Trade: Adult tabs atovaquone 250 mg + proguanil 100 mg. Pediatric tabs 62.5 mg + 25 mg.] ▶ Feces; LK ♀C ▶? $$$$$

MEFLOQUINE Malaria prophylaxis for chloroquine-resistant areas: 250 mg PO once a week from at least 2 weeks before exposure to 4 weeks after. Malaria treatment: 1250 mg PO single dose. Peds malaria prophylaxis: Give the following dose PO once a week starting at least 2 weeks before exposure to 4 weeks after: Dose based on wt: 5 mg/kg (prepared by pharmacist) for wt 9 kg or less; ¼ tab for wt greater than 9 to 19 kg; ½ tab for wt greater than 19 to 30 kg; ¾ tab for wt greater than 30 to 45 kg; 1 tab for wt greater than 45 kg. Peds malaria treatment: 20 to 25 mg/kg PO single dose or divided into 2 doses given 6 to 8 h apart. Take on full stomach. [Generic only: Tabs 250 mg.] ▶L ♀B ▶? $$ ■

PRIMAQUINE Prevention of relapse, *P. vivax/ovale* malaria: 0.5 mg/kg (up to 30 mg) base PO daily for 14 days. Do not use unless normal G6PD level. [Generic only: Tabs 26.3 mg (equiv to 15 mg base).] ▶L ♀– ▶– $$$ ■

QUININE (*Qualaquin*) Malaria: 648 mg PO three times per day. Peds: 25 to 30 mg/kg/day (up to 2 g/day) PO divided q 8 h. Treat for 3 days (Africa/South America) or 7 days (Southeast Asia). Also give 7-day course of doxycycline, tetracycline, or clindamycin. Nocturnal leg cramps: 325 mg PO at bedtime. FDA warns that risks exceed potential benefit for this indication. Can cause life-threatening adverse effects: Cinchonism with overdose; hemolysis with G6PD deficiency; hypersensitivity; thrombocytopenia; HUS/TTP; QT interval prolongation; many drug interactions. [Generic/Trade: Caps 324 mg.] ▶L ♀C ▶+? $$$$$ ■

Antimycobacterial Agents

NOTE: *Treat active mycobacterial infection with at least 2 drugs. See guidelines at www.thoracic.org/statements/ and www.aidsinfo.nih.gov.*

DAPSONE (*Aczone*) Pneumocystis pneumonia prophylaxis, leprosy: 100 mg PO daily. Pneumocystis pneumonia treatment: 100 mg PO daily with trimethoprim 5

(cont.)

mg/kg PO three times per day for 21 days. Acne (Aczone; $$$$$): Apply topically two times per day. [Generic only: Tabs 25, 100 mg. Trade only (Aczone): Topical gel 5% 30, 60, 90 g.] ▶LK ♀C ▶– $$$$

ETHAMBUTOL (*Myambutol*, *✦Etibi*) TB: 15 to 20 mg/kg PO daily. Dose with whole tabs based on estimated lean body weight: Give 800 mg PO daily for wt 40 to 55 kg, 1200 mg for wt 56 to 75 kg, 1600 mg for wt 76 to 90 kg. Peds: 15 to 20 mg/kg (up to 1 g) PO daily. [Generic/Trade: Tabs 100, 400 mg.] ▶LK ♀C but +▶+ $$$$

ISONIAZID (INH, *✦Isotamine*) Adults: 5 mg/kg (up to 300 mg) PO daily. Peds: 10 to 15 mg/kg (up to 300 mg) PO daily. Hepatotoxicity. Consider supplemental pyridoxine up to 50 mg per day to prevent neuropathy. [Generic only: Tabs 100, 300 mg. Syrup 50 mg/5 mL.] ▶LK ♀C but +▶+ $

PYRAZINAMIDE (PZA, *✦Tebrazid*) TB: 20 to 25 mg/kg (up to 2000 mg) PO daily. Dose with whole tabs based on estimated lean body weight: Give PO daily 1000 mg for 40 to 55 kg, 1500 mg for 56 to 75 kg, 2000 mg for 76 to 90 kg. Peds: 15 to 30 mg/kg (up to 2000 mg) PO daily. Hepatotoxicity. [Generic only: Tabs 500 mg.] ▶LK ♀C ▶? $$$$ ■

RIFABUTIN (*Mycobutin*) Mycobacterium avium complex disease, TB: 300 mg PO daily or 150 mg PO two times per day. Dosage reduction required with protease inhibitors. [Generic/Trade: Caps 150 mg.] ▶L ♀B ▶? $$$$$

***RIFAMATE* (isoniazid + rifampin)** TB: 2 caps PO daily on empty stomach. [Trade only: Caps isoniazid 150 mg + rifampin 300 mg.] ▶LK ♀C but +▶+ $$$$$ ■

RIFAMPIN (*Rifadin*, *✦Rofact*) TB: 10 mg/kg (up to 600 mg) PO/IV daily. Peds: 10 to 20 mg/kg (up to 600 mg) PO/IV daily. Neisseria meningitidis carriers: 600 mg PO two times per day for 2 days. Peds: Age younger than 1 mo: 5 mg/kg PO two times per day for 2 days. Age 1 mo or older: 10 mg/kg (up to 600 mg) PO two times per day for 2 days. IV and PO doses are the same. Take oral doses on empty stomach. Strong enzyme inducer; many drug interactions. [Generic/Trade: Caps 150, 300 mg. Pharmacists can make oral susp.] ▶L ♀C but +▶+ $$$$ ■

RIFAPENTINE (*Priftin*, RPT) Active pulmonary TB, age 12 yo and older: 600 mg PO two times per week for 2 months, then once weekly for 4 months. Use for continuation therapy only in selected HIV-negative patients. Latent TB, age 2 yo and older: Give with isoniazid both PO once weekly for 12 weeks. Use wt-based rifapentine dose of 300 mg for 10 to 14 kg; 450 mg for 14.1 to 25 kg; 600 mg for 25.1 to 32 kg; 750 mg for 32.1 to 50 kg; 900 mg for wt greater than 50 kg. Take with food. Intended for directly observed therapy. [Trade only: Tabs 150 mg.] ▶ Esterases, feces ♀C ▶? $$$$

***RIFATER* (isoniazid + rifampin + pyrazinamide)** TB, initial 2 months of treatment: 4 tabs PO daily for wt less than 45 kg, 5 tabs daily for wt 45 to 54 kg, 6 tabs daily for wt 55 kg or greater. Take PO on empty stomach. [Trade only: Tabs isoniazid 50 mg + rifampin 120 mg + pyrazinamide 300 mg.] ▶LK ♀C ▶? $$$$$ ■

Antiparasitics

ALBENDAZOLE (*Albenza*) Hydatid disease, neurocysticercosis: 15 mg/kg/day (up to 800 mg/day) PO divided in two doses for wt less than 60 kg; 400 mg PO two times per day for wt 60 kg or greater. [Trade only: Tabs 200 mg.] ▶L ♀C ▶? $$$$$

ATOVAQUONE (Mepron) Pneumocystis pneumonia. Treatment: 750 mg PO two times per day for 21 days. Prevention: 1500 mg PO daily. Take with meals. [Generic/Trade: Susp 750 mg/5 mL (210 mL). Trade only: foil pouch 750 mg/5 mL (5 mL).] ▶feces ♀C ▶? $$$$$

IVERMECTIN (Stromectol) Scabies: 200 mcg/kg PO on day 1 (3 mg for wt 15 to 24 kg, 6 mg for 25 to 35 kg, 9 mg for 36 to 50 kg, 12 mg for 51 to 65 kg, 15 mg for 66 to 79 kg); repeat dose in 7 to 14 days. Peds head lice: 200 or 400 mcg/kg PO on days 1 and 8. Single PO dose of 200 mcg/kg for strongyloidiasis, 150 mcg/kg for onchocerciasis. Not for children less than 15 kg. Take on empty stomach with water. [Generic/Trade: Tabs 3 mg.] ▶L ♀C ▶+ $$

NITAZOXANIDE (Alinia) Cryptosporidial or giardial diarrhea: 100 mg two times per day for age 1 to 3 yo; 200 mg two times per day for 4 to 11 yo; 500 mg two times per day for adults and children 12 yo or older. Give PO with food for 3 days. Use susp if younger than 12 yo. [Trade only: Oral susp 100 mg/5 mL (60 mL). Tabs 500 mg.] ▶L ♀B ▶? $$$$

PAROMOMYCIN Intestinal amebiasis: 25 to 35 mg/kg/day PO divided three times per day with or after meals. [Generic only: Caps 250 mg.] ▶Not absorbed ♀C ▶? $$$$$

PRAZIQUANTEL (Biltricide) Schistosomiasis: 20 mg/kg PO q 4 to 6 h for 3 doses. [Trade only: Tabs 600 mg.] ▶LK ♀B ▶– $$$$

PYRANTEL (Pin-X, Pinworm, ✦Combantrin) Pinworm, roundworm: 11 mg/kg (up to 1 g) PO single dose. Repeat in 2 weeks for pinworm. [OTC Trade only (Pin-X): Susp 144 mg/mL (equivalent to 50 mg/mL of pyrantel base) 30, 60 mL. Tabs 720.5 mg (equivalent to 250 mg of pyrantel base). OTC Generic only: Caps 180 mg (equivalent to 62.5 mg of pyrantel base).] ▶Not absorbed ♀– ▶? $

PYRIMETHAMINE (Daraprim) CNS toxoplasmosis in adults with AIDS. Acute therapy: For wt less than 60 kg give pyrimethamine 200 mg PO for first dose, then 50 mg PO once daily with sulfadiazine 1000 mg PO q 6 h and leucovorin 10 to 25 mg PO once daily (up to 50 mg once daily or two times per day). For wt 60 kg or greater give pyrimethamine 200 mg PO for first dose, then 75 mg PO once daily with sulfadiazine 1500 mg PO q 6 h and leucovorin 10 to 25 mg PO once daily (up to 50 mg once daily or two times per day). Treat for at least 6 weeks. Chronic maintenance therapy: Pyrimethamine 25 to 50 mg PO once daily with sulfadiazine 2000 to 4000 mg/day PO divided two to four times per day and leucovorin 10 to 25 mg PO once daily. Peds. Congenital toxoplasmosis, AAP regimen: 2 mg/kg PO once daily for 2 days, then 1 mg/kg PO once daily for 2 to 6 months, then 1 mg/kg three times weekly + sulfadiazine 50 mg/kg PO two times per day + leucovorin 10 mg PO once daily for 1 year. [Trade only: Tabs 25 mg.] ▶L ♀C ▶+ $$$$$

TINIDAZOLE (Tindamax) Adults: 2 g PO daily for 1 day for trichomoniasis or giardiasis, for 3 days for amebiasis. Bacterial vaginosis: 2 g PO once daily for 2 days or 1 g PO once daily for 5 days. Peds, age older than 3 yo: 50 mg/kg (up to 2 g) PO daily for 1 day for giardiasis, for 3 days for amebiasis. Take with food. [Generic/Trade: Tabs 250, 500 mg. Pharmacists can compound oral susp.] ▶KL ♀C ▶? $$ ■

Antiviral Agents—Anti-CMV

CIDOFOVIR CMV retinitis in AIDS: 5 mg/kg IV once a week for 2 weeks, then 5 mg/kg IV every other week. Severe nephrotoxicity. ▶K ♀C ▶– $$$$$ ▪

FOSCARNET (*Foscavir*) CMV retinitis: 60 mg/kg IV (over 1 h) q 8 h or 90 mg/kg IV (over 1.5 to 2 h) q 12 h for 2 to 3 weeks, then 90 to 120 mg/kg IV daily over 2 h. HSV infection: 40 mg/kg (over 1 h) q 8 to 12 h. Nephrotoxicity, seizures. ▶K ♀C ▶? $$$$$ ▪

GANCICLOVIR (*Cytovene*) CMV retinitis: Induction 5 mg/kg IV q 12 h for 14 to 21 days. Maintenance 6 mg/kg IV daily for 5 days per week. Myelosuppression. Potential carcinogen, teratogen. May impair fertility. ▶K ♀C ▶– $$$$$ ▪

VALGANCICLOVIR (*Valcyte*) CMV retinitis: 900 mg PO two times per day for 21 days, then 900 mg PO daily. Prevention of CMV disease in high-risk transplant patients: 900 mg PO daily given within 10 days post-transplant until 100 days post-transplant for heart or kidney/pancreas or 200 days for kidney transplant. See prescribing information for peds dose. Give with food. Impaired fertility, myelosuppression, potential carcinogen and teratogen. [Generic/Trade: Tabs 450 mg. Trade only: Oral soln 50 mg/mL.] ▶K ♀C ▶– $$$$$ ▪

Antiviral Agents—Anti-Hepatitis B

ADEFOVIR (*Hepsera*) Chronic hepatitis B, 12 yo and older: 10 mg PO daily. Nephrotoxic; lactic acidosis and hepatic steatosis; discontinuation may exacerbate hepatitis B; may result in HIV resistance in untreated HIV infection. [Generic/Trade: Tabs 10 mg.] ▶K ♀C ▶– $$$$$ ▪

ENTECAVIR (*Baraclude*) Chronic hepatitis B, 16 yo and older: 0.5 mg PO once daily if treatment-naive; give 1 mg if lamivudine- or telbivudine-resistant, history of viremia despite lamivudine treatment, decompensated liver disease, or HIV coinfected. Peds, age 2 yo and older. Treatment-naive: Give oral soln PO once daily at a dose of 3 mL for 10 to 11 kg; 4 mL for greater than 11 to 14 kg; 5 mL for greater than 14 to 17 kg; 6 mL for greater than 17 to 20 kg; 7 mL for greater than 20 to 23 kg; 8 mL for greater than 23 to 26 kg; 9 mL for greater than 26 to 30 kg; 10 mL or 0.5 mg tab for greater than 30 kg. Lamivudine-experienced: Give oral soln PO once daily at a dose of 6 mL for 10 to 11 kg; 8 mL for greater than 11 to 14 kg; 10 mL for greater than 14 to 17 kg; 12 mL for greater than 17 to 20 kg; 14 mL for greater than 20 to 23 kg; 16 mL for greater than 23 to 26 kg; 18 mL for greater than 26 to 30 kg; 20 mL or 1 mg tab for greater than 30 kg. Give on empty stomach. [Generic/Trade: Tabs 0.5, 1 mg. Trade only: Oral soln 0.05 mg/mL (210 mL).] ▶K ♀C ▶– $$$$$ ▪

TELBIVUDINE (*Tyzeka*, ✦*Sebivo*) Chronic hepatitis B, 16 yo and older: 600 mg PO once daily. [Trade only: Tabs 600 mg.] ▶K ♀B ▶– $$$$$ ▪

Antiviral Agents—Anti-Hepatitis C

NOTE: *Treatment recommendations for HCV can change rapidly. Refer to www.hcvguidelines.org for current recommendations.*

DACLATASVIR (*Daklinza*) Chronic hepatitis C. Genotype 1: 60 mg PO once daily with sofosbuvir 400 mg PO once daily for 12 weeks if no cirrhosis. If cirrhosis, treat for 24 weeks ± wt-based ribavirin (1000 mg/day PO for <75 kg; 1200 mg/day PO for 75 kg or greater). Genotype 2, intolerant to ribavirin: 60 mg PO once daily with sofosbuvir 400 mg PO once daily for 12 weeks; treat for 16 weeks if cirrhosis. Genotype 3: 60 mg PO once daily with sofosbuvir 400 mg PO once daily for 12 weeks if no cirrhosis. If cirrhosis, treat for 24 weeks ± wt-based ribavirin. Increase daclatasvir to 90 mg/day for moderate CYP3A4 inducers; reduce to 30 mg/day for strong CYP3A4 inhibitors (see cytochrome P450 table). Avoid strong CYP3A4 inducers. Cost of daclatasvir is $21,000/month. [Trade only: Tabs 30, 60 mg.] ▶L ♀? No data in women; no harm in animals ▶? $$$$$

HARVONI (ledipasvir + sofosbuvir) Chronic hepatitis C, genotype 1: 1 tab PO once daily without regard to meals. Treat for 12 weeks if treatment-naive or -experienced without cirrhosis, 24 weeks if treatment-experienced with cirrhosis. Can consider 8 weeks duration for treatment-naive HIV-negative patients without cirrhosis who have pre-treatment HCV RNA less than 6 million International Units/mL. Genotypes 4, 5, and 6: 1 tab PO once daily for 12 weeks. Warn patients that OTC antacids, H2 blockers, and proton pump inhibitors can reduce Harvoni levels. Cost is $33,750/month. [Trade only: Tabs ledipasvir 90 mg + sofosbuvir 400 mg.] ▶ Bile, LK ♀B ▶? $$$$$

RIBAVIRIN—ORAL (*Rebetol, Copegus, Ribasphere*) Combination therapy of chronic hepatitis C in adults: Daily dose of 1000 mg/day PO for wt less than 75 kg, 1200 mg/day PO for wt 75 kg or greater. Divide daily dose of ribavirin two times per day and give with food. Chronic hepatitis C, peds: Rebetol, age 3 yo and older: 15 mg/kg/day PO divided two times per day with peginterferon alfa-2b (PegIntron). Copegus, age 5 yo and older: 15 mg/kg/day PO divided two times per day with peginterferon alfa-2a (Pegasys). Can cause hemolytic anemia; dosage adjustments required based on Hb. [Generic/Trade: Caps 200 mg, Tabs 200 mg. Generic only: Tabs 400, 500, 600 mg. Trade only (Rebetol): Oral soln 40 mg/mL (100 mL).] ▶Cellular, K ♀X ▶– $$$$$ ■

SIMEPREVIR (*Olysio*, SMV, ✦*Galexos*) Chronic hepatitis C: Simeprevir dose for use only in combination regimens is 150 mg PO once daily with food. Genotype 1 (FDA approved and guideline-recommended for treatment-naive and -experienced patients): Simeprevir 150 mg + sofosbuvir 400 mg both PO once daily for 12 weeks if no cirrhosis. If cirrhosis and without Q80K polymorphism for genotype 1a, treat for 24 weeks ± wt-based ribavirin (1000 mg/day PO for <75 kg; 1200 mg/day PO for 75 kg or greater). Need for Q80K polymorphism screening in genotype 1a is unclear for this regimen in patients without cirrhosis. HCV treatment guideline no longer recommends FDA-approved regimen of simeprevir + wt-based ribavirin + peginterferon alfa. Cost of simeprevir is $22,120 per month. [Trade only: Caps 150 mg.] ▶L bile ♀ C for simeprevir without ribavirin, X for simeprevir with ribavirin ▶– $$$$$

SOFOSBUVIR (*Sovaldi*, SOF) Chronic hepatitis C: Dose of sofosbuvir for use only in combination regimens is 400 mg PO once daily without regard to food. HCV treatment guideline no longer recommends FDA-approved 12-week regimen of

(cont.)

sofosbuvir + peginterferon + ribavirin for genotype 1. Genotype 2: Sofosbuvir + wt-based ribavirin (1000 mg/day PO for wt less than 75 kg; 1200 mg/day PO for 75 kg or greater; dose divided two times per day) for 12 weeks (no cirrhosis) or 16 weeks (with cirrhosis). Genotype 3: Sofosbuvir + wt-based ribavirin + peginterferon alfa 2a 180 mcg SC once weekly for 12 weeks. Genotype 4: Sofosbuvir + wt-based ribavirin for 24 weeks. Sofosbuvir cost is $28,000/month. See daclasvir entry for daclatasvir-sofosbuvir regimens. See simeprevir entry for simeprevir-sofosbuvir regimens. [Trade only: Tabs 400 mg.] ▶LK ♀B for sofosbuvir, X for regimens that contain ribavirin ▶? $$$$$

TECHNIVIE (ombitasvir-paritaprevir-ritonavir) Chronic hepatitis C, genotype 4: 2 tabs PO once daily with breakfast for 12 weeks. Intended for use with ribavirin (1000 mg/day for wt less than 75 kg and 1200 mg/day for 75 kg or greater PO divided two times per day with food) in patients without cirrhosis. Many drug interactions. Cost of Technivie is $25,550 per month. [Trade only: Tabs ombitasvir 12.5 mg + paritaprevir 75 mg + ritonavir 50 mg.] ▶L ♀X ▶– $$$$$

VIEKIRA PAK (ombitasvir-paritaprevir-ritonavir + dasabuvir, ✦Holkira Pak) Chronic hepatitis C. Viekira Pak regimen is 2 tabs of ombitasvir-paritaprevir-ritonavir PO once each morning + dasabuvir 250 mg (1 tab) PO two times per day with a meal. Duration of therapy and need for ribavirin varies by genotype and cirrhosis. Genotype 1a, no cirrhosis: Viekira Pak + ribavirin for 12 weeks. Genotype 1a with cirrhosis: Viekira Pak + ribavirin for 24 weeks (may consider 12 weeks for some patients). Genotype 1b, no cirrhosis: Viekira Pak alone for 12 weeks. Genotype 1b with cirrhosis: Viekira Pak + ribavirin for 12 weeks. Ribavirin dose is 1000 mg/day for wt less than 75 kg and 1200 mg/day for wt 75 kg or greater PO divided two times per day with food. NOTE: Treatment guidelines does not recommend adding ribavirin for genotype 1b with cirrhosis. Cost of Viekira Pak is $27,773 per month. Many drug interactions. [Trade only: Tabs ombitasvir 12.5 mg + paritaprevir 75 mg + ritonavir 50 mg plus separate tabs dasabuvir 250 mg.] ▶L feces ♀B ▶? $$$$$

Antiviral Agents—Anti-Herpetic

ACYCLOVIR (*Zovirax, Sitavig*) Genital herpes: 400 mg PO three times per day for 7 to 10 days for 1st episode, or for 5 days for recurrent episodes. Chronic suppression of genital herpes: 400 mg PO two times per day; in HIV infection use 400 to 800 mg PO two to three times per day. See STD table. Zoster: 800 mg PO five times per day for 7 to 10 days. Chickenpox, age 2 yo to adult: 20 mg/kg (up to 800 mg) PO four times per day for 5 days. Adult IV: 5 to 10 mg/kg IV q 8 h, each dose over 1 h. Herpes encephalitis: 20 mg/kg IV q 8 h for 10 days for age 3 mo to 12 yo; 10 mg/kg IV q 8 h for 10 days for age 12 yo or older. Neonatal herpes: 20 mg/kg IV q 8 h for 21 days for disseminated/CNS disease, for 14 days for skin/mucous membrane infections. Sitavig for recurrent herpes labialis in immunocompetent adults: Apply buccal tab once to upper gum above incisor within 1 h of prodromal symptom onset; put slight pressure on upper lip for 30 seconds to ensure adhesion. Apply to side of mouth with herpes symptoms. [Generic/Trade: Caps 200 mg. Tabs 400, 800 mg. Susp 200 mg/5 mL. Buccal tab (Sitavig–$$$$): Trade only: 50 mg.] ▶K ♀B ▶+ $

ANTIMICROBIALS

FAMCICLOVIR (*Famvir*) First episode genital herpes: 250 mg PO three times per day for 7 to 10 days. Recurrent genital herpes: 1000 mg PO two times per day for 2 days; give 500 mg two times per day for 7 days if HIV infected. Chronic suppression of genital herpes: 250 mg PO two times per day; 500 mg PO two times per day if HIV-infected. See STD table. Recurrent herpes labialis: 1500 mg PO single dose; 500 mg two times per day for 7 days if HIV-infected. Zoster: 500 mg PO three times per day for 7 days. [Generic/Trade: Tabs 125, 250, 500 mg.] ▶K ♀B ▶? $$

VALACYCLOVIR (*Valtrex*) First episode genital herpes: 1 g PO two times per day for 10 days. Recurrent genital herpes: 500 mg PO two times per day for 3 days; if HIV infected, give 1 g PO two times per day for 5 to 10 days. Chronic suppression of genital herpes: 500 to 1000 mg PO daily; if HIV infected, give 500 mg PO two times per day. Reduction of genital herpes transmission in immunocompetent patients with no more than 9 recurrences per year: 500 mg PO daily for source partner, in conjunction with safer sex practices. See STD table. Herpes labialis, age 12 yo or older: 2 g PO q 12 h for 2 doses. Zoster: 1000 mg PO three times per day for 7 days. Chickenpox, age 2 to 18 yo: 20 mg/kg (max of 1 g) PO three times per day for 5 days. [Generic/Trade: Tabs 500, 1000 mg.] ▶K ♀B ▶+ $$$$

Antiviral Agents—Anti-HIV—CCR5 Antagonists

MARAVIROC (*Selzentry, MVC, ◆Celsentri*) 150 mg PO two times per day with strong CYP3A4 inhibitors (clarithromycin, itraconazole, ketoconazole, most protease inhibitors including ritonavir-boosted fosamprenavir); 300 mg PO two times per day with drugs that are not strong CYP3A4 inducers/inhibitors (NRTIs, tipranavir-ritonavir, nevirapine, raltegravir); rifabutin without a strong CYP3A4 inhibitor or inducer); 600 mg PO two times per day with strong CYP3A4 inducers (efavirenz, etravirine, rifampin, carbamazepine, phenobarbital, phenytoin). Do not give maraviroc with unboosted fosamprenavir. Tropism test before treatment; not for dual/mixed or CXCR4-tropic HIV infection. Hepatotoxicity with allergic features. [Trade only: Tabs 150, 300 mg.] ▶LK ♀B ▶– $$$$$ ■

Antiviral Agents—Anti-HIV—Combinations

ATRIPLA (*efavirenz + emtricitabine + tenofovir*) HIV infection, alone or in combination with other antiretrovirals: 1 tab PO once daily on empty stomach, preferably at bedtime. [Trade only: Tabs efavirenz 600 mg + emtricitabine 200 mg + tenofovir 300 mg.] ▶KL ♀D ▶– $$$$$ ■

COMBIVIR (*lamivudine + zidovudine*) Combination therapy of HIV infection: 1 tab PO two times per day for wt 30 kg or greater. [Generic/Trade: Tabs lamivudine 150 mg + zidovudine 300 mg.] ▶LK ♀C ▶– $$$$$ ■

COMPLERA (*emtricitabine + rilpivirine + tenofovir*) HIV infection, alone or in combination with other antiretrovirals in treatment-naive adults with baseline HIV RNA less than or equal to 100,000 copies/mL: 1 tab PO once daily with food. Also an option for some adults with HIV RNA less than 50 copies/mL on stable ritonavir-boosted protease inhibitor–containing regimen; monitor HIV RNA for virologic failure/rebound after switching to Complera. When coadministered with

(cont.)

rifabutin, give 1 tab Complera plus 25 mg rilpivirine PO once daily with a meal. [Trade only: Tabs emtricitabine 200 mg + rilpivirine 25 mg + tenofovir 300 mg.] ▶KL ♀B ▶- $$$$$ ■

EPZICOM (abacavir + lamivudine, *Kivexa*) Combination therapy of HIV infection: 1 tab PO daily. [Trade only: Tabs abacavir 600 mg + lamivudine 300 mg.] ▶LK ♀C ▶- $$$$$ ■

STRIBILD (elvitegravir + cobicistat + emtricitabine + tenofovir) HIV infection, treatment-naive: 1 tab PO once daily with food. Do not use Stribild with other antiretroviral drugs. Many drug interactions. [Trade only: Tabs elvitegravir 150 mg + cobicistat 150 mg + emtricitabine 200 mg + tenofovir 300 mg.] ▶KL ♀B ▶- $$$$$ ■

TRIUMEQ (abacavir + dolutegravir + lamivudine) HIV infection, alone or in combination with other drugs: 1 tab PO once daily. Coadministration with carbamazepine, efavirenz, fosamprenavir-ritonavir, tipranavir-ritonavir, or rifampin: Add dolutegravir 50 mg PO at least 12 hours after dose of Triumeq. Do not use Triumeq alone in patients with INSTI resistance substitutions or suspected INSTI resistance. [Trade only: Tabs abacavir 600 mg + dolutegravir 50 mg + lamivudine 300 mg.] ▶LK ♀C ▶- $$$$$ ■

TRIZIVIR (abacavir + lamivudine + zidovudine) HIV infection, alone (not a preferred regimen) or in combination with other agents: 1 tab PO two times per day. [Generic/Trade: Tabs abacavir 300 mg + lamivudine 150 mg + zidovudine 300 mg.] ▶LK ♀C ▶- $$$$$ ■

TRUVADA (emtricitabine + tenofovir) Combination therapy for HIV infection: 1 tab PO once daily in combination with other antiretroviral drugs. Pre-exposure prophylaxis (PrEP) of HIV in adults at high risk for sexually acquired HIV or injection drug users: 1 tab PO once daily. Screen for HIV q 3 months in patients taking it for PrEP. [Trade only: Tabs emtricitabine 200 mg + tenofovir 300 mg.] ▶K ♀B ▶- $$$$$ ■

Antiviral Agents—Anti-HIV—Integrase Strand Transfer Inhibitor

DOLUTEGRAVIR (*Tivicay*, DTG) Combination therapy of HIV, integrase strand inhibitor (INSTI)-naïve, adults or peds age 12 yo and older and wt 40 kg or greater: 50 mg PO once daily; increase to 50 mg PO two times per day if coadministered with carbamazepine, efavirenz, fosamprenavir-ritonavir, tipranavir-ritonavir, or rifampin. INSTI-experienced with INSTI resistance substitutions or suspected INSTI resistance, adults only: 50 mg PO two times per day. [Trade only: Tabs 50 mg.] ▶glucuronidation ♀B ▶- $$$$$

ELVITEGRAVIR (*Vitekta*, EVG) Combination therapy for HIV infection: Give elvitegravir with ritonavir-boosted protease inhibitor regimens listed here and additional antiretroviral drug. Elvitegravir 85 mg + atazanavir-ritonavir 300 mg-100 mg all PO once daily. Elvitegravir 85 mg PO once daily + lopinavir-ritonavir 400 mg-100 mg PO two times per day. Elvitegravir 150 mg PO once daily + darunavir-ritonavir 600 mg-100 mg PO two times per day. Elvitegravir 150 mg PO once daily + fosamprenavir-ritonavir 700 mg-100 mg PO two times per day. Elvitegravir 150 mg PO once daily + tipranavir-ritonavir 500 mg-200 mg per day.

(cont.)

PO two times per day. Take elvitegravir with food. [Trade only: Film-coated tabs 85, 150 mg.] ▶L glucuronidation ♀B ▶– $$$$$

RALTEGRAVIR (*Isentress*, RAL) Combination therapy of HIV infection. Adults: 400 mg PO two times per day. Increase to 800 mg PO two times per day if given with rifampin. Peds. Film-coated tabs, wt 25 kg or greater: 400 mg PO two times per day. Chew tabs, 11 kg or greater: Give PO two times per day at a dose of 75 mg for wt 11 to less than 14 kg; 100 mg for 14 to less than 20 kg; 150 mg for 20 to less than 28 kg; 200 mg for 28 to less than 40 kg; 300 mg for 40 kg or greater. Oral susp, age 4 weeks and older and wt 3 to 20 kg: Give PO two times per day at a dose of 20 mg for 3 to less than 4 kg; 30 mg for 4 to less than 6 kg; 40 mg for 6 to less than 8 kg; 60 mg for 8 to less than 11 kg; 80 mg for 11 to less than 14 kg; 100 mg for 14 to less than 20 kg. Do not substitute chew tab or susp for film-coated tabs. Give all formulations without regard to meals. [Trade only: Film-coated tabs 400 mg. Chewable tabs (contain phenylalanine): 25, 100 mg. Single-use packets of powder for oral susp: 100 mg/5 mL.] ▶glucuronidation ♀C ▶– $$$$$

Antiviral Agents—Anti-HIV—Non-Nucleoside Reverse Transcriptase Inhibitors

EFAVIRENZ (*Sustiva*, EFV) Combination therapy of HIV, adults and children wt 40 kg or greater: 600 mg PO once daily on an empty stomach, preferably at bedtime. With voriconazole: Use voriconazole 400 mg PO two times per day and efavirenz 300 mg PO once daily. With rifampin: Increase efavirenz to 800 mg PO once daily if wt is 50 kg or greater. Peds, age 3 mo or older and wt 3.5 to 40 kg: Consider antihistamine prophylaxis to prevent rash before starting. Give PO once daily at a dose of 100 mg for 3.5 to less than 5 kg; 150 mg for 5 to less than 7.5 kg; 200 mg for 7.5 to less than 15 kg; 250 mg for 15 to less than 20 kg; 300 mg for 20 to less than 25 kg; 350 mg for 25 to less than 32.5 kg; 400 mg for 32.5 to less than 40 kg. Take on empty stomach, preferably at bedtime. Capsule contents can be sprinkled on 1 to 2 teaspoons of food; do not give additional food for 2 h. [Trade only: Caps 50, 200 mg. Tabs 600 mg.] ▶L ♀D ▶– $$$$$

ETRAVIRINE (*Intelence*, ETR) Combination therapy for treatment-resistant HIV infection. Adults: 200 mg PO two times per day after meals. Peds, age 6 yo and older: Give PO two times per day after meals at 100 mg per dose for 16 to less than 20 kg; 125 mg per dose for 20 to less than 25 kg; 150 mg per dose for 25 to less than 30 kg; 200 mg per dose for 30 kg or greater. [Trade only: Tabs 25, 100, 200 mg.] ▶L ♀B ▶– $$$$$

NEVIRAPINE (*Viramune*, *Viramune XR*, NVP) Combination therapy for HIV: 200 mg PO daily for 14 days initially. If tolerated, increase to 200 mg PO two times per day or Viramune XR 400 mg PO once daily. Patients maintained on immediate-release tabs can switch directly to Viramune XR. Peds, age 15 days or older: 150 mg/m² PO once daily for 14 days, then 150 mg/m² two times per day (max dose 200 mg two times per day). Viramune XR, age 6 yo and older: 200 mg PO once daily for BSA 0.58 to 0.83 m²; 300 mg PO once daily for BSA 0.84 to 1.16 m²; 400 mg PO once daily for BSA 1.17 m² or greater. To reduce risk of rash, patients should receive immediate-release nevirapine 150 mg/m² once

(cont.)

daily (max 200 mg/day) for at least 14 days before conversion to Viramune XR. Patients already maintained on twice-daily immediate-release nevirapine can switch directly to Viramune XR. Severe skin reactions and hepatotoxicity. [Generic/Trade: Tabs 200 mg. Susp 50 mg/5 mL (240 mL). Extended-release tabs 400 mg. Trade only: Extended-release tabs (Viramune XR) 100 mg.] ▶LK ♀C ▶– $$$$$ ▪

RILPIVIRINE (*Edurant, RPV*) Combination therapy of HIV infection, treatment-naive adults with HIV RNA less than or equal to 100,000 copies/mL: 25 mg PO once daily with a meal. Dosage adjustment for rifabutin: Rilpivirine 50 mg PO once daily with a meal. [Trade only: Tabs 25 mg.] ▶L ♀B ▶– $$$$$

Antiviral Agents—Anti-HIV—Nucleoside/Nucleotide Reverse Transcriptase Inhibitors

ABACAVIR (*Ziagen, ABC*) Combination therapy for HIV. Adult: 300 mg PO two times per day or 600 mg PO daily. Peds: Oral soln, age 3 mo or older: 16 mg/kg (up to 600 mg/day) PO divided one or two times per day. Peds, tabs: 150 mg PO two times per day or 300 mg PO once daily for wt 14 to less than 20 kg; 150 mg PO q am and 300 mg PO q pm or 450 mg PO once daily for wt 20 to less than 25 kg; 300 mg PO two times per day or 600 mg PO once daily for wt 25 kg or greater. Potentially fatal hypersensitivity. HLA-B*5701 predisposes to hypersensitivity; screen before starting and avoid if positive test. Never rechallenge with abacavir after suspected reaction. [Generic/Trade: Tabs 300 mg scored. Trade only: Soln 20 mg/mL (240 mL).] ▶L ♀C ▶– $$$$$ ▪

DIDANOSINE (*Videx, Videx EC, DDI*) Combination therapy for HIV. Videx EC: Give 200 mg PO once daily for wt 20 to 24 kg; 250 mg PO once daily for wt 25 to 59 kg; 400 mg PO once daily for wt 60 kg or greater. Dosage reduction of Videx EC with tenofovir in adults: 200 mg for wt less than 60 kg; 250 mg for wt 60 kg or greater. Dosage reduction unclear with tenofovir if CrCl is less than 60 mL/min. Buffered powder, peds: 100 mg/m² PO two times per day for age 2 weeks to 8 mo; 120 mg/m² PO two times per day for age older than 8 mo (do not exceed adult dose). All formulations usually taken on empty stomach. [Generic/Trade: Delayed-release caps (Videx EC): 125, 200, 250, 400 mg. Pediatric powder for oral soln (buffered with antacid) 10 mg/mL. Generic only: Tabs for oral susp (chewable; buffered with antacid) 100, 150, 200 mg.] ▶LK ♀B ▶– $$$$$ ▪

EMTRICITABINE (*Emtriva, FTC*) Combination therapy for HIV. Adults: 200 mg cap or 240 mg oral soln PO once daily. Peds, oral soln: 3 mg/kg PO once daily for age 3 mo or younger; 6 mg/kg PO once daily (up to 240 mg) for age older than 3 mo. Can give 200 mg cap PO once daily if wt greater than 33 kg. [Trade only: Caps 200 mg. Oral soln 10 mg/mL (170 mL).] ▶K ♀B ▶– $$$$$ ▪

LAMIVUDINE (*Epivir, Epivir-HBV, 3TC, ✦Heptovir*) Epivir for HIV infection. Adults and teens older than 16 yo: 150 mg PO two times per day or 300 mg PO daily. Peds: 8 mg/kg (up to 300 mg/day) PO divided one or two times per day. Can use tabs if wt 14 kg or greater. Epivir-HBV for hepatitis B: Adults: 100 mg PO daily. Peds: 3 mg/kg (up to 100 mg) PO daily. [Generic/Trade: Tabs 100, 150 (scored), 300 mg. Oral soln 10 mg/mL. Trade only (Epivir-HBV, Heptovir): Oral soln 5 mg/mL.] ▶K ♀C ▶– $$$$$ ▪

ANTIMICROBIALS

TENOFOVIR (*Viread*, **TDF**) Combination therapy for HIV. Adults and adolescents: 300 mg PO daily. Peds, 2 yo and older: 8 mg/kg PO once daily (max 300 mg/day) as oral powder. Tabs for peds, wt 17 kg or greater: Give PO once daily at dose of 150 mg for wt 17 to less than 22 kg; 200 mg for wt 22 to less than 28 kg; 250 mg for wt 28 to less than 35 kg; 300 mg for wt 35 kg or greater. Chronic hepatitis B, adults and peds (age 12 yo and older and wt 35 kg or greater): 300 mg PO daily (7.5 scoops of power for those who cannot swallow tabs) without regard to meals. Mix powder with soft food (not liquid) and use immediately. [Trade only: Tabs 150, 200, 250, 300 mg. Oral powder 40 mg tenofovir/1 g scoop of powder, 60 g bottle.] ▶K ♀B ▶– $$$$$ ■

ZIDOVUDINE (*Retrovir*, **AZT**, **ZDV**) Combination therapy of HIV infection: 600 mg/day PO divided two or three times per day for wt 30 kg or greater. Peds dose based on wt: Give 24 mg/kg/day PO divided two or three times per day for wt 4 to 8 kg, 18 mg/kg/day PO divided two or three times per day for wt 9 to 29 kg. [Generic/Trade: Caps 100 mg. Syrup 50 mg/5 mL (240 mL). Generic only: Tabs 300 mg.] ▶LK ♀C ▶– $$$$$ ■

Antiviral Agents—Anti-HIV—Protease Inhibitors and Boosters

NOTE: *Many serious drug interactions: Always check before prescribing. Protease inhibitors and cobicistat inhibit CYP3A4. Contraindicated with alfuzosin, dronedarone, ergot alkaloids, lovastatin, pimozide, rifampin, rifapentine, salmeterol, high-dose sildenafil for pulmonary hypertension, simeprevir, simvastatin, St. John's wort, triazolam. Midazolam contraindicated in labeling; but can use single dose IV cautiously with monitoring for procedural sedation. Monitor INR with warfarin. Avoid inhaled/nasal budesonide/fluticasone with ritonavir/cobicistat if possible; increased corticosteroid levels can cause Cushing's syndrome/ adrenal suppression. Other protease inhibitors may increase budesonide/ fluticasone levels; find alternatives for long-term use. Reduce colchicine dose; do not coadminister colchicine and protease inhibitors in patients with renal or hepatic dysfunction. Adjust dose of bosentan or tadalafil for pulmonary hypertension. Reduce quetiapine dose to 1/6 of original dose if protease inhibitor or cobicistat is added; use lowest initial quetiapine dose if it is added to protease inhibitor or cobicistat. Erectile dysfunction: Single dose of sildenafil 25 mg q 48 h, tadalafil 5 mg (not more than 10 mg) q 72 h, or vardenafil initially 2.5 mg q 72 h. Protease inhibitor class adverse effects include spontaneous bleeding in hemophiliacs, hyperglycemia, hyperlipidemia, immune reconstitution syndrome, and fat redistribution. Coinfection with hepatitis C or other liver disease increases the risk of hepatotoxicity with protease inhibitors; monitor LFTs at least twice in 1st month of therapy, then q 3 months.*

ATAZANAVIR (*Reyataz*, **ATV**) Adults, therapy-naive: 400 mg PO once daily (without ritonavir if ritonavir-intolerant) OR 300 mg + ritonavir 100 mg PO both once daily. With tenofovir, therapy-naive: 300 mg + ritonavir 100 mg PO both once daily. With efavirenz, therapy-naive: 400 mg + ritonavir 100 mg PO both once daily. Do not give atazanavir with efavirenz in therapy-experienced patients. Adults, therapy-experienced: 300 mg + ritonavir 100 mg PO both once daily. Peds: Oral powder,

(cont.)

age 3 mo and older and wt 10 kg to less than 25 kg: 200 mg atazanavir powder (4 packets) with 80 mg ritonavir oral soln PO once daily for wt 10 kg to less than 15 kg; 250 mg atazanavir powder (5 packets) with 80 mg ritonavir oral soln PO once daily for wt 15 to less than 25 kg. Mix powder with food or beverage and give ritonavir immediately after. Oral capsules, age 6 yo or older: Atazanavir-ritonavir PO once daily 150/100 mg for wt 15 to less than 20 kg; 200/100 mg for wt 20 to less than 40 kg; 300/100 mg for 40 kg or greater. Peds, therapy-naive, ritonavir-intolerant, age 13 yo or older and wt 39 kg or greater: 400 mg PO once daily. Give caps with food. Give atazanavir 2 h before or 1 h after buffered didanosine. Do not give to infants less than 3 mo due to risk of kernicterus. [Trade only: Caps 150, 200, 300 mg. Powder packets (contain phenylalanine) 50 mg.] ▶L ♀B ▶– $$$$$

COBICISTAT (*Tybost*, COBI) Combination therapy for HIV infection: Cobicistat 150 mg + atazanavir 300 mg both PO once daily OR cobicistat 150 mg + darunavir 800 mg both once daily. Take cobicistat with food at the same time as atazanavir-darunavir. Dosage adjustment of cobicistat-atazanavir for efavirenz, treatment-naive patients: Cobicistat 150 mg + atazanavir 400 mg both PO once daily with food + efavirenz 600 mg PO once daily on an empty stomach, preferably at bedtime. Do not use cobicistat-atazanavir with efavirenz in treatment-experienced patients. Cobicistat is a strong CYP3A4 inhibitor that boosts atazanavir and darunavir levels (no antiviral activity). Many drug interactions! Not interchangeable with ritonavir; do not assume interactions are the same. [Trade only: Film-coated tabs 150 mg.] ▶L ♀B ▶– $$$$$

DARUNAVIR (*Prezista*, DRV) Therapy-naive or -experienced adults with no darunavir resistance substitutions: 800 mg + ritonavir 100 mg both PO once daily. Therapy-experienced adults with at least 1 darunavir resistance substitution: 600 mg + ritonavir 100 mg both PO two times per day. Peds: Treatment-naive or treatment-experienced without resistance substitutions, age 3 yo or older: Give darunavir + ritonavir both PO once daily according to wt: Darunavir 35 mg/kg + ritonavir 7 mg/kg for wt 10 to less than 15 kg; darunavir 600 mg + ritonavir 100 mg for wt 15 to less than 30 kg; darunavir 675 mg + ritonavir 100 mg for wt 30 to less than 40 kg; darunavir 800 mg + ritonavir 100 mg for wt 40 kg or greater. Treatment-experienced with at least 1 resistance substitution, age 3 yo or older: Give darunavir + ritonavir both two times per day according to wt: Darunavir 20 mg/kg + ritonavir 7 mg/kg for wt 10 to less than 15 kg; darunavir 375 mg + ritonavir 48 mg for wt 15 to less than 30 kg; darunavir 450 mg + ritonavir 60 mg for wt 30 to less than 40 kg; darunavir 600 mg + ritonavir 100 mg for wt 40 kg or greater. Take with food. [Trade only: Tabs 75, 150, 600, 800 mg. Susp 100 mg/mL (200 mL).] ▶L ♀B ▶– $$$$$

EVOTAZ (atazanavir + cobicistat) Combination therapy of HIV: 1 tab PO once daily with food. [Trade only: Tabs atazanavir 300 mg + cobicistat 150 mg.] ▶L ♀B ▶– $$$$$

FOSAMPRENAVIR (*Lexiva*, FPV, ✦*Telzir*) Therapy-naive adults: 1400 mg PO two times per day (without ritonavir) OR 1400 mg + ritonavir 100/200 mg PO both once daily OR 700 mg + ritonavir 100 mg PO both two times per day. Protease inhibitor–experienced adults: 700 mg + ritonavir 100 mg PO both two times per

ANTIMICROBIALS

day. Peds: Fosamprenavir-ritonavir for protease inhibitor–naive patients, 4 weeks of age or older, or protease inhibitor–experienced patients, 6 mo or older: Give PO two times per day according to wt: Fosamprenavir 45 mg/kg plus ritonavir 7 mg/kg for wt less than 11 kg; fosamprenavir 30 mg/kg plus ritonavir 3 mg/kg for wt 11 to less than 15 kg; fosamprenavir 23 mg/kg plus ritonavir 3 mg/kg for wt 15 to less than 20 kg; fosamprenavir 18 mg/kg plus ritonavir 3 mg/kg for wt 20 kg or greater. Do not exceed adult dose of fosamprenavir 700 mg plus ritonavir 100 mg both PO two times per day. For fosamprenavir-ritonavir, can use fosamprenavir tabs if wt 39 kg or greater and ritonavir caps if wt 33 kg or greater. Fosamprenavir monotherapy for protease inhibitor–naive patients, 2 yo or older: 30 mg/kg PO two times per day; can give 1400 mg as tabs PO two times per day if wt 47 kg or greater. Fosamprenavir is only for infants born at 38 weeks' gestation or more who have attained postnatal age of 28 days. Do not use once-daily dosing of fosamprenavir in children. Take tabs without regard to meals. Adults should take susp without food; children should take with food. [Trade only: Tabs 700 mg. Susp 50 mg/mL.] ▶L ♀C ▶– $$$$$

KALETRA (lopinavir + ritonavir, *LPV/R*) Combination therapy of HIV. Adults: 400/100 mg PO two times per day (tabs or oral soln). Can use 800/200 mg PO once daily in patients with less than 3 lopinavir resistance–associated substitutions. Coadministration with efavirenz, nevirapine, fosamprenavir, or nelfinavir: 500/125 mg tabs (use two 200/50 mg + one 100/25 mg tab) or 533/133 mg oral soln (6.5 mL) PO two times per day. Infants, age 14 days to 6 mo: Lopinavir 16 mg/kg PO two times per day. Peds age 6 mo to 12 yo: Lopinavir 12 mg/kg PO two times per day for wt less than 15 kg, use 10 mg/kg PO two times per day for wt 15 to 40 kg. Coadministration with efavirenz, nevirapine, fosamprenavir, or nelfinavir: Lopinavir 13 mg/kg PO two times per day for wt less than 15 kg, 11 mg/kg PO two times per day for wt 15 to 45 kg. Do not exceed adult dose in children. No once-daily dosing for pediatric or pregnant patients; coadministration with carbamazepine, phenobarbital, phenytoin, efavirenz, nevirapine, fosamprenavir, or nelfinavir; or in patients with 3 or more lopinavir resistance–associated substitutions. Give tabs without regard to meals; give oral soln with food. [Trade only (lopinavir-ritonavir): Tabs 200/50 mg, 100/25 mg. Oral soln 80/20 mg/mL (160 mL).] ▶L ♀C ▶– $$$$$

PREZCOBIX (darunavir + cobicistat) Combination therapy of HIV: 1 tab PO once daily with food. Genotypic testing recommended at baseline, especially for treatment-experienced patients. [Trade only: Tabs darunavir 800 mg + cobicistat 150 mg.] ▶L ♀C ▶– $$$$$

RITONAVIR (*Norvir, RTV*) Adult doses of 100 to 400 mg/day PO are used to boost levels of other protease inhibitors. See specific protease inhibitor entries for adult and pediatric boosting doses of ritonavir. Take ritonavir with food. [Trade only: Caps 100 mg, tabs 100 mg. Oral soln 80 mg/mL (240 mL).] ▶L ♀B ▶– $$$$$ ■

SAQUINAVIR (*Invirase, SQV*) Combination therapy for HIV infection: Regimens must contain ritonavir. Saquinavir 1000 mg + ritonavir 100 mg both PO two times per day within 2 h after meals. Saquinavir 1000 mg + Kaletra 400/100 mg PO both two times per day. [Trade only: Caps 200 mg. Tabs 500 mg.] ▶L ♀B ▶– $$$$$

TIPRANAVIR (*Aptivus*, TPV) Treatment-experienced patients with resistance to multiple protease inhibitors: 500 mg boosted by ritonavir 200 mg PO two times per day with food. Peds: 14 mg/kg with 6 mg/kg ritonavir PO two times per day; do not exceed adult dose. Hepatotoxicity. [Trade only: Caps 250 mg. Oral soln 100 mg/mL (95 mL in unit-of-use amber glass bottle).] ▶Feces ♀C ▶– $$$$$ ■

Antiviral Agents—Anti-Influenza

AMANTADINE Parkinsonism: 100 mg PO two times per day. Max 300 to 400 mg/day divided three to four times per day. Prevention/treatment of influenza A: 5 mg/kg/day up to 150 mg/day divided two times per day for age 1 to 9 yo and any child wt less than 40 kg. Give 100 mg PO two times per day for adults and children age 10 yo or older; reduce to 100 mg PO daily if age 65 yo or older. The CDC generally recommends against amantadine/rimantadine for treatment/prevention of influenza A in the United States due to high levels of resistance. [Generic only: Caps 100 mg. Tabs 100 mg. Syrup 50 mg/5 mL (480 mL).] ▶K ♀C ▶? $$$$

OSELTAMIVIR (*Tamiflu*) Influenza A/B: For treatment, give each dose two times per day for 5 days starting within 2 days of symptom onset. For prevention, give each dose once daily for 10 days starting within 2 days of exposure. For adults each dose is 75 mg. For peds, age 1 yo or older, each dose is 30 mg for wt 15 kg or less; 45 mg for wt 16 to 23 kg; 60 mg for wt 24 to 40 kg; and 75 mg for wt greater than 40 kg or age 13 yo or older. Influenza treatment in infants age 2 weeks old to 1 yo: 3 mg/kg/dose PO two times per day for 5 days. Influenza prophylaxis in infants 3 to 11 mo: 3 mg/kg PO once daily. Due to limited data, prophylaxis is not recommended for infants younger than 3 mo unless the situation is critical. Can take with food to improve tolerability. See influenza table. [Trade only: Caps 30, 45, 75 mg. Susp 6 mg/mL (60 mL) with 10 mL dosing device. Pharmacist can also compound susp (6 mg/mL).] ▶LK ♀C, but + ▶? $$$$

PERAMIVIR (*Rapivab*) Influenza, uncomplicated in adults: 600 mg IV single dose infused over 15 to 30 minutes. See influenza table. ▶K ♀C ▶? $$$$$

RIMANTADINE (*Flumadine*) Treatment or prevention of influenza A in adults: 100 mg PO two times per day. Reduce dose to 100 mg PO once daily for age older than 65 yo. Peds influenza A prophylaxis: 5 mg/kg (up to 150 mg/day) PO once daily for age 1 to 9 yo. Use adult dose for age 10 yo or older. The CDC generally recommends against amantadine/rimantadine for treatment/prevention of influenza A in the United States due to high levels of resistance. [Generic/Trade: Tabs 100 mg. Pharmacist can compound suspension.] ▶LK ♀C ▶– $$

ZANAMIVIR (*Relenza*) Influenza A/B treatment: 2 puffs two times per day for 5 days for adults and children 7 yo or older. Influenza A/B prevention: 2 puffs once daily for 10 days for adults and children 5 yo or older starting within 2 days of exposure. Do not use if chronic airway disease. See influenza table. [Trade only: Rotadisk inhaler 5 mg/puff (20 puffs).] ▶K ♀C ▶? $$$

INFLUENZA TREATMENT AND CHEMOPREVENTION: CDC RECOMMENDATIONS

	Treatment[a] (Duration of 5 days) for oseltamivir/ zanamivir	Prevention[b] (Duration of 7 to 10 days post-exposure)
OSELTAMIVIR (*Tamiflu*)		
Adults and adolescents age 13 years and older		
	75 mg PO bid	75 mg PO once daily
Children, 1 year of age and older[c]		
Body weight ≤15 kg	30 mg PO bid	30 mg PO once daily
Body weight >15 to 23 kg	45 mg PO bid	45 mg PO once daily
Body weight >23 to 40 kg	60 mg PO bid	60 mg PO once daily
Body weight >40 kg	75 mg PO bid	75 mg PO once daily
Infants, newborn to 11 months of age[c]		
Age 3 to 11 months old[d]	3 mg/kg/dose PO bid	3 mg/kg/dose PO once daily
Age younger than 3 months old[e]	3 mg/kg/dose PO bid	Not for routine prophylaxis in infants <3 months old
ZANAMIVIR (*Relenza*)[f]		
Adults and children (7 years and older for treatment, 5 years and older for prophylaxis)		
	10 mg (two 5-mg inhalations) bid	10 mg (two 5-mg inhalations) once daily
PERAMIVIR (*Rapivab*)		
Adults with uncomplicated influenza[g]		
	600 mg IV over15 to 30 minutes as single dose	N/A (NOTE: Peramivir is not used for prevention of influenza)

(cont.)

Antimicrobials **47**

INFLUENZA TREATMENT AND CHEMOPREVENTION: CDC RECOMMENDATIONS (continued)

Adapted from http://www.cdc.gov/flu/professionals/antivirals/summary-clinicians.htm. bid=two times per day

a For treatment, start antiviral drugs as soon as possible; do not wait for lab test confirmation. Starting within 2 days of symptom onset is ideal, but starting later may help severe/complicated/hospitalized cases. Consider treating longer if patients remain severely ill after 5 days of treatment, especially if immunosuppressed. Patients at high risk of influenza complications should be treated, including age less than 2 years or at least 65 years old; chronic pulmonary, cardiovascular (except hypertension only), renal, hepatic, hematologic, metabolic, neurologic/ neurodevelopment disorders; immunosuppressed or HIV; pregnant or within 2 weeks postpartum; child or adolescent on long-term aspirin; native American/ Alaskan native; morbid obesity; resident of nursing home or chronic care facility.

b For chemoprophylaxis, duration is 10 days after household exposure, and 7 days after most recent known exposure in other situations. For long-term care facilities and hospitals, prophylaxis should last a minimum of 14 days and up to 7 days after the most recent case was identified.

c If Tamiflu suspension is unavailable, pharmacists can compound 6 mg/mL suspension from package insert recipe. Capsule contents of 30, 45, and 75 mg capsules can be mixed with sweetened liquid. Unit of measure is mL for 10 mL Tamiflu suspension oral dispenser; make sure units of measure in dosing instructions match dosing device provided. Tamiflu is FDA-approved for treatment of influenza in infants 2 weeks of age and older and prevention of influenza in children 1 year of age and older.

d AAP (http://pediatrics.aappublications.org/content/early/2014/09/17/peds.2014-2413) recommends that infants age 9 to 11 mo receive oseltamivir 3.5 mg/kg/dose PO twice daily for treatment and 3.5 mg/kg/dose PO once daily for prevention. This is based on pharmacokinetic data that suggests a higher dose is needed for adequate oseltamivir exposure in this age group. There is no data to suggest the higher dose is more effective or causes more adverse effects than the usual dose.

e This dose is not intended for premature infants. Immature renal function may lead to slow clearance and high concentrations of oseltamivir in this age group.

f Zanamivir should not be used by patients with underlying pulmonary disease. Do not use Relenza in a nebulizer or ventilator; lactose in the formulation may clog the device.

g IV peramivir is FDA-approved for uncomplicated influenza in adults. Peramivir 600 mg IV once daily for 5 days (10 mg/kg up to 600 mg once daily for children age 6 yo and older) had no benefit in a randomized clinical trial of hospitalized patients with influenza. CDC recommends PO/NG oseltamivir for influenza in hospitalized patients. In patients who cannot tolerate or absorb PO/NG oseltamivir (due to gastric stasis, malabsorption, or GI bleeding), consider IV peramivir or investigational IV zanamivir. In oseltamivir-resistant influenza, consider IV zanamivir. Contact gskclinicalsupportHD@gsk.com, or call 1-877-626-8019 or 1-866-341-9160 (24 h/day) for availability of IV zanamivir.

Antiviral Agents—Other

INTERFERON ALFA-2B (Intron A) Chronic hepatitis B: 5 million units/day or 10 million units three times per week SC/IM for 16 weeks if HBeAg+, for 48 weeks if HBeAg−. [Trade only: Powder/soln for injection 10, 18, 50 million units/vial. Soln for injection 18, 25 million units/multidose vial. Multidose injection pens 3, 5, 10 million units/0.2 mL (1.5 mL), 6 doses/pen.] ▶K ♀C ▶?+ $$$$$

PALIVIZUMAB (Synagis) Prevention of respiratory syncytial virus pulmonary disease in high-risk infants: 15 mg/kg IM once monthly for a max of 5 doses per RSV season. ▶L ♀C ▶? $$$$$

PEGINTERFERON ALFA-2A (*Pegasys*) See www.hcvguidelines.org for current treatment recommendations; few regimens include peginterferon anymore. Combination therapy of chronic hepatitis C: 180 mcg SC in abdomen or thigh once a week. Hepatitis B: 180 mcg SC in abdomen or thigh once a week for 48 weeks. Peds: Chronic hepatitis C, age 5 yo or older: 180 mcg/1.73 m^2 (max dose of 180 mcg) SC once weekly with PO ribavirin for 24 weeks (genotype 2 or 3) or 48 weeks (genotype 1 or 4). May cause or worsen severe autoimmune, neuropsychiatric, ischemic, and infectious diseases. Frequent clinical and lab monitoring. [Trade only: 180 mcg/1 mL soln in single-use vial; 180 mcg/0.5 mL prefilled syringe; 180 mcg/0.5 mL, 135 mcg/0.5 mL auto-injector.] ▶LK ♀C ▶– $$$$$ ■

PEGINTERFERON ALFA-2B (*PegIntron*) See www.hcvguidelines.org for current treatment recommendations; few regimens include peginterferon anymore. Chronic hepatitis C: 1.5 mcg/kg SC weekly with ribavirin and other HCV drugs. Peds, age 3 yo and older: 60 mcg/m^2 SC once a week with ribavirin 15 mg/kg/day PO divided two times per day. May cause or worsen severe autoimmune, neuropsychiatric, ischemic, and infectious diseases. Frequent clinical and lab monitoring. [Trade only: 50, 80, 120, 150 mcg/ 0.5 mL single-use vials with diluent, 2 syringes, and alcohol swabs.] ▶K? ♀C ▶– $$$$$ ■

Carbapenems

NOTE: *Carbapenems can dramatically reduce valproic acid levels; use another antibiotic (preferred) or add a supplemental anticonvulsant in valproate-treated patients.*

DORIPENEM (*Doribax*) Complicated intra-abdominal infection, complicated UTI/pyelonephritis: 500 mg IV q 8 h. Not indicated for ventilator-associated bacterial pneumonia due to higher mortality rate. ▶K ♀B ▶? $$$$$

ERTAPENEM (*Invanz*) 1 g IV/IM q 24 h. Prophylaxis, colorectal surgery: 1 g IV 1 h before incision. Peds, younger than 13 yo: 15 mg/kg IV/IM q 12 h (up to 1 g/day). Infuse IV over 30 min. ▶K ♀B ▶? $$$$$

MEROPENEM (*Merrem IV*) Complicated skin infection, 3 mo and older: 10 mg/kg up to 500 mg IV q 8 h; use 500 mg IV for adults and peds with wt greater than 50 kg. Complicated skin infection caused by *P. aeruginosa*, 3 mo and older: 20 mg/kg IV q 8 h up to 1 g IV q 8 h; use 1 g IV q 8 h for adults and peds with wt greater than 50 kg. Complicated intra-abdominal infection. Age 3 mo and older: 20 mg/kg up to 1 g IV q 8 h; use 1 g IV q 8 h for adults and peds with wt greater than 50 kg. Age 2 weeks to less than 3 mo: 20 mg/kg IV q 8 h if gestational age less than 32 weeks; 30 mg/kg IV q 8 h if gestational age 32 weeks and older. Age less than 2 weeks: 20 mg/kg IV q 12 h if gestational age less than 32 weeks; 20 mg/kg IV q 8 h if gestational age 32 weeks and older. Peds meningitis, 3 mo and older: 40 mg/kg IV q 8 h for age 3 mo or older; 2 g IV q 8 h for wt greater than 50 kg. Anthrax: See table. ▶K ♀B ▶? $$$$$

PRIMAXIN (imipenem-cilastatin) 250 to 1000 mg IV q 6 to 8 h. Peds, age older than 3 mo: 15 to 25 mg/kg IV q 6 h. Seizures (especially if given with ganciclovir, elderly with renal dysfunction, or cerebrovascular or seizure disorder). ▶K ♀C ▶? $$$$$

CEPHALOSPORINS: GENERAL ANTIMICROBIAL SPECTRUM

1st generation	Gram-positive (including *S. aureus*); basic Gram-negative coverage
2nd generation	diminished *S. aureus*, improved Gram-negative coverage compared to 1st generation; some with anaerobic coverage
3rd generation	further diminished *S. aureus*, further improved Gram-negative coverage compared to 1st and 2nd generation; some with pseudomonal coverage and diminished Gram-positive coverage
4th generation	same as 3rd generation plus coverage against *Pseudomonas*
5th generation	Gram-negative coverage similar to 3rd generation; also active against *S. aureus* (including MRSA) and *S. pneumoniae*

ANTIMICROBIALS

Cephalosporins—1st Generation

CEFADROXIL 1 to 2 g/day PO once daily or divided two times per day. Peds: 30 mg/kg/day divided two times per day. Group A streptococcal pharyngitis: 30 mg/kg/day to max of 1 g/day PO divided once or twice daily for 10 days. [Generic only: Tabs 1 g. Caps 500 mg. Susp 250, 500 mg/5 mL.] ▶K ♀B ▶+ $$$

CEFAZOLIN 0.5 to 1.5 g IM/IV q 6 to 8 h. Peds: 25 to 50 mg/kg/day divided q 6 to 8 h (up to 100 mg/kg/day for severe infections). ▶K ♀B ▶+ $$

CEPHALEXIN (*Keflex*) 250 to 500 mg PO four times per day. Peds: 25 to 50 mg/kg/day. Group A streptococcal pharyngitis: 20 mg/kg/dose to max of 500 mg/dose PO two times per day for 10 days. Not for otitis media, sinusitis. [Generic/Trade: Caps 250, 500, 750 mg. Generic only: Tabs 250, 500 mg. Susp 125, 250 mg/5 mL.] ▶K ♀B ▶? $$

Cephalosporins—2nd Generation

CEFACLOR (★*Ceclor*) 250 to 500 mg PO three times per day. Peds: 20 to 40 mg/kg/day PO divided three times per day. Group A streptococcal pharyngitis (2nd line to penicillin): 20 mg/kg/day PO divided two times per day for 10 days. Serum sickness–like reactions with repeated use. [Generic only: Caps 250, 500 mg. Susp 125, 187, 250, 375 mg per 5 mL. Extended-release tab: 500 mg.] ▶K ♀B ▶? $$$$

CEFOXITIN 1 to 2 g IM/IV q 6 to 8 h. Peds: 80 to 160 mg/kg/day IV divided q 4 to 8 h. ▶K ♀B ▶+ $

CEFPROZIL 250 to 500 mg PO two times per day. Peds: Otitis media: 15 mg/kg/dose PO two times per day. Group A streptococcal pharyngitis (2nd line to penicillin): 7.5 mg/kg/dose PO two times per day for 10 days. [Generic only: Tabs 250, 500 mg. Susp 125, 250 mg/5 mL.] ▶K ♀B ▶+ $$$$

CEFUROXIME (*Zinacef, Ceftin*) Adults: 750 to 1500 mg IM/IV q 8 h. 250 to 500 mg PO two times per day. Peds: 50 to 100 mg/kg/day IV divided q 6 to 8 h; not for meningitis; 20 to 30 mg/kg/day susp PO divided two times per day. [Generic/Trade: Tabs 250, 500 mg. Susp 125, 250 mg/5 mL.] ▶K ♀B ▶? $$$$

Cephalosporins—3rd Generation

CEFDINIR (*Omnicef*) 14 mg/kg/day up to 600 mg/day PO once daily or divided two times per day. See otitis media table. [Generic only: Caps 300 mg. Susp 125, 250 mg/5 mL.] ▶K ♀B ▷? $$$$

CEFDITOREN (*Spectracef*) 200 to 400 mg PO two times per day with food. [Generic/Trade: Tabs 200, 400 mg.] ▶K ♀B ▷? $$$$$

CEFIXIME (*Suprax*) 400 mg PO once daily. Gonorrhea (not pharyngeal): 400 mg PO single dose + azithromycin 1 g PO single dose. CDC now considers cefixime 2nd-line for treatment of gonorrhea and requires test-of-cure. See STD table. Peds: 8 mg/kg/day once daily or divided two times per day. Use only susp/chew tabs for otitis media (better blood levels). See acute sinusitis table. [Generic/Trade: Susp 100, 200 mg/5 mL. Trade only: Susp 500 mg/5 mL. Chewable tabs 100, 200 mg. Tabs 400 mg. Caps 400 mg.] ▶K/Bile ♀B ▷? $$$$

CEFOTAXIME (*Claforan*) Usual dose: 1 to 2 g IM/IV q 6 to 8 h. Peds: 50 to 180 mg/kg/day IM/IV divided q 4 to 6 h. AAP dose for pneumococcal meningitis: 225 to 300 mg/kg/day IV divided q 6 to 8 h. ▶KL ♀B ▷+ $$$$

CEFPODOXIME 100 to 400 mg PO two times per day. Peds: 10 mg/kg/day divided two times per day. See acute sinusitis and otitis media tables. [Generic: Tabs 100, 200 mg. Susp 50, 100 mg/5 mL.] ▶K ♀B ▷? $$$$

CEFTAZIDIME (*Fortaz, Tazicef*) 1 g IM/IV or 2 g IV q 8 to 12 h. Peds: 30 to 50 mg/kg IV q 8 h. ▶K ♀B ▷+ $$$$

CEFTIBUTEN (*Cedax*) 400 mg PO once daily. Peds: 9 mg/kg (up to 400 mg) PO once daily. [Trade only: Caps 400 mg. Susp 90 mg/5 mL.] ▶K ♀B ▷? $$$$$

CEFTRIAXONE (*Rocephin*) 1 to 2 g IM/IV q 24 h. Meningitis: 2 g IV q 12 h. Gonorrhea: 250 mg IM plus azithromycin 1 g PO both single dose. See STD table. Peds: 50 to 75 mg/kg/day (up to 2 g/day) divided q 12 to 24 h. Peds meningitis: 100 mg/kg/day (up to 4 g/day) IV divided q 12 to 24 h. Otitis media: 50 mg/kg up to 1 g IM single dose. May dilute in 1% lidocaine for IM. See acute sinusitis and otitis media tables. Contraindicated in neonates who require (or are expected to require) IV calcium (including calcium in TPN) due to reports of fatal lung/kidney precipitation of calcium ceftriaxone. In other patients, do not give ceftriaxone and calcium-containing solns simultaneously, but sequential administration is acceptable if lines are flushed with a compatible fluid between infusions. ▶K/Bile ♀B ▷+ $

Cephalosporins—4th Generation

***AVYCAZ* (ceftazidime-avibactam)** Complicated intra-abdominal infection (in combination with metronidazole), complicated UTI, pyelonephritis: 2.5 g IV q 8 h infused over 2 h. Avycaz 2.5 g = 2 g ceftazidime + 0.5 g avibactam. ▶K ♀B ▷? $$$$$

CEFEPIME (*Maxipime*) 0.5 to 2 g IM/IV q 12 h. Peds: 50 mg/kg IV q 8 to 12 h. ▶K ♀B ▷? $$$$

***ZERBAXA* (ceftolozane-tazobactam)** Complicated intra-abdominal infections (in combination with metronidazole), complicated UTI , pyelonephritis: 1.5 g IV q 8 h infused over 1 h. Zerbaxa 1.5 g = 1 g ceftolozane + 0.5 g tazobactam. ▶K ♀B ▷? $$$$$

Cephalosporins—5th Generation

CEFTAROLINE (*Teflaro*) Community-acquired bacterial pneumonia, acute bacterial skin and skin structure infections: 600 mg IV q 12 h infused over 1 h. ▶K ♀B ▶? $$$$$

Glycopeptides

DALBAVANCIN (*Dalvance*) Gram-positive skin infections, including MRSA: 1000 mg followed 1 week later by 500 mg. Infuse IV over 30 minutes. Rapid infusion can cause "red man" syndrome. ▶K ♀C ▶? $$$$$

ORITAVANCIN (*Orbactiv*) Gram-positive skin infections, including MRSA: 1200 mg IV single dose infused over 3 h. Increased INR with warfarin. ▶K feces ♀C ▶? $$$$$

TELAVANCIN (*Vibativ*) Complicated skin infections including MRSA: 10 mg/kg IV once daily for 7 to 14 days. Hospital-acquired/ventilator-associated *S. aureus* pneumonia (not 1st-line): 10 mg/kg IV once daily for 7 to 21 days. Infuse over 1 h. Teratogenic; get serum pregnancy test before use in women of childbearing potential. Nephrotoxic; monitor renal function. Do not use if CrCl is 50 mL/min or lower unless potential benefit exceeds risk. Not approved in children. ▶K ♀C ▶? $$$$$ ■

VANCOMYCIN (*Vancocin*) Usual adult dose: 15 to 20 mg/kg IV q 8 to 12 h; consider loading dose of 25 to 30 mg/kg for severe infection. Infuse over 1 h; infuse over 1.5 to 2 h if dose greater than 1 g. Peds: 10 to 15 mg/kg IV q 6 h. *C. difficile* diarrhea: 40 mg/kg/day PO up to 2 g/day divided four times per day for at least 10 days. IV administration ineffective for this indication. Dose depends on severity and complications, see table for management of *C. difficile* infection in adults. [Generic/Trade: Caps 125, 250 mg.] ▶K ♀C ▶? $$$$$

Macrolides

AZITHROMYCIN (*Zithromax, Zmax*) Usual dose: 10 mg/kg (up to 500 mg) PO on day 1, then 5 mg/kg (up to 250 mg) daily for 4 days. Usual IV dose for adults: 500 mg IV once daily. Azithromycin is a poor option for otitis media and sinusitis due to pneumococcal and *H. influenzae* resistance; see otitis media and sinusitis treatment tables for alternatives. Otitis media: 30 mg/kg PO single dose or 10 mg/kg PO daily for 3 days. Peds sinusitis: 10 mg/kg PO daily for 3 days. Group A streptococcal pharyngitis (2nd-line to penicillin): 12 mg/kg (up to 500 mg) PO daily for 5 days. Adult acute sinusitis or exacerbation of chronic bronchitis: 500 mg PO daily for 3 days. Zmax for community-acquired pneumonia, acute sinusitis: 60 mg/kg (up to 2 g) PO single dose on empty stomach; give adult dose of 2 g for wt 34 kg or greater. Chlamydia (including pregnancy), chancroid: 1 g PO single dose. See STD table. Prevention of disseminated *Mycobacterium avium* complex disease: 1200 mg PO once a week. Pertussis treatment/post-exposure prophylaxis: 10 mg/kg PO once daily for 5 days for infants age younger than 6 mo; 10 mg/kg (max 500 mg) PO on day 1, then 5 mg/kg (max 250 mg) PO once daily for 4 days for children 6 mo and older; 500 mg PO on day 1, then 250 mg PO daily for 4 days for adolescents and

(cont.)

adults. [Generic/Trade: Tabs 250, 500, 600 mg. Susp 100, 200 mg/5 mL. Packet 1000 mg. Z-Pak: #6, 250 mg tab. Tri-Pak: #3, 500 mg tab. Trade only: Extended-release oral susp (Zmax): 2 g in 60 mL single-dose bottle.] ▶L ♀B ▶? $$

CLARITHROMYCIN (*Biaxin*) Usual dose. Adult: 250 to 500 mg PO two times per day. Peds: 7.5 mg/kg PO two times per day. *H. pylori*: See table in GI section. See table for prophylaxis of bacterial endocarditis. *Mycobacterium avium* complex disease prevention: 7.5 mg/kg up to 500 mg PO two times per day. [Generic/Trade: Tabs 250, 500 mg. Extended-release tab 500 mg. Susp 125, 250 mg/5 mL.] ▶KL ♀C ▶? $$$

ERYTHROMYCIN BASE (*Ery-Tab, P.C.E., ✦Eryc*) Adult: 250 to 500 mg PO four times per day, 333 mg PO three times per day, or 500 mg PO two times per day. Peds: 30 to 50 mg/kg/day PO divided four times per day. [Generic only: Tabs 250, 500 mg. Delayed-release caps 250 mg. Trade only: Delayed-release tabs (Ery-Tab, PCE) 250, 333, 500 mg.] ▶L ♀B ▶+ $$$$

ERYTHROMYCIN ETHYL SUCCINATE (*EES, EryPed*) Adult: 400 mg PO four times per day. Peds: 30 to 50 mg/kg/day PO divided four times per day. [Generic/Trade: Tabs 400 mg. Trade only: Susp 200, 400 mg/5 mL.] ▶L ♀B ▶+ $

ERYTHROMYCIN LACTOBIONATE (*Erythrocin IV*) Adult: 15 to 20 mg/kg/day (max 4 g) IV divided q 6 h. Peds: 15 to 50 mg/kg/day IV divided q 6 h. ▶L ♀B ▶+ $$$$$

FIDAXOMICIN (*Dificid*) C. difficile–associated diarrhea: 200 mg PO two times per day for 10 days. [Trade only: 200 mg tabs.] ▶minimal absorption ♀B ▶? $$$$$

PENICILLINS — GENERAL ANTIMICROBIAL SPECTRUM

1st generation	Most streptococci; oral anaerobic coverage
2nd generation	Most streptococci; *S. aureus* (but not MRSA)
3rd generation	Most streptococci; basic Gram-negative coverage
4th generation	*Pseudomonas*

Penicillins—1st Generation—Natural

BENZATHINE PENICILLIN (*Bicillin L-A*) Usual dose: 1.2 million units IM for adults and peds wt greater than 27 kg; 600,000 units IM for peds wt 27 kg or less. Give single dose for group A streptococcal pharyngitis. Give IM q month for secondary prevention of rheumatic fever (q 3 weeks for high-risk patients). See STD table for treatment of syphilis in adults. Dose lasts 2 to 4 weeks. [Trade only: For IM use, 600,000 units/mL; 1, 2, 4 mL syringes.] ▶K ♀B ▶? $$$

BICILLIN C-R (procaine penicillin + benzathine penicillin) For IM use. Not for treatment of syphilis. [Trade only: For IM use 300/300 and 450/150 (Peds) thousand units/mL procaine/benzathine penicillin (600,000 units/mL); 2 mL syringe.] ▶K ♀B ▶? $$$$

PENICILLIN G Pneumococcal pneumonia and severe infections: 250,000 to 400,000 units/kg/day (8 to 12 million units/day in adult) IV divided q 4 to 6 h. Pneumococcal meningitis: 250,000 to 400,000 units/kg/day (24 million units/day in adult) in 4 to 6 divided doses. Anthrax: See table. ▸K ♀B ▶? $$$$

PENICILLIN V Adult: 250 to 500 mg PO four times per day. Peds: 25 to 50 mg/kg/day divided two to four times per day. AHA doses for pharyngitis: 250 mg (peds 27 kg or less) or 500 mg (adults and peds greater than 27 kg) PO two to three times per day for 10 days. Anthrax: See table. [Generic only: Tabs 250, 500 mg. Oral soln 125, 250 mg/5 mL.] ▸K ♀B ▶? $

PROCAINE PENICILLIN 0.6 to 1 million units IM daily (peak 4 h, lasts 24 h). [Generic: For IM use, 600,000 units/mL; 1, 2 mL syringes.] ▸K ♀B ▶? $$$$$ ■

Penicillins—2nd Generation—Penicillinase-Resistant

DICLOXACILLIN Adult: 250 to 500 mg PO four times per day. Peds: 12.5 to 25 mg/kg/day PO divided four times per day. [Generic only: Caps 250, 500 mg.] ▸KL ♀B ▶? $$

NAFCILLIN Adult: 1 to 2 g IM/IV q 4 h. Peds: 50 to 200 mg/kg/day IM/IV divided q 4 to 6 h. ▸L ♀B ▶? $$$$$

OXACILLIN Adult: 1 to 2 g IM/IV q 4 to 6 h. Peds: 150 to 200 mg/kg/day IM/IV divided q 4 to 6 h. ▸KL ♀B ▶? $$$$$

Penicillins—3rd Generation—Aminopenicillins

AMOXICILLIN (*Moxatag*) Usual dose: 250 to 500 mg PO three times per day, or 500 to 875 mg PO two times per day. High-dose for community-acquired pneumonia, acute sinusitis: 1 g PO three times per day. See table for management of acute sinusitis in adults and children. Lyme disease: 500 mg PO three times per day for 14 days for early disease, for 28 days for Lyme arthritis. Chlamydia in pregnancy (CDC alternative regimen): 500 mg PO three times per day for 7 days. See STD table. AHA dosing for group A streptococcal pharyngitis: 50 mg/kg (max 1 g) PO once daily for 10 days. Group A streptococcal pharyngitis/tonsillitis: 775 mg ER tab (Moxatag) PO for 10 days for age 12 yo or older. Peds AAP otitis media: 80 to 90 mg/kg/day divided two times per day. Give 5 to 7 days of therapy for age 6 yo and older with mild to moderate symptoms, 7 days for age 2 to 5 yo with mild to moderate symptoms, and 10 days for age younger than 2 yo and children with severe symptoms. See table for management of acute otitis media in children. Peds infections other than otitis media: 40 mg/kg/day PO divided three times per day or 45 mg/kg/day divided two times per day. [Generic only: Caps 250, 500 mg. Tabs 500, 875 mg. Chewable tabs 125, 200, 250, 400 mg. Susp 125, 250 mg/5 mL. Susp 200, 400 mg/5 mL. Trade only: Extended-release tab (Moxatag) 775 mg.] ▸K ♀B ▶+ $

AMOXICILLIN-CLAVULANATE (*Augmentin, Augmentin ES-600, Augmentin XR, ✦Clavulin*) Adults, usual dose: 500 to 875 mg PO two times per day or 250 to 500 mg three times per day. Augmentin XR: 2 tabs PO q 12 h with meals. See table for management of acute sinusitis in adults and children. Peds, usual dose: 45 mg/kg/day PO divided two times per day or 40 mg/kg/day divided three times

(cont.)

per day. Community-acquired pneumonia, otitis media, sinusitis: 90 mg/kg/day PO divided two times per day (max dose of 2 g PO two times per day for age 5 yo and older). Treat pneumonia for up to 10 days; sinusitis for 10 to 14 days. For oral therapy of acute otitis media, AAP recommends 5 to 7 days of therapy for children 6 yo and older with mild to moderate symptoms, 7 days for children 2 to 5 yo with mild to moderate symptoms, and 10 days for children younger than 2 yo and those with severe symptoms. See table for management of acute otitis media in children. [Generic/Trade: (amoxicillin-clavulanate) Tabs 250/125, 500/125, 875/125 mg. Chewables, Susp 200/28.5, 400/57 mg per tab or 5 mL, 250/62.5 mg per 5 mL. (ES) Susp 600/42.9 mg per 5 mL. Extended-release tabs 1000/62.5 mg. Trade only: Susp 125/31.25 per 5 mL, 250/62.5 mg per 5 mL.] ▶K ♀B ▷? $$$

AMPICILLIN Usual dose: 1 to 2 g IV q 4 to 6 h. Sepsis, meningitis: 150 to 200 mg/kg/day IV divided q 3 to 4 h. Peds: 100 to 400 mg/kg/day IM/IV divided q 4 to 6 h. [Generic only: Caps 250, 500 mg. Susp 125, 250 mg/5 mL.] ▶K ♀B ▷? $$$$$

UNASYN (ampicillin-sulbactam) Adult: 1.5 to 3 g IM/IV q 6 h. Peds: 100 to 400 mg/kg/day of ampicillin divided q 6 h. ▶K ♀B ▷? $$$

Penicillins—4th Generation—Extended Spectrum

PIPERACILLIN-TAZOBACTAM (Zosyn, ✦Tazocin) Adult: 3.375 to 4.5 g IV q 6 h. Peds appendicitis or peritonitis: 80 mg/kg IV q 8 h for age 2 to 9 mo, 100 mg/kg piperacillin IV q 8 h for age older than 9 mo, use adult dose for wt greater than 40 kg. ▶K ♀B ▷? $$$$$

QUINOLONES: GENERAL ANTIMICROBIAL SPECTRUM

1st generation	1st generation quinolones are no longer available
2nd generation	Gram-negative (including *Pseudomonas*); *S. aureus* (but not MRSA or pneumococcus); some atypicals
3rd generation	Gram-negative (including *Pseudomonas*); Gram-positive, including pneumococcus and *S. aureus* (but not MRSA); expanded atypical coverage
4th generation	Same as 3rd generation plus enhanced coverage of pneumococcus, decreased *Pseudomonas* activity

Quinolones—2nd Generation

CIPROFLOXACIN (Cipro, Cipro XR) 200 to 400 mg IV q 8 to 12 h. 250 to 750 mg PO two times per day. Simple UTI: 250 mg PO two times per day for 3 days or Cipro XR 500 mg PO daily for 3 days. Cipro XR for pyelonephritis or complicated UTI: 1000 mg PO daily for 7 to 14 days. Plague: 400 mg IV q 8 to 12 h or 500 to 750 mg PO q 12 h for 14 days. Peds. Complicated UTI, pyelonephritis, 1 to 17 yo: 6 to 10 mg/kg (max 400 mg/dose) IV q 8 h, then 10 to 20 mg/kg (max 750 mg/dose) PO q 12 h. Plague, birth to 17 yo: 10 mg/kg IV q8 to 12h or 15 mg/kg (max 500 mg) PO q 8

(cont.)

to 12 h for 10 to 21 days. Anthrax: See table. [Generic/Trade: Tabs 100, 250, 500, 750 mg. Extended-release tabs 500, 1000 mg. Oral susp 250, 500 mg/5 mL.] ▶LK ♀C but teratogenicity unlikely ▶? + $ ■

OFLOXACIN Adult: 200 to 400 mg PO two times per day. [Generic only: Tabs 200, 300, 400 mg.] ▶LK ♀C ▶? + $$$ ■

Quinolones—3rd Generation

LEVOFLOXACIN (*Levaquin*) IV and PO doses are the same. Usual adult dose: 250 to 750 mg daily. Simple UTI: 250 mg once daily for 3 days. Complicated UTI or pyelonephritis: 250 mg once daily for 10 days or 750 mg once daily for 5 days. Community-acquired pneumonia: 750 mg once daily for 5 days or 500 mg once daily for 7 to 14 days. See table for management of acute sinusitis in adults and children. Plague: 500 mg once daily for 10 to 14 days. Peds. Community-acquired pneumonia: 8 to 10 mg/kg two times per day for age 6 mo to 5 yo; 8 to 10 mg/kg once daily (max 750 mg/day) for age 5 to 16 yo. Plague, age 6 mo and older: Treat for 10 to 14 days with 8 mg/kg (max 250 mg/dose) two times per day if wt less than 50 kg; 500 mg once daily if wt greater than 50 kg. Anthrax: See table. [Generic only: Tabs 250, 500, 750 mg. Oral soln 25 mg/mL.] ▶KL ♀C ▶? $$$ ■

Quinolones—4th Generation

GEMIFLOXACIN (*Factive*) Community-acquired pneumonia, acute exacerbation of chronic bronchitis: 320 mg PO daily for 5 days (bronchitis), or 5 to 7 days (pneumonia). [Trade only: Tabs 320 mg.] ▶Feces, K ♀C ▶− $$$$$ ■

MOXIFLOXACIN (*Avelox*) 400 mg PO/IV daily for 5 days (chronic bronchitis exacerbation), 5 to 14 days (complicated intra-abdominal infection), 7 days (uncomplicated skin infections), 10 days (acute sinusitis), 7 to 14 days (community-acquired pneumonia), 7 to 21 days (complicated skin infections). See tables for management of acute sinusitis and anthrax. [Generic/Trade: Tabs 400 mg.] ▶LK ♀C ▶− $$$$ ■

Sulfonamides

TRIMETHOPRIM-SULFAMETHOXAZOLE (*Bactrim*, *Septra*, *Sulfatrim Pediatric*, *cotrimoxazole*, *TMP-SMX*) Adult usual dose: 1 tab PO two times per day, double-strength (DS, 160 mg/800 mg) or single-strength (SS, 80 mg/400 mg). Peds usual dose: 1 mL/kg/day susp PO divided two times per day (up to 20 mL PO two times per day). Use adult dose for wt greater than 40 kg. TMP-SMX is a poor option for otitis media and sinusitis due to high pneumococcus and *H. influenzae* resistance rates; see otitis media and sinusitis treatment tables for alternatives. Community-acquired MRSA skin infections. Adults: 1 to 2 DS tabs PO two times per day for 7 to 10 days; 2 DS tabs PO two times per day for wt 100 kg or BMI of 40 or greater. Peds: 1 to 1.5 mL/kg/day PO divided two times per day. Pneumocystis pneumonia treatment: 15 to 20 mg/kg/day (based on TMP) IV divided q 6 to 8 h or PO divided three times per day for 21 days total. Pneumocystis pneumonia prophylaxis, adults: 1 DS tab PO daily. Risk of hyperkalemia increased by high doses, renal impairment, and drug interactions. [Generic/Trade: Tabs 80 mg TMP/400 mg SMX (SS), 160 mg TMP/800 mg SMX (DS). Susp 40 mg TMP/200 mg SMX per 5 mL. 20 mL susp = 2 SS tabs = 1 DS tab.] ▶K ♀C ▶+ $

ANTIMICROBIALS

Tetracyclines

NOTE: *Tetracyclines can cause photosensitivity and pseudotumor cerebri (avoid with isotretinoin which is also linked to pseudotumor cerebri). Increased INR with warfarin. May increase risk of ergotism with ergot alkaloids. Avoid in children younger than 8 yo due to risk of teeth-staining.*

DEMECLOCYCLINE Usual dose: 150 mg PO four times per day or 300 mg PO two times per day on empty stomach. SIADH: 600 to 1200 mg/day PO given in 3 to 4 divided doses. [Generic/Trade: Tabs 150, 300 mg.] ▶K, feces ♀D ▶?+ $$$$

DOXYCYCLINE (*Doryx, Monodox, Oracea, Vibramycin, Acticlate, Adoxa, ✦Doxycin*) Usual dose: 100 mg PO two times per day on 1st day, then 50 mg two times per day or 100 mg daily. Severe infections: 100 mg PO/IV two times per day. See table for management of acute sinusitis. Community-acquired MRSA skin infections: 100 mg PO two times per day. Lyme disease: 100 mg PO two times per day for 14 days for early disease, for 28 days for Lyme arthritis. Chlamydia, nongonococcal urethritis: 100 mg PO two times per day for 7 days. See STD table. Doryx for chlamydia urethritis/cervicitis: 200 mg PO once daily for 7 days. Acne: Up to 100 mg PO two times per day. Oracea ($$$$$) for inflammatory rosacea: 40 mg PO once q am on empty stomach. Periodontitis: 20 mg PO two times per day. Malaria prophylaxis: 2 mg/kg/day up to 100 mg PO daily starting 1 to 2 days before exposure until 4 weeks after. [Monohydrate salt. Generic/Trade: Caps ($$) 50, 75, 100, 150 mg. Tabs ($$$) 50, 75, 100, 150 mg. Susp (Vibramycin) 25 mg/5 mL. Trade only: Delayed-release caps 40 mg (Oracea $$$$$). Generic: Delayed-release caps 40 mg ($$$$$). Hyclate salt. Tabs: Trade only: 75, 150 mg (Acticlate-$$$$$). Generic: 20 mg. Generic only: 100 mg. Caps: Generic only: 50 mg. Generic/Trade: 100 mg. Delayed-release tabs: Generic only: 75, 100 mg. Generic/Trade: 150 mg. Trade only: 200 mg (Doryx $$$$$). Delayed-release caps: Generic only: 75, 100 mg. Calcium salt. Trade only: Syrup (Vibramycin Calcium) 50 mg/5 mL. Monohydrate formulations may have better GI tolerability than hyclate formulations.] ▶LK ♀D ▶?+ varies by therapy

MINOCYCLINE (*Minocin, Solodyn*) Usual dose: 200 mg IV/PO initially, then 100 mg q 12 h. Community-acquired MRSA skin infections: 200 mg PO 1st dose, then 100 mg PO two times per day for 5 to 10 days. Acne (traditional dosing): 50 mg PO two times per day. Solodyn ($$$$$) for inflammatory acne in adults and children 12 yo and older: 1 mg/kg PO once daily. [Generic/Trade: Caps, Tabs ($) 50, 75, 100 mg. Extended-release tabs ($$$$$) 45, 90, 135 mg. Trade only: Extended-release tabs (Solodyn-$$$$$) 55 , 65, 80, 105, 115 mg.] ▶LK ♀D ▶?+ $$

Other Antimicrobials

AZTREONAM (*Azactam, Cayston*) Gram-negative infections: Adults: 0.5 to 2 g IM/IV q 6 to 12 h. Peds: 30 mg/kg IV q 6 to 8 h. Cystic fibrosis respiratory symptoms, age 7 yo and older: 1 vial Cayston nebulized three times per day for 28 days, followed by cycle of 28 days off treatment. [Trade only (Cayston): 75 mg/vial with diluent for inhalation.] ▶K ♀B ▶+ $$$$$

CHLORAMPHENICOL Usual dose, adult and peds: 50 to 100 mg/kg/day IV divided q 6 h. Aplastic anemia. ▶LK ♀C ▶– $$$$$ ■

CLINDAMYCIN (*Cleocin*, *♦Dalacin C*) Usual adult dose: 150 to 450 mg PO four times per day. 600 to 900 mg IV q 8 h. Community-acquired MRSA skin infections: 300 to 450 mg PO three times per day for 5 to 10 days for adults; 10 to 13 mg/kg/dose PO q 6 to 8 h (max 40 mg/kg/day) for peds. Peds usual dose: 20 to 40 mg/kg/day IV divided q 6 to 8 h or give 8 to 25 mg/kg/day susp PO divided q 6 to 8 h. See tables for management of anthrax, and acute sinusitis and otitis media in children. [Generic/Trade: Caps 75, 150, 300 mg. Oral soln 75 mg/5 mL (100 mL).] ▶L ♀B ▶?+ $ ■

DAPTOMYCIN (*Cubicin*) Complicated skin infections (including MRSA): 4 mg/kg IV daily for 7 to 14 days. *S. aureus* bacteremia (including MRSA): 6 mg/kg IV daily for at least 2 to 6 weeks. Infuse over 30 min. Not for pneumonia (inactivated by surfactant). Not approved in children. ▶K ♀B ▶? $$$$$

FOSFOMYCIN (*Monurol*) Simple UTI: One 3 g packet PO single dose. [Trade only: 3 g packet of granules.] ▶K ♀B ▶? $$$

LINEZOLID (*Zyvox*, *♦Zyvoxam*) Pneumonia, complicated skin infections (including MRSA), vancomycin-resistant *E. faecium* infections: 10 mg/kg (up to 600 mg) IV/PO q 8 h for age younger than 12 yo, 600 mg IV/PO q 12 h for adults and age 12 yo or older. Anthrax: See table. Myelosuppression, drug interactions due to MAO inhibition. Limit tyramine foods to less than 100 mg/meal. [Generic/Trade: Tabs 600 mg. Susp 100 mg/5 mL.] ▶Oxidation/K ♀C ▶? $$$$$

METRONIDAZOLE (*Flagyl, Flagyl ER*, *♦Nidazol*) Bacterial vaginosis: 500 mg PO two times per day or Flagyl ER 750 mg PO daily for 7 days. Trichomoniasis: 2 g PO single dose for patient and sex partners (may be used in pregnancy per CDC). See STD table. *H. pylori*: See table in GI section. Anaerobic bacterial infections: Load 1 g or 15 mg/kg IV, then 500 mg or 7.5 mg/kg (up to 4 g/day) IV/PO q 6 to 8 h, each IV dose over 1 h. Peds: 7.5 mg/kg IV q 6 h. *C. difficile*–associated diarrhea: Adults: 500 mg PO three times per day for 10 to 14 days. Peds: 30 mg/kg/day PO divided four times per day for 10 to 14 days. See table for management of *C. difficile* infection in adults. Giardia: 250 mg (5 mg/kg/dose for peds) PO three times per day for 5 to 7 days. [Generic/Trade: Tabs 250, 500 mg. Trade only: Caps 375 mg. Extended-release tab: 750 mg.] ▶KL ♀B ▶?- $

NITROFURANTOIN (*Furadantin, Macrodantin, Macrobid*) Uncomplicated UTI: 50 to 100 mg PO four times per day for 7 days. Peds: 5 to 7 mg/kg/day divided four times per day. Macrobid for uncomplicated UTI: 100 mg PO two times per day for 7 days. Take nitrofurantoin with food. [Generic/Trade: Caps (Macrodantin) 25, 50, 100 mg. Caps (Macrobid) 100 mg. Susp (Furadantin) 25 mg/5 mL.] ▶KL ♀B ▶+ $$

RIFAXIMIN (*Xifaxan*) Traveler's diarrhea: 200 mg PO three times per day for 3 days. Prevention of recurrent hepatic encephalopathy ($$$$$): 550 mg PO two times per day. Irritable bowel syndrome with diarrhea: 550 mg PO three times per day for 14 days. Can retreat up to 2 times if recurrence. [Trade only: Tabs 200, 550 mg.] ▶Feces ♀C ▶? $$$$

SYNERCID (quinupristin + dalfopristin) Complicated streptococcal/staphylococcal skin infection: 7.5 mg/kg IV q 12 h, each dose over 1 h. MRSA bacteremia (2nd line): 7.5 mg/kg IV q 8 h. Not active against *E. faecalis*. ▶Bile ♀B ▶? $$$$$

TEDIZOLID (*Sivextro*) Skin infections, including MRSA: 200 mg IV/PO once daily for 6 days. Infuse IV over 1 hour. [Trade only: Tabs 200 mg.] ▶L ♀C ▶? $$$$$

TELITHROMYCIN (*Ketek*) Community-acquired pneumonia: 800 mg PO daily for 7 to 10 days. No longer indicated for acute sinusitis or acute exacerbation of chronic bronchitis (risks exceed potential benefit). Contraindicated in myasthenia gravis. [Trade only: Tabs 300, 400 mg.] ▶LK ♀C ▶? $$$$ ■

TIGECYCLINE (*Tygacil*) Complicated skin infections, complicated intra-abdominal infections, community-acquired pneumonia: 100 mg IV 1st dose, then 50 mg IV q 12 h. Infuse over 30 to 60 min. Mortality higher with tigecycline than comparators; do not use unless there are no alternatives. Not indicated for hospital-acquired or ventilator-associated pneumonia or diabetic foot infection. ▶Bile, K ♀D ▶?+ $$$$$ ■

TRIMETHOPRIM (*Primsol*, *✦Proloprim*) 100 mg PO two times per day or 200 mg PO daily. Risk of hyperkalemia increased by high doses, renal impairment, and drug interactions. [Generic only: Tabs 100 mg. Trade only (Primsol): Oral soln 50 mg/5 mL.] ▶K ♀C ▶– $

CARDIOVASCULAR

ACE INHIBITOR DOSING

ACE INHIBITOR DOSING	HTN		Heart Failure	
	Initial	Max/day	Initial	Max/day
benazepril (Lotensin)	10 mg daily*	80 mg	—	—
captopril (Capoten)	25 mg bid/tid	450 mg	6.25 mg tid	450 mg
enalapril (Vasotec)	5 mg daily*	40 mg	2.5 mg bid	40 mg
fosinopril (Monopril)	10 mg daily*	80 mg	5-10 mg daily	40 mg
lisinopril (Zestril/ Prinivil)	10 mg daily	80 mg	2.5-5 mg daily	40 mg
moexipril (Univasc)	7.5 mg daily*	30 mg	—	—
perindopril (Aceon)	4 mg daily*	16 mg	2 mg daily	16 mg
quinapril (Accupril)	10-20 mg daily*	80 mg	5 mg bid	40 mg
ramipril (Altace)	2.5 mg daily*	20 mg	1.25-2.5 mg bid	10 mg
trandolapril (Mavik)	1-2 mg daily*	8 mg	1 mg daily	4 mg

bid=two times per day; tid=three times per day.

Data taken from prescribing information and *Circulation* 2013;128:e240-e327.

* May require bid dosing for 24-h BP control.

CARDIAC PARAMETERS AND FORMULAS

Cardiac output (CO) = heart rate × CVA volume [normal 4 to 8 L/min]

Cardiac index (CI) = CO/BSA [normal 2.8 to 4.2 L/min/m^2]

MAP (mean arterial pressure) = [(SBP – DBP)/3] + DBP [normal 80 to 100 mmHg]

SVR (systemic vascular resistance) = (MAP – CVP) × (80)/CO [normal 800 to 1200 dyne x sec/cm^5]

PVR (pulmonary vasc resisistance) = (PAM – PCWP) × (80)/CO [normal 45 to 120 dyne x sec/cm^5]

QTc = QT/square root of RR [normal 0.38 to 0.42]

Right atrial pressure (central venous pressure) [normal 0 to 8 mmHg]

Pulmonary artery systolic pressure (PAS) [normal 20 to 30 mmHg]

Pulmonary artery diastolic pressure (PAD) [normal 10 to 15 mmHg]

Pulmonary capillary wedge pressure (PCWP) [normal 8 to 12 mmHg (post-MI ~16 mmHg)]

LIPID CHANGE BY CLASS/AGENT[1]

Drug class/agent	LDL-C	HDL-C	TG
Atorvastatin + ezetimibe[2]	↓ 53–61%	↑ 5–9%	↓ 30–40%
Bile acid sequestrants[3]	↓ 15–30%	↑ 3–5%	No change or ↑
Cholesterol absorption inhibitor[4]	↓ 18%	↑ 1%	↓ 8%
Fibrates[5]	↓ 5–20%	↑ 10–20%	↓ 20–50%
Lovastatin + ext'd release niacin[6]*	↓ 30–42%	↑ 20–30%	↓ 32–44%
Niacin[7]*	↓ 5–25%	↑ 15–35%	↓ 20–50%
Omega3 fatty acids[8]	↓ 5% or ↑ 44%	↓ 4% or ↑ 9%	↓ 27–45%
Statins[9]	↓ 18–63%	↑ 5–15%	↓ 7–35%
Simvastatin + ezetimibe[10]	↓ 45–59%	↑ 6–10%	↓ 23–31%

LDL-C= low density lipoprotein cholesterol. HDL-C = high density lipoprotein cholesterol. TG = triglycerides.

[1] Adapted from prescribing information.

[2] Liptruzet® (10/10–10/80 mg).

[3] Cholestyramine (4–16 g), colestipol (5–20 g), colesevelam (2.6–3.8 g).

[4] Ezetimibe (10 mg). When added to statin therapy, will ↓ LDL-C 25%, ↑ HDL-C 3%, ↓ TG 14% in addition to statin effects.

[5] Fenofibrate (145–200 mg), gemfibrozil (600 mg two times per day).

[6] Advicor® (20/1000–40/2000 mg).

[7] Extended release nicotinic acid (Niaspan® 1–2 g), immediate release (crystalline) nicotinic acid (1.5–3g), sustained release nicotinic acid (Slo-Niacin® 1–2 g).

[8] Epanova® (4 g), Lovaza® (4 g), Vascepa® (4 g)

[9] Atorvastatin (10–80 mg), fluvastatin (20–80 mg), lovastatin (20–80 mg), pravastatin (20–80 mg), rosuvastatin (5–40 mg), simvastatin (20–40 mg).

[10] Vytorin® (10/10–10/40 mg).

*Lowers lipoprotein a.

CHOLESTEROL TREATMENT RECOMMENDATIONS (AGES ≥21 YEARS)

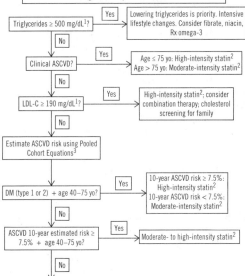

Lifestyle changes should be initiated in all patients; reinforce lifestyle changes at each patient encounter.

Triglycerides ≥ 500 mg/dL[1]? — **Yes** → Lowering triglycerides is priority. Intensive lifestyle changes. Consider fibrate, niacin, Rx omega-3

No ↓

Clinical ASCVD? — **Yes** → Age ≤ 75 yo: High-intensity statin[2]
Age > 75 yo: Moderate-intensity statin[2]

No ↓

LDL-C ≥ 190 mg/dL[1]? — **Yes** → High-intensity statin[2]; consider combination therapy; cholesterol screening for family

No ↓

Estimate ASCVD risk using Pooled Cohort Equations[3]

DM (type 1 or 2) + age 40–75 yo? — **Yes** → 10-year ASCVD risk ≥ 7.5%: High-intensity statin[2]
10-year ASCVD risk < 7.5%: Moderate-intensity statin[2]

No ↓

ASCVD 10-year estimated risk ≥ 7.5% + age 40–75 yo? — **Yes** → Moderate- to high-intensity statin[2]

No ↓

Benefit of statin therapy is less clear.

Recalculate 10-year ASCVD risk every 4–6 years for patients aged 40–75 yo without clinical ASCVD or DM + LDL-C 70-189 mg/dL + not receiving statin therapy.

Assess risk factors + 30-year or lifetime ASCVD risk in those 20-59 yo with low 10-year ASCVD risk.

Consider benefits, risks, drug–drug interactions, adverse effects, and patient preferences before initiating statin therapy.

[1] Rule out secondary causes. If non-fasting triglycerides ≥ 500 mg/dL, then a fasting lipid panel is needed.

(cont.)

CARDIOVASCULAR

CHOLESTEROL TREATMENT RECOMMENDATIONS (AGES ≥ 21 YEARS) (*continued*)

[2]High-intensity statin = atorvastatin 40, 80 mg; rosuvastatin 20, 40 mg. Moderate-intensity statin is acceptable if patient is not a candidate for high-intensity statin therapy. Moderate-intensity statin = atorvastatin 10, 20 mg; fluvastatin 40 mg twice daily, fluvastatin XL 80 mg; lovastatin 40 mg; pitavastatin 2, 4 mg; pravastatin 40, 80 mg; rosuvastatin 5, 10 mg; simvastatin 20, 40 mg.

[3]Calculator available: http://tools.cardiosource.org/ASCVD-Risk-Estimator/

ASCVD = atherosclerotic cardiovascular disease (includes coronary heart disease, stroke, and peripheral artery disease.) DM = Diabetes mellitus. LCL-C = low-density lipoprotein cholesterol. Rx = prescription strength.

Adapted from: *J Am Coll Cardiol*. 2014; 63(25_PA), *Circulation*. 2011; 123: 2292–2333.

HTN THERAPY FOR ADULTS ≥ 18 YEARS OLD

Patient Information		BP target (mm Hg)	Preferred therapy	Comments
All patients with CKD (with or without DM)	Any age	< 140/90	Start ACEI or ARB; alone or in combination with drug from another class[1]	Implement lifestyle interventions; reinforce adherence during patient encounters. Drug treatment strategy based on response and tolerance: Either, titrate first drug to max dose before adding second; add second drug before reaching max dose of first drug; or start with 2 drug classes separately or as fixed dose combinations.[2,3]
Nonblack (no CKD)	Any age + DM	< 140/90	Start ACEI, ARB, CCB, or thiazide; alone or combination[1]	
	Age < 60 yo (no DM or CKD)	< 140/90		
	Age ≥ 60 yo (no DM or CKD)	< 150/90		
Black (no CKD)	Any age + DM	< 140/90	Start CCB or thiazide; alone or combination[1]	
	Age < 60 yo (no DM or CKD)	< 140/90		
	Age ≥ 60 yo (no DM or CKD)	< 150/90		

(cont.)

HTN THERAPY FOR ADULTS ≥ 18 YEARS OLD (continued)

[1] Do not combine ACEI and ARB therapy.

[2] Consider starting with 2 drugs when SBP is > 160 mmHg and/or DBP is > 100 mm Hg, or if SBP is > 20 mm Hg above goal and/or DBP is > 10 mm Hg above goal. If goal BP is not achieved with 2 drugs, select a third drug from the list. Titrate prn.

[3] If needed, may add another drug (eg, beta-blocker, aldosterone antagonist, others) and/or refer to physician with HTN management expertise.

ACEI = angiotensin converting enzyme inhibitor; ARB = angiotensin-receptor blocker;

CCB = calcium-channel blocker; CKD = chronic kidney disease.

SELECTED DRUGS THAT MAY PROLONG THE QT INTERVAL

alfuzosin	dronedarone*	isradipine	promethazine
amiodarone*	droperidol*	lapatinib	quetiapine
anagrelide*	eribulin	leuprolide	quinidine*
arsenic trioxide*	erythromycin*	levofloxacin*	ranolazine
atazanavir	escitalopram*	lithium	risperidone
azithromycin*	famotidine	methadone*	saquinavir
bedaquiline	felbamate	mirabegron	sevoflurane*
chloroquine*	fingolimod	mirtazapine	sotalol*
chlorpromazine*	flecainide*	moexipril/HCTZ	sunitinib
cisapride*	fluconazole	moxifloxacin*	tacrolimus
citalopram*	foscarnet	nicardipine	tamoxifen
clarithromycin*	fosphenytoin	nilotinib	telithromycin
clozapine	gatifloxacin	ofloxacin	thioridazine*
cocaine*	gemifloxacin	olanzapine	tizanidine
dexmedetomidine*	granisetron	ondansetron*	tolterodine
disopyramide*	halofantrine*	oxytocin	vandetanib
dofetilide*	haloperidol*	paliperidone	vardenafil
dolasetron	ibutilide*	pentamidine*	venlafaxine
	iloperidone	perflutren lipid microspheres	ziprasidone
		pimozide*	
		procainamide*	

NOTE: This table may not include all drugs that prolong the QT interval or cause torsades. Risk of drug-induced QT prolongation may be increased in women, elderly, hypokalemia, hypomagnesemia, bradycardia, starvation, CHF, and CNS injuries. Hepatorenal dysfunction and drug interactions can increase the concentration of QT interval-prolonging drugs. Coadministration of QT interval prolonging drugs can have additive effects. Avoid these (and other) drugs in congenital prolonged QT syndrome (www.crediblemeds.org).

*Torsades reported in product labeling/case reports.

HIGH- AND MODERATE-INTENSITY STATIN DOSES

Statin	High-intensity dose (lowers LDL-C at least 50%)	Moderate-intensity dose (lowers LDL-C 30% to 50%)
atorvastatin	40, 80 mg	10, 20 mg
fluvastatin XL	n/a	80 mg
fluvastatin	n/a	40 mg twice daily
lovastatin	n/a	40 mg
pitavastatin	n/a	2, 4 mg
pravastatin	n/a	40, 80 mg
rosuvastatin	20, 40 mg	5, 10 mg
simvastatin	n/a	20, 40 mg

LDL-C=low density lipoprotein cholesterol. Will see ~6% decrease in LDL-C with every doubling of dose.

Adapted from J Am Coll Cardiol. 2014; 63(25_PA).

THROMBOLYTIC THERAPY FOR ST-SEGMENT ELEVATION MI (STEMI)

Indications (if high-volume cath lab unavailable)	Clinical history and presentation strongly suggestive of MI within 12 h plus at least 1 of the following: 1 mm ST elevation in at least 2 contiguous leads; new left BBB; or 2 mm ST depression in V1-4 suggestive of true posterior MI.
Absolute contraindications	Previous intracranial hemorrhage; known cerebral vascular lesion (arteriovenous malformation); known malignant intracranial neoplasm; recent (<3 months) ischemic CVA (except acute ischemic CVA <4.5 h); aortic dissection; active bleeding or bleeding diathesis (excluding menses); significant closed head or facial trauma (<3 months); intracranial or intraspinal surgery (<2 months); severe uncontrolled HTN (unresponsive to emergency therapy); for streptokinase: prior exposure (<6 months).
Relative contraindications	Severe uncontrolled HTN (>180/110 mm Hg) on presentation or chronic severe HTN; prior ischemic CVA (>3 months), dementia, other intracranial pathology; traumatic/prolonged (>10 min) cardiopulmonary resuscitation; major surgery (<3 weeks); recent (within 2–4 weeks) internal bleeding; puncture of noncompressible vessel; pregnancy; active peptic ulcer disease; current use of anticoagulants.

Reference: *Circulation* 2013;127:e362-425

ACE Inhibitors

NOTE: *See also Antihypertensive Combinations. Contraindicated in pregnancy or with history of angioedema. Do not use with aliskiren in patients with DM or CrCl < 60 mL/min. Avoid combined use with renin-angiotensin system inhibitors (i.e. angiotensin receptor blockers, aliskiren); increases risk of renal impairment, hypotension, and hyperkalemia. Hyperkalemia possible, especially if used with other drugs that increase K⁺ (heparin, K⁺ sparing diuretics, K⁺ supplements, salt substitutes containing K⁺) and in patients with heart failure, DM, or renal impairment. Concomitant NSAID, including selective COX-2 inhibitors, may further deteriorate renal function and decrease antihypertensive effects.*

BENAZEPRIL (*Lotensin*) HTN: Start 10 mg PO daily, usual maintenance dose 20 to 40 mg PO daily or divided two times per day, max 80 mg/day. [Generic/Trade: Tabs, unscored 5, 10, 20, 40 mg.] ▶LK ♀D ▶? $$ ■

CAPTOPRIL (*Capoten*) HTN: Start 25 mg PO two to three times per day, usual maintenance dose 25 to 150 mg two to three times per day, max 450 mg/day. Heart failure: Start 6.25 to 12.5 mg PO three times per day, usual dose 50 to 100 mg PO three times per day, max 450 mg/day. Diabetic nephropathy: 25 mg PO three times per day. [Generic only: Tabs, scored 12.5, 25, 50, 100 mg.] ▶LK ♀D ▶+ $$$ ■

CILAZAPRIL (✦*Inhibace*) Canada only. HTN: 1.25 to 10 mg PO daily. [Generic/Trade: Not available in US. Tabs, scored 1, 2.5, 5 mg.] ▶LK ♀D ▶? $ ■

ENALAPRIL (**enalaprilat**, *Vasotec, Epaned*) HTN: Start 5 mg PO daily, usual maintenance dose 10 to 40 mg PO daily or divided two times per day, max 40 mg/day. If oral therapy not possible, can use enalaprilat 1.25 mg IV q 6 h over 5 min, and increase up to 5 mg IV q 6 h if needed. Renal impairment or concomitant diuretic therapy: Start 2.5 mg PO daily. Heart failure: Start 2.5 mg PO two times per day, usual dose 10 to 20 mg PO two times per day, max 40 mg/day. [Generic/Trade: Tabs, scored 2.5, 5 mg, unscored 10, 20 mg. Trade only: Oral Soln 1 mg/mL (Epaned-$$$$$).] ▶LK ♀D ▶+ $$ ■

FOSINOPRIL HTN: Start 10 mg PO daily, usual maintenance dose 20 to 40 mg PO daily or divided two times per day, max 80 mg/day. Heart failure: Start 5 to 10 mg PO daily, usual dose 20 to 40 mg PO daily, max 40 mg/day. [Generic only: Tabs, scored 10 mg, unscored 20, 40 mg.] ▶LK ♀D ▶? $$ ■

LISINOPRIL (*Prinivil, Zestril*) HTN: Start 10 mg PO daily, usual maintenance dose 20 to 40 mg PO daily, max 80 mg/day. Heart failure, acute MI: Start 2.5 to 5 mg PO daily, usual dose 5 to 20 mg PO daily, max dose 40 mg. [Generic/Trade: Tabs, unscored (Zestril) 2.5, 5, 10, 20, 30, 40 mg. Tabs, scored (Prinivil) 10, 20, 40 mg.] ▶K ♀D ▶? $ ■

MOEXIPRIL (*Univasc*) HTN: Start 7.5 mg PO daily, usual maintenance dose 7.5 to 30 mg PO daily or divided two times per day, max 30 mg/day. [Generic: Tabs scored 7.5, 15 mg.] ▶LK ♀D ▶? $$ ■

PERINDOPRIL (*Aceon*, ✦*Coversyl*) HTN: Start 4 mg PO daily, usual maintenance dose 4 to 8 mg PO daily or divided two times per day, max 16 mg/day. Reduction

(cont.)

CARDIOVASCULAR

of cardiovascular events in stable CAD: Start 4 mg PO daily for 2 weeks, max 8 mg/day. Elderly (age older than 65 yo): 4 mg PO daily, max 8 mg/day. [Generic/Trade: Tabs scored 2, 4, 8 mg.] ▶K ♀D ▶? $$$ ■

QUINAPRIL (*Accupril*) HTN: Start 10 to 20 mg PO daily (start 10 mg/day if elderly), usual maintenance dose 20 to 80 mg PO daily or divided two times per day, max 80 mg/day. Heart failure: Start 5 mg PO two times per day, usual maintenance dose 10 to 20 mg two times per day. [Generic/Trade: Tabs scored 5, unscored 10, 20, 40 mg.] ▶LK ♀D ▶? $$ ■

RAMIPRIL (*Altace*) HTN: 2.5 mg PO daily, usual maintenance dose 2.5 to 20 mg PO daily or divided two times per day, max 20 mg/day. Heart failure post-MI: Start 2.5 mg PO two times per day, usual maintenance dose 5 mg PO two times per day. Reduce risk of MI, CVA, death from cardiovascular causes: 2.5 mg PO daily for 1 week, then 5 mg daily for 3 weeks, increase as tolerated to max 10 mg/day. [Generic/Trade: Caps 1.25, 2.5, 5, 10 mg.] ▶LK ♀D ▶? $ ■

TRANDOLAPRIL (*Mavik*) HTN: Start 1 mg PO daily, usual maintenance dose 2 to 4 mg PO daily or divided two times per day, max 8 mg/day. Heart failure/post-MI: Start 1 mg PO daily, usual maintenance dose 4 mg PO daily. Renal impairment or concomitant diuretic therapy: Start 0.5 mg PO daily. [Generic/Trade: Tabs, scored 1 mg, unscored 2, 4 mg.] ▶LK ♀D ▶? $ ■

Aldosterone Antagonists

NOTE: *Hyperkalemia possible, especially if used concomitantly with other drugs that increase K+ (including K+ containing salt substitutes) and in patients with heart failure, DM, or renal impairment.*

EPLERENONE (*Inspra*) HTN: Start 50 mg PO daily; max 50 mg two times per day. Improve survival of stable patients with LV systolic dysfunction (LVEF 40% or less) and heart failure post MI: Start 25 mg PO daily; titrate to target dose 50 mg daily within 4 weeks, if tolerated. [Generic/trade: Tabs, unscored 25, 50 mg.] ▶L ♀B ▶? $$$$

SPIRONOLACTONE (*Aldactone*) HTN: 50 to 100 mg PO daily or divided two times per day (usual dose 25 to 50 mg daily according to ASH-ISH guidelines). Edema: 25 to 200 mg/day. Hypokalemia: 25 to 100 mg PO daily. Primary hyperaldosteronism, maintenance: 100 to 400 mg/day PO. Heart failure, NYHA III or IV: 25 to 50 mg PO daily. [Generic/Trade: Tabs, unscored 25 mg, scored 50, 100 mg.] ▶LK ♀D ▶+ $ ■

Angiotensin Receptor Blockers (ARBs)

NOTE: *See also Antihypertensive Combinations. Contraindicated in pregnancy. Avoid use with aliskiren in patients with DM or CrCl < 60 mL/min. Avoid combined use with renin-angiotensin system inhibitors (i.e. ACE inhibitors, aliskiren); increases risk of renal impairment, hypotension, and hyperkalemia. Hyperkalemia possible, especially if used with other drugs that increase K+ (heparin, K+ sparing diuretics, K+ supplements, salt substitutes containing K+) and in patients with heart failure, DM, or renal impairment. Concomitant*

(cont.)

NSAID, including selective COX-2 inhibitors, may further deteriorate renal function and decrease antihypertensive effects. May increase lithium levels.

AZILSARTAN (*Edarbi*) HTN: 80 mg daily. [Trade only: Tabs, unscored 40, 80 mg.] ▶L – ♀D ▶? $$$$ ■

CANDESARTAN (*Atacand*) HTN: Start 16 mg PO daily, max 32 mg/day. Heart failure (NYHA II–IV and LVEF 40% or less): Start 4 mg PO daily, max 32 mg/day. [Generic/Trade: Tabs 4, 8, 16, 32 mg.] ▶K ♀D ▶? $$$ ■

EPROSARTAN (*Teveten*) HTN: Start 600 mg PO daily, max 900 mg/day given daily or divided two times per day. [Generic/Trade: Tabs, unscored 600 mg.] ▶Fecal excretion ♀D ▶? $$$$ ■

IRBESARTAN (*Avapro*) HTN: Start 150 mg PO daily, max 300 mg/day. Type 2 diabetic nephropathy: Start 150 mg PO daily, target dose 300 mg daily. [Generic/Trade: Tabs, unscored 75, 150, 300 mg.] ▶L ♀D ▶? $ ■

LOSARTAN (*Cozaar*) HTN: Start 50 mg PO daily, max 100 mg/day given daily or divided two times per day. Volume-depleted patients or history of hepatic impairment: Start 25 mg PO daily. CVA risk reduction in patients with HTN and LV hypertrophy (may not be effective in black patients): Start 50 mg PO daily. If need more BP reduction add HCTZ 12.5 mg PO daily, then increase losartan to 100 mg/day, then increase HCTZ to 25 mg/day. Type 2 diabetic nephropathy: Start 50 mg PO daily, target dose 100 mg daily. [Generic/Trade: Tabs, unscored 25, 50, 100 mg.] ▶L ♀D ▶? $ ■

OLMESARTAN (*Benicar*, ✦*Olmetec*) HTN: Start 20 mg PO daily, max 40 mg/day. [Trade only: Tabs, unscored 5, 20, 40 mg.] ▶K ♀D ▶? $$$$ ■

TELMISARTAN (*Micardis*) HTN: Start 40 mg PO daily, max 80 mg/day. Cardiovascular risk reduction: Start 80 mg PO daily, max 80 mg/day. [Generic/Trade: Tabs, unscored 20, 40, 80 mg.] ▶L ♀D ▶? $$$$ ■

VALSARTAN (*Diovan*) HTN: Start 80 to 160 mg PO daily, max 320 mg/day. Heart failure: Start 40 mg PO two times per day, target dose 160 mg two times per day. Reduce mortality/morbidity post-MI with LV systolic dysfunction/failure: Start 20 mg PO two times per day, target dose 160 mg two times per day. [Generic/Trade: Tabs, scored 40 mg, unscored 80, 160, 320 mg.] ▶L ♀D ▶? $$$$ ■

Antiadrenergic Agents

CLONIDINE (*Catapres, Catapres-TTS, Kapvay, ✦Dixarit*) HTN, immediate-release: Start 0.1 mg PO two times per day, usual maintenance dose 0.2 to 0.6 mg/day in 2 to 3 divided doses, max 2.4 mg daily. Rebound HTN with abrupt discontinuation, taper dose slowly. HTN, transdermal (Catapres-TTS): Start 0.1 mg/24 h patch once a week, titrate to desired effect, max effective dose 0.6 mg/24 h (two 0.3 mg/24 h patches). Transdermal Therapeutic System (TTS) is designed for 7-day use so that a TTS-1 delivers 0.1 mg/day for 7 days. May supplement 1st dose of TTS with oral for 2 to 3 days while therapeutic level is achieved. ADHD (6 to 17 yo), extended-release (Kapvay): Start 0.1 mg PO at bedtime; may increase by 0.1 mg/day each week; give two times per day with equal or higher dose at bedtime, max 0.4 mg daily. ADHD, immediate-release (unapproved peds): Start 0.05 mg PO at

(cont.)

bedtime, titrate based on response over 8 weeks to max 0.2 mg/day (for wt less than 45 kg) or to max 0.4 mg/day (for wt 45 kg or greater) in 2 to 4 divided doses. Tourette syndrome (unapproved peds and adult): 3 to 5 mcg/kg/day PO divided two to four times per day. Opioid withdrawal, adjunct: 0.1 to 0.3 mg PO three to four times per day or 0.1 to 0.2 mg PO q 4 h for 3 days tapering off over 4 to 10 days. Alcohol withdrawal, adjunct: 0.1 to 0.2 mg PO q 4 h prn. Smoking cessation: Start 0.1 mg PO two times per day, increase 0.1 mg/day at weekly intervals to 0.75 mg/day as tolerated; transdermal (Catapres TTS): 0.1 to 0.2 mg/24 h patch once a week for 2 to 3 weeks after cessation. Menopausal flushing: 0.1 to 0.4 mg/day PO divided two to three times per day. Transdermal system applied weekly: 0.1 mg/day. May cause dizziness, drowsiness, or lightheadedness. Monitor for bradycardia when taking concomitant digitalis, nondihydropyridine calcium channel blockers, or beta-blockers. [Generic/Trade: Tabs, immediate-release, unscored (Catapres) 0.1, 0.2, 0.3 mg. Transdermal weekly patch ($$$$$) 0.1 mg/day (TTS-1), 0.2 mg/day (TTS-2), 0.3 mg/day (TTS-3). Tabs, extended-release, unscored ($$$$$) 0.1 mg. Trade only: Tabs, extended-release, unscored (Kapvay-$$$$$) 0.2 mg.] ▶LK ♀C ▶? $

DOXAZOSIN (*Cardura, Cardura XL*) BPH, immediate-release: Start 1 mg PO at bedtime, max 8 mg/day. BPH, extended-release (not approved for HTN): 4 mg PO q am with breakfast, max 8 mg/day. HTN, immediate-release: Start 1 mg PO at bedtime, max 16 mg/day. Take 1st dose at bedtime to minimize orthostatic hypotension. [Generic/Trade: Tabs, scored 1, 2, 4, 8 mg. Trade only (Cardura XL): Tabs, extended-release, 4, 8 mg.] ▶L ♀C ▶? $$ ■

GUANFACINE (*Tenex, ✦Intuniv XR*) HTN: Start 1 mg PO at bedtime, max 3 mg/day. [Generic/Trade: Tabs, unscored 1, 2 mg.] ▶K ♀B ▶? $

METHYLDOPA HTN: Start 250 mg PO 2 to 3 times daily, max 3000 mg/day. May be used to manage BP during pregnancy. [Generic only: Tabs, unscored 250, 500 mg.] ▶LK ♀B ▶+ $

PRAZOSIN (*Minipress*) HTN: Start 1 mg PO two to three times per day, max 40 mg/day. Take 1st dose at bedtime to minimize orthostatic hypotension. [Generic/Trade: Caps 1, 2, 5 mg.] ▶L ♀C ▶? $$ ■

RESERPINE HTN: Start 0.05 to 0.1 mg PO daily or 0.1 mg PO every other day, max dose 0.25 mg/day. [Generic only: Tabs, scored 0.1, 0.25 mg.] ▶LK ♀C ▶— $$

TERAZOSIN HTN: Start 1 mg PO at bedtime, usual effective dose 1 to 5 mg PO daily or divided two times per day, max 20 mg/day. Take 1st dose at bedtime to minimize orthostatic hypotension. BPH: Start 1 mg PO at bedtime, usual effective dose 10 mg/day, max 20 mg/day. [Generic only: Caps 1, 2, 5, 10 mg.] ▶LK ♀C ▶? $$ ■

Antidysrhythmics/Cardiac Arrest

ADENOSINE (*Adenocard*) PSVT conversion (not A-fib): Adult and peds wt 50 kg or greater: 6 mg rapid IV and flush, preferably through a central line. If no response after 1 to 2 min, then 12 mg. A 3rd dose of 12 mg may be given prn. Peds wt less than 50 kg: Initial dose 50 to 100 mcg/kg, subsequent doses 100 to 200 mcg/kg q 1 to 2 min prn up to a max single dose of 300 mcg/kg or 12 mg, whichever is less. Half-life is less than 10 sec. Give doses by rapid IV push followed by NS flush.

(cont.)

Need higher dose if on theophylline or caffeine, lower dose if on dipyridamole or carbamazepine ▶plasma ♀C▶? $

AMIODARONE (*Pacerone, Cordarone*) Proarrhythmic. Life-threatening ventricular arrhythmia without cardiac arrest: Load 150 mg IV over 10 min, then 1 mg/min for 6 h, then 0.5 mg/min for 18 h. Mix in D5W. Oral loading dose 800 to 1600 mg PO daily for 1 to 3 weeks, reduce to 400 to 800 mg PO daily for 1 month when arrhythmia is controlled, reduce to lowest effective dose thereafter, usually 200 to 400 mg PO daily. Photosensitivity with oral therapy. Pulmonary and hepatic toxicity. Hypo- or hyperthyroidism possible. Coadministration of fluoroquinolones, macrolides, loratadine, trazodone, azoles, or Class IA and antiarrhythmic drugs may prolong QTc. May increase digoxin levels; discontinue digoxin or decrease dose by 50%. May increase INR with warfarin; decrease warfarin dose by 33 to 50%. Do not use with grapefruit juice. Do not use with simvastatin dose greater than 20 mg/day, lovastatin dose greater than 40 mg/day; may increase atorvastatin level; increases risk of myopathy and rhabdomyolysis. Caution with beta-blockers and calcium channel blockers. IV therapy may cause hypotension. Contraindicated in cardiogenic shock and in profound/symptomatic bradycardia (whether from AV block or sinus-node dysfunction) in the absence of a functioning pacemaker. [Trade only (Pacerone): Tabs, unscored 100 mg. Generic/Trade: Tabs, scored 200, 400 mg.] ▶L ♀D▶– $$$$ ■

ATROPINE (*AtroPen*) Bradyarrhythmia/CPR: 0.5 to 1 mg IV q 3 to 5 min to max 0.04 mg/kg (3 mg). Peds: 0.02 mg/kg/dose, minimum single dose 0.1 mg, max cumulative dose 1 mg. Treatment of muscarinic symptoms of insecticide or nerve agent poisonings: Mild symptoms: 1 injection of 2 mg auto-injector pen, 2 additional injections after 10 min may be given in rapid succession if severe symptoms develop. Severe symptoms: 3 injections of 2 mg pen in rapid succession. Administer in mid-lateral thigh. Max 3 injections. [Trade only: Prefilled auto-injector pen: 0.25 mg (yellow), 0.5 mg (blue), 1 mg (dark red), 2 mg (green).] ▶K ♀C▶– $

DIGOXIN (*Lanoxin, Digitek, ✦Toloxin*) Proarrhythmic. Systolic heart failure/rate control of chronic A-fib: Age from 70 yo: 0.25 mg PO daily; age 70 yo or older: 0.125 mg PO daily; impaired renal function: 0.0625 to 0.125 mg PO daily. Rapid A-fib: Total loading dose (TLD), 10 to 15 mcg/kg IV/PO, give in 3 divided doses q 6 to 8 h; give ~50% TLD for 1 dose, then ~25% TLD for 2 doses (eg, 70 kg with normal renal function: 0.5 mg, then 0.25 mg q 6 to 8 h for 2 doses). Impaired renal function, 6 to 10 mcg/kg IV/PO TLD, given in 3 divided doses of 0.125 to 0.375 mg IV/PO daily. Consider patient-specific characteristics (lean/ ideal wt, CrCl, age, concomitant disease states, concomitant medications, and factors likely to alter pharmacokinetic/dynamic profile of digoxin) when dosing; see prescribing information for alterations based on wt, renal function, or drug interactions. Assess electrolytes, renal function, levels periodically. Adjust dose based on response and therapeutic serum levels; the risk of adverse events increases when the serum level is more than 1.2 ng/mL. Nausea, vomiting, visual disturbances, and cardiac arrhythmias may indicate toxicity. [Generic/Trade: Tabs, scored (Lanoxin, Digitek) 0.125, 0.25 mg. Generic only: elixir 0.05 mg/mL.] ▶KL ♀C▶+ $

DIGOXIN IMMUNE FAB (*Digibind, DigiFab*) Digoxin toxicity: Acute ingestion of known amount: 1 vial binds approximately 0.5 mg digoxin. Acute ingestion of unknown amount: 10 vials IV, may repeat once. Toxicity during chronic therapy: 6 vials usually adequate; one formula is: Number vials = (serum dig level in ng/mL) × (kg)/100. ▶K ♀C▶? $$$$$

DISOPYRAMIDE (*Norpace, Norpace CR*) Proarrhythmic. Rarely indicated, consult cardiologist. Ventricular arrhythmia: 400 to 800 mg PO daily in divided doses (immediate-release is divided q 6 h: extended-release is divided q 12 h). [Generic/Trade: Caps, immediate-release 100, 150 mg. Trade only: Caps, extended-release 100, 150 mg.] ▶KL ♀C▶ ■

DOFETILIDE (*Tikosyn*) Proarrhythmic. Conversion of A-fib/flutter: Specialized dosing based on CrCl and QTc interval. Available only to hospitals and prescribers who have received appropriate dosing and treatment-initiation education. [Trade only: Caps, 0.125, 0.25, 0.5 mg.] ▶KL ♀C▶ $$$$$ ■

DRONEDARONE (*Multaq*) Proarrhythmic. Reduce hospitalization risk for patients with atrial fib who are in sinus rhythm and have a history of paroxysmal or persistent atrial fib: 400 mg PO two times per day with morning and evening meals. Do not use with permanent atrial fibrillation, NYHA Class IV heart failure or NYHA Class II to III heart failure with recent decompensation requiring hospitalization or referral to heart failure clinic, 2nd or 3rd degree AV block or sick sinus syndrome without functioning pacemaker, bradycardia less than 50 bpm, QTc Bazett interval greater than 500 msec, liver or lung toxicity related to previous amiodarone use, severe hepatic impairment, pregnancy, lactation, grapefruit juice, drugs or herbals that increase QT interval, Class I or III antiarrhythmic agents, potent inhibitors of CYP3A4 enzyme system (clarithromycin, itraconazole, ketoconazole, nefazodone, ritonavir, voriconazole), or inducers of CYP3A4 enzyme system (carbamazepine, phenytoin, phenobarbital, rifampin, St. John's wort). Correct hypo/hyperkalemia and hypomagnesemia before giving. Monitor ECG q 3 months; if in atrial fib, then either discontinue dronedarone or cardiovert. May initiate or worsen heart failure symptoms. May be associated with hepatic injury; discontinue if hepatic injury is suspected. Serum creatinine may increase during 1st weeks, but does not reflect change in renal function; reversible when discontinued. Monitor renal function periodically. Give with appropriate antithrombotic therapy. May increase INR when used with warfarin. May increase dabigatran level. May increase digoxin level; discontinue digoxin or decrease dose by 50%. Use cautiously with beta-blockers (BB) and calcium channel blockers (CCB); initiate lower doses of BB or CCB; initiate at low dose and monitor ECG. Do not use with more than 10 mg of simvastatin. May increase level of sirolimus, tacrolimus, or CYP3A4 substrates with narrow therapeutic index. [Trade only: Tabs, unscored 400 mg.] ▶L ♀X▶ $$$$$ ■

FLECAINIDE Proarrhythmic. Prevention of paroxysmal atrial fib/flutter or PSVT, with symptoms and no structural heart disease: Start 50 mg PO q 12 h, may increase by 50 mg two times per day q 4 days, max 300 mg/day. Use with AV nodal slowing agent (beta-blocker, verapamil, diltiazem) to minimize risk of 1:1 atrial flutter. Life-threatening ventricular arrhythmias without structural heart disease: Start

(cont.)

100 mg PO q 12 h, may increase by 50 mg two times per day q 4 days, max 400 mg/day. With CrCl less than 35 mL/min: Start 50 mg PO two times per day. [Generic: Tabs, unscored 50, scored 100, 150 mg.] ▶K ♀C ▶– $$$$ ■

IBUTILIDE (*Corvert*) Proarrhythmic. Recent onset A-fib/flutter: 0.01 mg/kg up to 1 mg IV over 10 min, may repeat once if no response after 10 min. Keep on cardiac monitor at least 4 h. ▶K ♀C ▶? $$$$$ ■

ISOPROTERENOL (*Isuprel*) Refractory bradycardia or 3rd degree AV block: bolus method: 0.02 to 0.06 mg IV: infusion method, dilute 2 mg in 250 mL D5W (8 mcg/mL); a rate of 37.5 mL/h delivers 5 mcg/min. Peds infusion method: 0.05 to 2 mcg/kg/min. Using the same concentration as adult for a 10 kg child, a rate of 8 mL/h delivers 0.1 mcg/kg/min. ▶LK ♀C ▶? $$$$$

LIDOCAINE (*Xylocaine, Xylocard*) Ventricular arrhythmia: Load 1 mg/kg IV, then 0.5 mg/kg q 8 to 10 min prn to max 3 mg/kg. IV infusion: 4 g in 500 mL D5W (8 mg/mL) run at rate of 7.5 to 30 mL/h to deliver 1 to 4 mg/min. Peds: 20 to 50 mcg/kg/min. ▶LK ♀B ▶? $

MEXILETINE (*Mexitil*) Proarrhythmic. Rarely indicated, consult cardiologist. Ventricular arrhythmia: Start 200 mg PO q 8 h with food or antacid, max dose 1200 mg/day. [Generic only: Caps 150, 200, 250 mg.] ▶L ♀C ▶– $$$$ ■

PROCAINAMIDE Proarrhythmic. Ventricular arrhythmia: Loading dose: 100 mg IV q 10 min or 20 mg/min (150 mL/h) until QRS widens more than 50%, dysrhythmia suppressed, hypotension, or total of 17 mg/kg or 1000 mg delivered. Infusion: dilute 2 g in 250 mL D5W (8 mg/mL) rate of 15 to 45 mL/h to deliver 2 to 6 mg/min. ▶LK ♀C ▶? $$ ■

PROPAFENONE (*Rythmol, Rythmol SR*) Proarrhythmic. Prevention of paroxysmal atrial fib/flutter or PSVT, with symptoms and no structural heart disease: Start (immediate-release) 150 mg PO q 8 h, may increase after 3 to 4 days to 225 mg PO q 8 h, max 900 mg/day. Prolong time to recurrence of symptomatic atrial fib without structural heart disease: 225 mg SR PO q 12 h, may increase after 5 days to 325 mg SR PO q 12 h, max 425 mg SR PO q 12 h. Consider using with AV nodal blocking agent (beta-blocker, verapamil, diltiazem) to minimize risk of 1:1 atrial flutter. Do not use with amiodarone, quinidine, or the combination of CYP3A4 and CYP2D6 inhibitors or CYP2D6 deficiency). May increase digoxin, warfarin, beta-blocker levels. CYP1A2, 2D6, or 3A4 inhibitors; cimetidine; fluoxetine may increase level. Rifampin reduces level. Orlistat reduces level; taper orlistat withdrawal in patients stabilized on propafenone. Concomitant lidocaine increases risk of CNS side effects. [Generic/Trade: Tabs, immediate-release scored 150, 225 mg. Caps, sustained-release, (SR-$$$$$) 225, 325, 425 mg. Generic only: Tabs, immediate-release, scored 300 mg.] ▶L ♀C ▶? $$ ■

QUINIDINE Proarrhythmic. Arrhythmia: Gluconate, extended-release: 324 to 648 mg PO q 8 to 12 h; sulfate, immediate-release: 200 to 400 mg PO q 6 to 8 h; sulfate, extended-release: 300 to 600 mg PO q 8 to 12 h. [Generic only: Gluconate, Tabs ($$$$), extended-release, unscored 324 mg. Sulfate, Tabs ($), scored immediate-release 200, 300 mg, Tabs, extended-release, ($$$$) 300 mg.] ▶LK ♀C ▶+ $ ■

SODIUM BICARBONATE Severe acidosis: 1 mEq/kg IV up to 50 to 100 mEq/dose. ▶K ♀C ▷? $

SOTALOL (*Betapace, Betapace AF, Sotylize, ✦Rylosol*) Proarrhythmic. Ventricular arrhythmia (Sotylize, Betapace): Start 80 mg PO two times per day, Sotylize max 320 mg/day, Betapace max 640 mg/day. A-fib/A-flutter (Sotylize, Betapace AF): Start 80 mg PO two times per day, Sotylize max 160 mg/day, Betapace AF max 640 mg/day. Initiate or re-initiate this product in a facility with cardiac resuscitation capacity, continuous EKG and CrCl monitoring. Do not substitute Betapace for Betapace AF. Adjust dose if CrCl less than 60 mL/min. [Generic/Trade: Tabs, scored 80, 120, 160, 240 mg. Tabs, scored (Betapace AF) 80, 120, 160 mg. Trade only: 5 mg/mL (Sotylize).] ▶K ♀B ▷– $$$$ ■

Antihypertensive Combinations

NOTE: *In general, establish dose using component drugs first. See component drugs for metabolism, pregnancy, and lactation.*

Antihypertensive Combinations

BY TYPE:	
ACEI + Diuretic	*Accuretic, Capozide, Inhibace Plus, Lotensin HCT, Monopril HCT, Prinzide, Uni-retic, Vaseretic, Zestoretic*
ACEI + CCB	*Lotrel, Prestalia, Tarka*
ARB + Diuretic	*Atacand HCT, Atacand Plus, Avalide, Benicar HCT, Diovan HCT, Edarbyclor, Hyzaar, Micardis HCT, Micardis Plus, Teveten HCT*
ARB + CCB	*Azor, Exforge, Twynsta*
ARB + CCB + Diuretic	*Exforge HCT, Tribenzor*
Beta-blocker + Diuretic	*Corzide, Dutoprol, Inderide, Lopressor HCT, Tenoretic, Ziac*
CCB + Statin	*Caduet*
Direct Renin Inhibitor + CCB	*Tekamlo*
Direct Renin Inhibitor + CCB + Diuretic	*Amturnide*
Direct Renin Inhibitor + Diuretic	*Rasilez HCT, Tekturna HCT*
Diuretic combinations	*Aldactazide, Maxzide, Moduret, Moduretic, Triazide*
Diuretic + Miscellaneous Antihypertensive	*Aldoril, Clorpres, Minizide*

(cont.)

Antihypertensive Combinations (*continued*)

ACEI=ACE Inhibitor ARB=angiotensin receptor blocker CCB=calcium channel blocker

BY NAME: *Accuretic* (quinapril + HCTZ): Generic/Trade: Tabs, scored 10/12.5, 20/12.5, unscored 20/25 mg. *Aldactazide* (spironolactone + HCTZ): Generic/Trade: Tabs, unscored 25/25, scored 50/50 mg. *Aldoril* (methyldopa + HCTZ): Generic: Tabs, unscored 250/15, 250/25 mg. *Amturnide* (aliskiren + amlodipine + HCTZ): Trade only: Tabs, unscored 150/5/12.5, 300/5/12.5, 300/5/25, 300/10/12.5, 300/10/25 mg. *Atacand* HCT (candesartan + HCTZ, *Atacand Plus*): Generic/Trade: Tab, unscored 16/12.5, 32/12.5, 32/25 mg. *Avalide* (irbesartan + HCTZ): Generic/Trade: Tabs, unscored 150/12.5, 300/12.5 mg. *Azor* (amlodipine + olmesartan): Trade only: Tabs, unscored 5/20, 5/40, 10/20, 10/40 mg. *Benicar HCT* (olmesartan + HCTZ): Trade only: Tabs, unscored 20/12.5, 40/12.5, 40/25 mg. *Caduet* (amlodipine + atorvastatin): Generic/Trade: 2.5/10, 2.5/20, 2.5/40, 5/10, 5/20, 5/40, 5/80, 10/10, 10/20, 10/40, 10/80 mg. *Capozide* (captopril + HCTZ): Generic only: Tabs, scored 25/15, 25/25, 50/15, 50/25 mg. *Clorpres* (clonidine + chlorthalidone): Generic/Trade: Tabs, scored 0.1/15, 0.2/15, 0.3/15 mg. *Corzide* (nadolol + bendroflumethiazide): Generic/Trade: Tabs 40/5, 80/5 mg. *Diovan HCT* (valsartan + HCTZ): Generic/Trade: Tabs, unscored 80/12.5, 160/12.5, 160/25, 320/12.5, 320/25 mg. *Dutoprol* (metoprolol succinate + HCTZ): Trade only: Tabs, unscored 25/12.5, 50/12.5, 100/12.5 mg. *Dyazide* (triamterene + HCTZ): Generic/Trade: Caps, (Dyazide) 37.5/25, (generic only) 50/25 mg. *Edarbyclor* (azilsartan + chlorthalidone): Trade only: Tabs, unscored 40/12.5, 40/25 mg. *Exforge* (amlodipine + valsartan): Generic/Trade: Tabs, unscored 5/160, 5/320, 10/160, 10/320 mg. *Exforge HCT* (amlodipine + valsartan + HCTZ): Generic/Trade: Tabs, unscored 5/160/12.5, 5/160/25, 10/160/12.5, 10/160/25, 10/320/25 mg. *Hyzaar* (losartan + HCTZ): Generic/Trade: Tabs, unscored 50/12.5, 100/12.5, 100/25 mg. *Inderide* (propranolol + HCTZ): Generic only: Tabs, scored 40/25, 80/25 mg. *Inhibace Plus* (cilazapril + HCTZ): Generic/Trade: Tabs, scored 5/12.5 mg. *Lopressor HCT* (metoprolol tartrate + HCTZ): Generic/Trade: Tabs, scored 50/25, 100/25 mg. Generic: Tabs, scored 100/50 mg. *Lotensin HCT* (benazepril + HCTZ): Generic/ Trade: Tabs, scored 5/6.25, 10/12.5, 20/12.5, 20/25 mg. *Lotrel* (amlodipine + benazepril): Generic/Trade: Cap, 2.5/10, 5/10, 5/20, 10/20 mg, 5/40, 10/40 mg. *Maxzide* (triamterene + HCTZ, Triazide): Generic/Trade: Tabs, scored (Maxzide-25) 37.5/25 (Maxzide) 75/50 mg. *Micardis HCT* (telmisartan + HCTZ, *Micardis Plus*): Generic/Trade: Tabs, unscored 40/12.5, 80/12.5, 80/25 mg. *Minizide* (prazosin + polythiazide): Trade only: Caps, 1/0.5, 2/0.5, 5/0.5 mg. *Moduretic* (amiloride + HCTZ, *Moduret*): Generic only: Tabs, scored 5/50 mg. *Monopril HCT* (fosinopril + HCTZ): Generic only: Tabs, unscored 10/12.5, scored 20/12.5 mg. *Prestalia* (perindopril + amlodipine): Trade: Tabs, unscored 3.5/2.5, 7/5, 14/10mg. *Prinzide* (lisinopril + HCTZ): Generic/Trade: Tabs, unscored 10/12.5, 20/12.5, 20/25 mg. *Tarka* (trandolapril + verapamil): Trade only: Tabs, unscored 2/180, 1/240, 2/240, 4/240 mg. *Tekamlo* (aliskiren + amlodipine): Trade only: Tabs, unscored 150/5, 150/10, 300/5, 300/10 mg. *Tekturna HCT* (aliskiren + HCTZ, Rasilez HCT): Trade only: Tabs, unscored 150/12.5, 150/25, 300/12.5, 300/25 mg. *Tenoretic* (atenolol + chlorthalidone): Generic/Trade: Tabs, scored 50/25, unscored 100/25 mg. *Teveten HCT* (eprosartan + HCTZ): Trade only: Tabs, unscored 600/12.5, 600/25 mg. *Tribenzor* (amlodipine + olmesartan + HCTZ): Trade only: Tabs, unscored 5/20/12.5, 5/40/12.5, 5/40/25,10/40/12.5,10/40/25 mg. *Twynsta* (amlodipine + telmisartan): Generic/Trade: Tabs, unscored 5/40, 5/80, 10/40, 10/80 mg. *Uniretic* (moexipril + HCTZ): Generic/Trade: Tabs, unscored 7.5/12.5, 15/25 mg. Generic: Tabs, scored 7.5/12.5 mg. *Vaseretic* (enalapril + HCTZ): Generic/Trade: Tabs, unscored 5/12.5, 10/25 mg. *Zestoretic* (lisinopril HCTZ): Generic/Trade: Tabs, unscored 10/12.5, 20/12.5, 20/25 mg. *Ziac* (bisoprolol + HCTZ): Generic/Trade: Tabs, unscored 2.5/6.25, 5/6.25, 10/6.25 mg.

CARDIOVASCULAR

Antihypertensives—Other

ALISKIREN (*Tekturna*, *✦Rasilez*) HTN: 150 mg PO daily, max 300 mg/day. Contraindicated in pregnancy or with ACE inhibitors or angiotensin receptor blockers in patients with DM. Avoid use with ACE inhibitors or angiotensin receptor blockers, particularly in patients with CRCl less than 60 mL/min; increases risk of renal impairment, hypotension, and hyperkalemia. Do not use with cyclosporine or itraconazole. Concomitant NSAID, including selective COX-2 inhibitors, may further deteriorate renal function and decrease antihypertensive effects. Hyperkalemia possible, especially if used concomitantly with other drugs that increase K^+ (including K^+-containing salt substitutes) and in patients with heart failure, DM, or renal impairment. Monitor potassium and renal function periodically. [Trade only: Tabs, unscored 150, 300 mg.] ▶LK ♀D ▶–? $$$$ ■

ENTRESTO (**sacubitril + valsartan**) Reduce cardiovascular death and hospitalization for heart failure with chronic heart failure (NYHA Class II–IV) and reduced ejection fraction: Start 49/51 mg PO two times per day, double dose after 2 to 4 weeks as tolerated, target maintenance dose 97/103 mg PO two times daily. Patients not currently taking ACE inhibitor or angiotensin receptor blocker or previously taking low dose of these agents, severe renal impairment (eGFR less than 30mL/min/1.73 m^2), moderate hepatic impairment (Child-Pugh B): Start 24/26 mg PO two times per day, double dose after 2 to 4 weeks as tolerated; target maintenance dose 97/103 mg PO two times daily. Usually given with other heart failure therapies, in place of ACE inhibitor or other angiotensin receptor blocker. If switching from ACE inhibitor, allow 36 hours washout period between administration of the drugs. Do not use with severe hepatic impairment. Contraindicated with pregnancy, concomitant ACE inhibitor, concomitant aliskiren in patients with DM, or previous angioedema with ACE inhibitor or angiotensin receptor blocker. Combined use with renin-angiotensin system inhibitors (ie, ACE inhibitors, aliskiren, other angiotensin receptor blocker) increases risk of renal impairment, hypotension, and hyperkalemia. Hyperkalemia possible, especially if used concomitantly with other drugs that increase K^+ (including K^+-containing salt substitutes) and in patients with heart failure, DM, or renal impairment. Concomitant NSAID, including selective COX-2 inhibitors, may further deteriorate renal function and decrease antihypertensive effects. May increase lithium levels. [Trade: Tabs, unscored 24/26, 49/51, 97/103 mg.] ▶esterases ♀D ▶– $$$$$ ■

FENOLDOPAM (*Corlopam*) Severe HTN: 10 mg in 250 mL D5W (40 mcg/mL), start at 0.1 mcg/kg/min titrate q 15 min, usual effective dose 0.1 to 1.6 mcg/kg/min. ▶LK ♀B ▶? $$$$

HYDRALAZINE (*Apresoline*) Hypertensive emergency: 10 to 20 mg IV or 10 to 50 mg IM, repeat prn. HTN: Start 10 mg PO two to four times per day, max 300 mg/day. Headaches, peripheral edema, systemic lupus erythematosus–like syndrome. [Generic only: Tabs, unscored 10, 25, 50, 100 mg.] ▶LK ♀C ▶+ $$$

NITROPRUSSIDE (*Nitropress*) Hypertensive emergency: Dilute 50 mg in 250 mL D5W (200 mcg/mL), rate of 6 mL/h for 70 kg adult delivers starting dose of 0.3 mcg/kg/min. Max 10 mcg/kg/min. Protect from light. Cyanide toxicity with high

(cont.)

doses (10 mcg/kg/min), hepatic/renal impairment, and prolonged infusions (longer than 3 to 7 days); check thiocyanate levels. ▶RBCs ♀C ▶– $$$$$ ■

PHENTOLAMINE (*Regitine*, *✦Rogitine*) Extravasation: 5 to 10 mg in 10 mL NS, inject 1 to 5 mL SC (in divided doses) around extravasation site. ▶plasma ♀C ▶? $$$$

Antihyperlipidemic Agents—Bile Acid Sequestrants

CHOLESTYRAMINE (*Questran, Questran Light, Prevalite, ✦Olestyr*) Elevated LDL-C: Powder: Start 4 g PO daily to two times per day before meals, increase up to max 24 g/day. [Generic/Trade: Powder for oral susp, 4 g cholestyramine resin/9 g powder (Questran), 4 g cholestyramine resin/5 g powder (Questran Light), 4 g cholestyramine resin/5.5 g powder (Prevalite). Each available in bulk powder and single-dose packets.] ▶Not absorbed ♀C ▶+ $$$$

COLESEVELAM (*Welchol, ✦Lodalis*) LDL-C reduction or glycemic control of type 2 diabetes: 3.75 g once daily or 1.875 g PO two times per day, max 3.75 g/day. Give with meal and 4 to 8 ounces of water, fruit juice, or diet soft drink. 3.75 g is equivalent to 6 tabs; 1.875 g is equivalent to 3 tabs. Powder packets contain phenylalanine. [Trade only: Tabs, unscored 625 mg. Powder single-dose packets 3.75 g.] ▶Not absorbed ♀B ▶+ $$$$$

COLESTIPOL (*Colestid, Colestid Flavored*) Elevated LDL-C: Tabs: Start 2 g PO daily to two times per day with full glass of liquid, max 16 g/day. Granules: Start 5 g PO daily to two times per day, max 30 g/day. Mix granules in at least 90 mL of non-carbonated liquid. Administer other drugs at least 1 h before or 4 to 6 h after colestipol. [Generic/Trade: Tabs 1 g. Granules for oral susp, 5 g/7.5 g powder. Available in bulk powder and individual packets] ▶Not absorbed ♀B ▶+ $$$

Antihyperlipidemic Agents—Fibrates

NOTE: *Contraindicated with active liver disease, gall bladder disease, and/or severe renal impairment (see prescribing information and guidelines for product specific information). Evaluate renal function (SrCr and estimated glomerular filtration rate [eGFR] based on creatinine) at baseline, within 3 months after initiation, q 6 months thereafter. Monitor LFTs (baseline, periodically). Increased risk of myopathy and rhabdomyolysis when used with a statin or colchicine. May cause paradoxical decrease in HDL. May increase cholesterol excretion into bile, leading to cholelithiasis. May increase the effect of warfarin; monitor INR. Take either at least 2 h before or 4 h after bile acid sequestrants.*

BEZAFIBRATE (*✦Bezalip SR*) Canada only. Hyperlipidemia/hypertriglyceridemia: 400 mg of sustained-release PO daily. [Canada Trade only: Sustained-release tab 400 mg.] ▶K ♀D ▶– $$$

FENOFIBRATE (*TriCor, Antara, Fenoglide, Lipofen, Triglide, ✦Lipidil Micro, Lipidil Supra, Lipidil EZ*) Hypertriglyceridemia: TriCor tabs: 48 to 145 mg PO daily, max 145 mg daily. Antara: 30 to 90 mg PO daily; max 130 mg daily. Fenoglide: 40 to 120 mg PO daily; max 120 mg daily. Lipofen: 50 to 150 mg PO daily, max 150 mg

(cont.)

daily. Triglide: 50 to 160 mg PO daily, max 160 mg daily. Generic tabs: 54 to 160 mg, max 160 mg daily. Generic caps: 67 to 200 mg PO daily; max 200 mg daily. Hypercholesterolemia/mixed dyslipidemia: TriCor tabs: 145 mg PO daily. Antara: 130 mg PO daily. Fenoglide: 120 mg daily. Lipofen: 150 mg daily. Triglide: 160 mg daily. Generic tabs: 160 mg daily. Generic caps 200 mg daily. Reduce dose for mild to moderate renal insufficiency. All formulations, except Antara, TriCor, and Triglide, should be taken with food. May consider concomitant therapy with a low- or moderate-intensity statin if the benefits from CVD risk reduction or triglyceride lowering (when 500 mg/dL or more) outweigh the risk of adverse effects. May increase serum creatinine level without changing eGFR. [Generic only: Tabs, unscored 54, 160 mg. Generic caps 67, 134, 200 mg. Generic/Trade: Tabs (TriCor), unscored 48, 145 mg. Caps, (Antara) 30, 90 mg. Trade only: (Fenoglide) unscored 40, 120 mg. Tabs (Lipofen), unscored 50, 150 mg. Tabs (Triglide), unscored 50, 160 mg.] ▶LK ♀C ▶– $$$

FENOFIBRIC ACID (*Fibricor, TriLipix*) Hypertriglyceridemia: Fibricor: 35 to 105 mg PO daily, max 105 mg daily. Trilipix: 45 to 135 mg PO daily, max 135 mg daily. Hypercholesterolemia/mixed dyslipidemia: Fibricor: 105 mg PO daily. Trilipix: 135 mg PO daily. Renal impairment: Fibricor: 35 mg PO daily. TriLipix: 45 mg PO daily. May increase serum creatinine level without changing eGFR. [Trade only: Caps (Trilipix) delayed-release 45, 135 mg. Tabs (Fibricor) 35, 105 mg. Generic only: Tabs 35, 105 mg.] ▶LK ♀C ▶– $$$

GEMFIBROZIL (*Lopid*) Hypertriglyceridemia/primary prevention of CAD: 600 mg PO two times per day 30 min before meals. Do not use with statin; increases risk of myopathy and rhabdomyolysis. [Generic/Trade: Tabs, scored 600 mg.] ▶LK ♀C ▶? $

Antihyperlipidemic Agents—HMG-CoA Reductase Inhibitors ("Statins") and combinations

NOTE: *Each statin has restricted maximum doses that are lower than typical maximum doses when used with certain interacting medications; see prescribing information for complete information. Consider patient characteristics that may modify the decision to use higher intensity statin therapy, including history of hemorrhagic stroke or Asian descent.* **Muscle Issues:** *Evaluate muscle symptoms before initiating statin therapy and at each follow-up visit. Measure creatinine kinase before starting statin, if patient at risk for adverse muscle events. Risk of muscle issues increases with advanced age (65 yo or older), female gender, uncontrolled hypothyroidism, low vitamin D level, renal impairment, higher statin doses, history of muscle disorders, and concomitant use of certain medicines (eg, fibrates, niacin 1 gram or more, colchicine, or ranolazine). Teach patients to report promptly unexplained muscle pain, tenderness, or weakness; rule out common causes; discontinue if myopathy diagnosed or suspected. Obtain creatine kinase, TSH, vitamin D level when patient complains of muscle soreness, tenderness, weakness, or pain.* **Hepatoxicity:** *Monitor ALT before initiating statin therapy and as clinically indicated thereafter. Discontinue statin with persistent ALT elevations more than 3 times the*

(cont.)

upper limit of normal or objective evidence of liver injury. **Diabetes:** *Measure A1c before starting statin, if diabetes status unknown. Statins may increase the risk of hyperglycemia and type 2 diabetes in patients with risk factors for diabetes; benefit usually outweighs risk.* **Cognition:** *The 2013 ACC/AHA cholesterol guidelines expert panel did not find evidence that statins adversely affect cognition. If patient complains of confusion or memory impairment while on statin therapy, consider all possible causes, including other drugs (eg, sleep aides, analgesics, OTC antihistamines) and medical conditions (eg, depression, anxiety, sleep apnea) that affect memory.*

ADVICOR (**lovastatin + niacin**) Hyperlipidemia: 1 tab PO at bedtime, max 40/2000 mg/day. [Trade only: Tabs, unscored extended-release lovastatin/niacin 20/500, 20/750, 20/1000, 40/1000 mg. See component drugs for other dose restrictions.] ▶LK ♀X ▶– $$$$

ATORVASTATIN (**Lipitor**) Hyperlipidemia/prevention of cardiovascular events: Start 10 to 40 mg PO daily, max 80 mg/day. Do not give with cyclosporine or tipranavir + ritonavir. Use with caution and lowest dose necessary with lopinavir + ritonavir. Do not exceed 20 mg/day when given with clarithromycin, itraconazole, other protease inhibitors (saquinavir + ritonavir, darunavir + ritonavir, fosamprenavir, or fosamprenavir + ritonavir). Do not exceed 40 mg/day when given with boceprevir or nelfinavir. [Generic/Trade: Tabs, unscored 10, 20, 40, 80 mg.] ▶L ♀X ▶– $

CADUET (**amlodipine + atorvastatin**) Simultaneous treatment of HTN and hypercholesterolemia: Establish dose using component drugs first. See component drugs for other dose restrictions. Dosing interval: Daily. [Generic/Trade: Tabs, 2.5/10, 2.5/20, 2.5/40, 5/10, 5/20, 5/40, 5/80, 10/10, 10/20, 10/40, 10/80 mg.] ▶L ♀X ▶– $$$$

FLUVASTATIN (**Lescol, Lescol XL**) Hyperlipidemia: Start 20 to 80 mg PO at bedtime, max 80 mg daily (XL) or divided two times per day. Post-percutaneous coronary intervention: 80 mg of extended-release PO daily, max 80 mg daily. Do not exceed 20 mg/day when given with cyclosporine or fluconazole. [Generic/Trade: Caps 20, 40 mg. Trade only: Tab, extended-release, unscored 80 mg.] ▶L ♀X ▶– $$$$

LIPTRUZET (**ezetimibe + atorvastatin**) Hyperlipidemia: Start 10/10 or 10/20 mg PO daily, max 10/80 mg/day. See component drug for other dose restrictions. [Trade only: Tabs, unscored ezetimibe/atorvastatin 10/10, 10/20, 10/40, 10/80 mg.] ▶L – ♀X ▶– $$$$

LOVASTATIN (**Mevacor, Altoprev**) Hyperlipidemia/prevention of cardiovascular events: Start 20 mg PO q pm, max 80 mg/day daily or divided two times per day. Do not use with boceprevir, clarithromycin, cobicistat-containing products, cyclosporine, erythromycin, gemfibrozil, grapefruit juice, HIV protease inhibitors, itraconazole, ketoconazole, nefazodone, posaconazole, telithromycin or voriconazole; increases risk of myopathy. Do not exceed 20 mg/day when used with danazol, diltiazem, dronedarone, verapamil, or CrCl less than 30 mL/min. Do not exceed 40 mg/day when used with amiodarone. [Generic/Trade: Tabs, unscored 20, 40 mg. Generic only: Tabs, unscored 10 mg. Trade only: Tabs, extended-release (Altoprev) 20, 40, 60 mg.] ▶L ♀X ▶– $$$

CARDIOVASCULAR

PITAVASTATIN (*Livalo*) Hyperlipidemia: Start 2 mg PO at bedtime, max 4 mg daily. CrCl 15 to 59 mL/min or on dialysis: Max start 1 mg PO daily, max 2 mg daily. Do not use with cyclosporine. Do not exceed 1 mg/day when given with erythromycin. Do not exceed 2 mg/day when given with rifampin. [Trade only: Tabs 1, 2, 4 mg.] ▶L - ♀X ▶– $$$$$

PRAVASTATIN (*Pravachol*) Hyperlipidemia/prevention of cardiovascular events: Start 40 mg PO daily, max 80 mg/day. Do not exceed 20 mg/day when given with cyclosporine. Do not exceed 40 mg/day when given with clarithromycin. [Generic/Trade: Tabs, unscored 10, 20, 40, 80 mg.] ▶L ♀X ▶– $$$

ROSUVASTATIN (*Crestor*) Hyperlipidemia/slow progression of atherosclerosis/primary prevention of cardiovascular disease: Start 10 to 20 mg PO daily, max 40 mg/day. Renal impairment (CrCl less than 30 mL/min and not on hemodialysis): Start 5 mg PO daily, max 10 mg/day. Asians: Start 5 mg PO daily. When given with atazanavir with or without ritonavir, lopinavir with ritonavir, or simeprevir, do not exceed 10 mg/day. When given with cyclosporine, do not exceed 5 mg/day. Avoid using with gemfibrozil; if used concomitantly, do not exceed 10 mg/day. When given with colchicine, do not exceed 5 mg/day. [Trade only: Tabs, unscored 5, 10, 20, 40 mg.] ▶L ♀X ▶– $$$$$

SIMCOR (simvastatin + niacin) Hyperlipidemia: 1 tab PO at bedtime with a low-fat snack, max 40/2000 mg/day. If niacin-naive or switching from immediate-release niacin, start: 20/500 mg PO q pm. If receiving extended-release niacin, do not start with more than 40/2000 mg PO q pm. Do not use with boceprevir, clarithromycin, cyclosporine, danazol, diltiazem, erythromycin, fenofibrate, gemfibrozil, grapefruit juice, HIV protease inhibitors, itraconazole, ketoconazole, nefazodone, posaconazole, strong CYP3A4 inhibitors, telithromycin, verapamil; increases risk of myopathy. Do not exceed 20/1000 mg/day when used in Chinese patients or with amiodarone, amlodipine, or ranolazine; increases risk of myopathy. Immediate-release aspirin or NSAID 30 min prior may decrease niacin-flushing reaction. Niacin may worsen glucose control, peptic ulcer disease, gout, headaches, and menopausal flushing. Swallow whole; do not break, chew, or crush. [Trade only: Tabs, unscored extended-release simvastatin/niacin 20/500, 20/750, 20/1000, 40/500, 40/1000 mg.] ▶LK ♀X ▶– $$$

SIMVASTATIN (*Zocor*) Do not initiate therapy with or titrate to 80 mg/day; only use 80 mg/day in patients who have taken this dose for more than 12 months without evidence of muscle toxicity. Hyperlipidemia: Start 10 to 20 mg PO q pm, max 40 mg/day. Reduce cardiovascular mortality/events in high risk for coronary heart disease event: Start 40 mg PO q pm, max 40 mg/day. Severe renal impairment: Start 5 mg/day, closely monitor. Chinese patients: Do not exceed 20 mg/day with niacin 1 g or more daily. Do not use with boceprevir, clarithromycin, cobicistat-containing products, cyclosporine, danazol, erythromycin, gemfibrozil, grapefruit juice, HIV protease inhibitors, itraconazole, ketoconazole, nefazodone, posaconazole, strong CYP3A4 inhibitors, telithromycin, voriconazole; increases risk of myopathy. Do not exceed 10 mg/day when used with diltiazem, dronedarone, or verapamil. Do not exceed 20 mg/day when used with amiodarone, amlodipine or ranolazine. Do not exceed 20 mg/day when used with lomitapide; if patient has

(cont.)

been on simvastatin 80 mg/day for at least 1 year without muscle toxicity, do not exceed 40 mg/day when used with lomitapide. [Generic/Trade: Tabs, unscored 5, 10, 20, 40, 80 mg.] ▶L ♀X ▶– $

VYTORIN (ezetimibe + simvastatin) Hyperlipidemia: Start 10/10 or 10/20 mg PO q pm, max 10/40 mg/day. Restrict the use of the 10/80 mg dose to patients who have taken it at least 12 months without muscle toxicity. See simvastatin monograph for other dose restrictions. [Trade only: Tabs, unscored ezetimibe/ simvastatin 10/10, 10/20, 10/40, 10/80 mg.] ▶L ♀X ▶– $$$$

Antihyperlipidemic Agents—Omega Fatty Acids

NOTE: *FDA-approved fish oil. Swallow whole. May prolong bleeding time, may potentiate warfarin. Monitor AST/ALT if hepatic impairment. Use caution in patients with known hypersensitivity to fish and/or shellfish.*

ICOSAPENT ETHYL (*Vascepa*) Hypertriglyceridemia (500 mg/dL or above): 2 caps PO twice daily. Contains EPA. [Trade only: Caps 1 g.] ▶L ♀C ▶? $$$$$

OMEGA-3-ACID ETHYL ESTERS (*Omtryg, Lovaza*) Hypertriglyceridemia (500 mg/dL or above): 4 caps PO daily or divided two times per day. Contains EPA + DHA. [Generic/Trade (Lovaza): 1 g cap. Trade only (Omtryg): 1.2 g cap.] ▶L ♀C ▶? $$$$$

OMEGA-3-CARBOXYLIC ACIDS (*Epanova*) Hypertriglyceridemia (500 mg/dL or above): 2 to 4 capsules PO daily. Contains EPA + DHA. [Trade only: Caps 1 g.] ▶L ♀C ▶? $$$$$

Antihyperlipidemic Agents—Other

ALIROCUMAB (*Praluent*) Reduce LDL-C as adjunct to diet and maximally tolerated statin with heterozygous familial hypercholesterolemia or clinical atherosclerotic cardiovascular disease: Start 75 mg SC q 2 weeks; max 150 mg q 2 weeks. Human monoclonal antibody. Give in abdomen, upper arm, or thigh. ▶N/A ♀? ▶? $$$$$

EVOLOCUMAB (*Repatha*) Reduce LDL-C as adjunct to diet and maximally tolerated statin with heterozygous familial hypercholesterolemia or clinical atherosclerotic cardiovascular disease: 140 mg SC every 2 weeks or 420 mg SQ once monthly. Reduce LDL-C as adjunct to diet and other lipid lowering therapies with homozygous familial hypercholesterolemia: 420 mg SQ once monthly. Human monoclonal antibody. Give in abdomen, upper arm, or thigh. ▶N/A ♀? ▶? $$$$$ ∎

EZETIMIBE (*Zetia, ✦Ezetrol*) Hyperlipidemia: 10 mg PO daily. [Trade only: Tabs, unscored 10 mg.] ▶L ♀C ▶? $$$$

Antiplatelet Drugs

ABCIXIMAB (*ReoPro*) Platelet aggregation inhibition, percutaneous coronary intervention: 0.25 mg/kg IV bolus via separate infusion line before procedure, then 0.125 mcg/kg/min (max 10 mcg/min) IV infusion for 12 h. ▶plasma ♀C ▶? $$$$$

CARDIOVASCULAR

AGGRENOX (acetylsalicylic acid + dipyridamole) Prevention of CVA after TIA/CVA: 1 cap PO two times per day. Headache is a common adverse effect. [Trade only: Caps, 25 mg aspirin/200 mg extended-release dipyridamole.] ▶LK ♀D ▶? $$$$$

CANGRELOR (*Kengreal*) Adjunct to percutaneous coronary intervention (PCI) to reduce thrombotic events, including periprocedural MI, repeat coronary revascularization, and stent thrombosis, in patients who have not been treated with P2Y12 platelet inhibitor and glycoprotein IIb/IIIa inhibitor: Load 30 mcg/kg IV prior to PCI, then IV infusion 4 mcg/kg/min for at least 2 hours or duration of procedure, whichever is longer. Use dedicated IV line. Maintain platelet inhibition with oral P2Y12 inhibitor: Give clopidogrel or prasugrel loading dose immediately after discontinuing cangrelor infusion, or give ticagrelor loading dose during cangrelor infusion or immediately after discontinuing infusion. ▶degraded chemically ♀C ▶? $$$$$

CLOPIDOGREL (*Plavix*) Reduction of thrombotic events, recent acute MI/CVA, established peripheral arterial disease: 75 mg PO daily. Non-ST segment elevation acute coronary syndrome: 300 to 600 mg loading dose, then 75 mg PO daily in combination with aspirin. ST segment elevation MI: Start with/without 300 mg loading dose, then 75 mg PO daily in combination with aspirin, with/without thrombolytic. Allergic cross-reactivity may occur among thienopyridines (clopidogrel, prasugrel, ticlopidine). Avoid drugs that are strong or moderate CYP2C19 inhibitors (eg, omeprazole, esomeprazole, cimetidine, etravirine, felbamate, fluconazole, fluoxetine, fluvoxamine, ketoconazole, voriconazole). Concomitant aspirin, SSRI, or SNRI increases bleeding risk. [Generic/Trade: Tabs, unscored 75, 300 mg.] ▶LK ♀B ▶? $ ■

DIPYRIDAMOLE (*Persantine*) Antithrombotic: 75 to 100 mg PO four times per day. [Generic/Trade: Tabs, unscored 25, 50, 75 mg.] ▶L ♀B ▶? $$$

EPTIFIBATIDE (*Integrilin*) Acute coronary syndrome: Load 180 mcg/kg IV bolus, then infuse 2 mcg/kg/min for up to 72 h. Discontinue infusion prior to CABG. Percutaneous coronary intervention: Load 180 mcg/kg IV bolus just before procedure, followed by infusion of 2 mcg/kg/min and a 2nd 180 mcg/kg IV bolus 10 min after the first bolus. Continue infusion for up to 18 to 24 h (minimum 12 h) after procedure. CrCl less than 50 mL/min not on dialysis: Reduce infusion rate to 1 mcg/kg/min. Dialysis: contraindicated. Thrombocytopenia possible; monitor platelets. ▶K ♀B ▶? $$$$$

PRASUGREL (*Effient*) Reduction of thrombotic events after acute coronary syndrome managed with percutaneous coronary intervention (PCI): 60 mg loading dose, then 10 mg PO daily in combination with aspirin. Wt less than 60 kg: Consider lower maintenance dose of 5 mg PO daily. May cause significant, fatal bleeding. Do not use with active bleeding or history of TIA or CVA. Generally not recommended for patients 75 yo and older. Risk factors for bleeding: Body wt less than 60 kg, propensity to bleed, concomitant medications that increase bleeding risk. Allergic cross-reactivity may occur among thienopyridines (clopidogrel, prasugrel, ticlopidine). [Trade only: Tabs, unscored 5, 10 mg.] ▶LK ♀B ▶? $$$$$ ■

TICAGRELOR (*Brilinta*) Reduction of thrombotic events in patients with acute coronary syndrome (MI or unstable angina): 180 mg loading dose, then 90

(cont.)

mg PO two times daily in combination with aspirin. After any initial dose, use with aspirin 75 to 100 mg max per day. Do not use with history of intracranial hemorrhage, active bleeding, severe hepatic impairment, strong CYP3A inhibitors, or CYP3A inducers. Monitor digoxin levels when initiating or changing ticagrelor therapy. Do not use with strong CYP3A inhibitors (eg, clarithromycin, HIV protease inhibitors, itraconazole, ketoconazole, nefazodone, telithromycin, voriconazole), CYP3A inducers (eg, carbamazepine, dexamethasone, phenobarbital, phenytoin, rifampin), or severe hepatic impairment. P-glycoprotein inhibitors (eg, cyclosporine) increase ticagrelor levels. [Trade only: Tabs, unscored 90 mg.] ▶L - ♀C ▶? $$$$$ ■

TICLOPIDINE Due to high incidence of neutropenia and thrombotic thrombocytopenia purpura, other antiplatelet agents preferred. Platelet aggregation inhibition/reduction of thrombotic CVA: 250 mg PO twice daily with food. Allergic cross-reactivity may occur among thienopyridines (clopidogrel, prasugrel, ticlopidine). [Generic: Tabs, unscored 250 mg.] ▶L ♀B ▶? $$$$ ■

TIROFIBAN (Aggrastat) Non-ST segment elevation acute coronary syndromes: Give 25 mcg/kg within 5 min, then 0.15 mcg/kg/min for up to 18 h. Renal impairment (CrCl 60 mL/min or less): Give 25 mcg/kg within 5 min, then 0.075 mcg/kg/min. ▶K ♀B ▶? $$$$$

VORAPAXAR (Zontivity) Reduction of thrombotic events in patients with history of MI or with peripheral artery disease: 2.08 mg PO daily. Do not use with active bleeding or history of CVA or stroke. Avoid use with strong CYP3A inhibitors or inducers. Store in original container with desiccant. [Trade only: Tabs, unscored 2.08 mg.] ▶L ♀B ▶– $$$$$ ■

Beta-Blockers

NOTE: See also Antihypertensive Combinations. Not first line for HTN (unless concurrent angina, post MI, or heart failure with reduced ejection fraction). Atenolol may be less effective for HTN than other beta-blockers. Non-selective beta-blockers, including carvedilol and labetalol, are contraindicated with asthma; use agents with beta-1 selectivity and monitor cautiously; beta-1 selectivity diminishes at high doses. Contraindicated with acute decompensated heart failure, sick sinus syndrome without pacer, cardiogenic shock, heart block greater than first degree, or severe bradycardia. Agents with intrinsic sympathomimetic activity (eg, pindolol) are contraindicated post acute MI. Abrupt cessation may precipitate angina, MI, arrhythmias, tachycardia, rebound HTN; or with thyrotoxicosis, thyroid storm; discontinue by tapering over 1 to 2 weeks. Do not routinely stop chronic beta-blocker therapy prior to surgery. Discontinue beta-blocker several days before discontinuing concomitant clonidine to minimize the risk of rebound HTN. Patients actively using cocaine should avoid beta-blockers with unopposed alpha-adrenergic vasoconstriction, because this will promote coronary artery vasoconstriction/spasm (carvedilol or labetalol have additional alpha-1-blocking effects and are safer). Concomitant amiodarone, disopyramide, clonidine, digoxin, or nondihydropyridine calcium channel blockers may increase risk of bradycardia. Monitor heart failure

(cont.)

exacerbation and hypotension (particularly orthostatic) when titrating dose. May increase blood sugar or mask tachycardia occurring with hypoglycemia. May aggravate psoriasis or symptoms of arterial insufficiency. Intraoperative floppy iris syndrome may occur during cataract surgery, if patient is on or has previously taken agents with alpha-1 blocking activity.

ACEBUTOLOL (*Sectral, ✦Rhotral*) HTN: Start 400 mg PO daily or 200 mg PO two times per day, max 1200 mg/day. Beta-1 receptor selective; has mild intrinsic sympathomimetic activity. [Generic/Trade: Caps 200, 400 mg.] ▶LK ♀B ▶– $$ ■

ATENOLOL (*Tenormin*) Acute MI: 50 to 100 mg PO daily or in divided doses. HTN: Start 25 to 50 mg PO daily or divided two times per day, max 100 mg/day. Beta-1 receptor selective. May be less effective for HTN and lowering CV event risk than other beta-blockers. [Generic/Trade: Tabs, unscored 25, 100 mg; scored, 50 mg.] ▶K ♀D ▶– $ ■

BETAXOLOL (*Kerlone*) HTN: Start 5 to 10 mg PO daily, max 20 mg/day. Beta-1 receptor selective. [Generic/Trade: Tabs, scored 10 mg; unscored 20 mg.] ▶LK ♀C ? $ ■

BISOPROLOL (*Zebeta, ✦Monocor*) HTN: Start 2.5 to 5 mg PO daily, max 20 mg/day. Highly beta-1 receptor selective. [Generic/Trade: Tabs, scored 5 mg; unscored 10 mg.] ▶LK ♀C ? $$ ■

CARVEDILOL (*Coreg, Coreg CR*) Heart failure, immediate-release: Start 3.125 mg PO two times per day, double dose q 2 weeks as tolerated up to max of 25 mg two times per day (for wt 85 kg or less) or 50 mg two times per day (for wt greater than 85 kg). Heart failure, sustained-release: Start 10 mg PO daily, double dose q 2 weeks as tolerated up to max of 80 mg/day. LV dysfunction following acute MI, immediate-release: Start 3.125 to 6.25 mg PO two times per day, double dose q 3 to 10 days as tolerated to max of 25 mg two times per day. LV dysfunction following acute MI, sustained-release: Start 10 to 20 mg PO daily, double dose q 3 to 10 days as tolerated to max of 80 mg/day. HTN, immediate-release: Start 6.25 mg PO two times per day, double dose q 7 to 14 days as tolerated to max 50 mg/day. HTN, sustained-release: Start 20 mg PO daily, double dose q 7 to 14 days as tolerated to max 80 mg/day. Take with food to decrease orthostatic hypotension. Give Coreg CR in the morning. Alpha-1, beta-1, and beta-2 receptor blocker. [Generic/Trade: Tabs, immediate-release, unscored 3.125, 6.25, 12.5, 25 mg. Trade only: Caps, extended-release 10, 20, 40, 80 mg.] ▶L ♀C ▶? $$$ ■

ESMOLOL (*Brevibloc*) SVT/HTN emergency: Load 500 mcg/kg over 1 min (dilute 5 g in 500 mL to make a soln of 10 mg/mL and give 3.5 mL to deliver 35 mg bolus for 70 kg patient), then start infusion 50 to 200 mcg/kg/min (42 mL/h delivers 100 mcg/kg/min for 70 kg patient). Half-life is 9 min. Beta-1 receptor selective. ▶K ♀C ▶? $$$$$ ■

LABETALOL (*Trandate*) HTN: Start 100 mg PO two times per day, max 2400 mg/day. HTN emergency: Start 20 mg IV slow injection, then 40 to 80 mg IV q 10 min prn up to 300 mg or IV infusion 0.5 to 2 mg/min. Peds: Start 0.3 to 1 mg/kg/dose (max 20 mg). May be used to manage BP during pregnancy. Alpha-1, beta-1, and beta-2 receptor blocker. [Generic/Trade: Tabs, scored 100, 200, 300 mg.] ▶LK ♀C ▶+ $$$ ■

METOPROLOL (*Lopressor, Toprol-XL, ✦Betaloc*) Acute MI: 50 to 100 mg PO q 12 h; or 5-mg increments IV q 5 to 15 min up to 15 mg followed by oral therapy. HTN (immediate-release): Start 100 mg PO daily or in divided doses, increase prn up to 450 mg/day; may require multiple daily doses to maintain 24 h BP control. HTN (extended-release): Start 25 to 100 mg PO daily, increase prn up to 400 mg/day. Heart failure: Start 12.5 to 25 mg (extended-release) PO daily, double dose q 2 weeks as tolerated to max 200 mg/day. Angina: Start 50 mg PO two times per day (immediate-release) or 100 mg PO daily (extended-release), increase prn up to 400 mg/day. IV to PO conversion: 1 mg IV is equivalent to 2.5 mg PO (divided four times per day). Immediate-release form is metoprolol tartrate; extended-release form is metoprolol succinate. The immediate-release and extended-release products may not give same clinical response on mg:mg basis; monitor response and side effects when interchanging between metoprolol products. Extended-release tabs may be broken in half, but do not chew or crush. Beta-1 receptor selective. Take with food. [Generic/Trade: Tabs, immediate release, tartrate, scored 50, 100 mg, extended-release, succinate, 25, 50, 100, 200 mg. Generic only: Tabs, extended-release, tartrate, scored 25 mg.] ▶L ♀C ▶? $$ ■
NADOLOL (*Corgard*) HTN: Start 20 to 40 mg PO daily, max 320 mg/day. Prevent rebleeding esophageal varices: 40 to 160 mg PO daily; titrate dose to reduce heart rate to 25% below baseline. Beta-1 and beta-2 receptor blocker. [Generic/Trade: Tabs, scored 20, 40, 80 mg.] ▶K ♀C ▶– $$$$
NEBIVOLOL (*Bystolic*) HTN: Start 5 mg PO daily, max 40 mg/day. At doses of 10 mg or less or for extensive metabolizers: beta-1 receptor selective. At doses greater than 10 mg or poor metabolizers: beta-1 and beta-2 receptor blocker. [Trade only: Tabs, unscored 2.5, 5, 10, 20 mg.] ▶L ♀C ▶– $$$ ■
PINDOLOL HTN: Start 5 mg PO two times per day, max 60 mg/day. Has intrinsic sympathomimetic activity (partial beta-agonist activity); beta-1 and beta-2 receptor blocker. [Generic only: Tabs, scored 5, 10 mg.] ▶K ♀B ▶? $$$
PROPRANOLOL (*Inderal, Inderal LA, InnoPran XL*) HTN: Start 20 to 40 mg PO two times per day or 60 to 80 mg PO daily, max 640 mg/day; extended-release (Inderal LA) max 640 mg/day; extended-release (InnoPran XL) 80 mg at bedtime (10 pm), max 120 mg at bedtime (chronotherapy). Supraventricular tachycardia or rapid atrial fibrillation/flutter: 1 mg IV q 2 min. Max of 2 doses in 4 h. Migraine prophylaxis: Start 40 mg PO two times per day or 80 mg PO daily (extended-release) max 240 mg/day. Prevent rebleeding esophageal varices: 20 to 180 mg PO two times per day; titrate dose to reduce heart rate to 25% below baseline. Beta-1 and beta-2 receptor blocker. [Generic/Trade: Caps, extended-release 60, 80, 120, 160 mg. Generic only: Soln 20, 40 mg/5 mL. Tabs, scored 10, 20, 40, 60, 80 mg. Trade only: (InnoPran XL at bedtime) 80, 120 mg.] ▶L ♀C ▶+ $$ ■
TIMOLOL (*Blocadren*) HTN: Start 10 mg PO two times per day, max 60 mg/day. Beta-1 and beta-2 receptor blocker. [Generic only: Tabs, 5, 10, 20 mg.] ▶LK ♀C ▶+ $$$ ■

CARDIOVASCULAR

Calcium Channel Blockers (CCBs)—Dihydropyridines

NOTE: *See also Antihypertensive Combinations. Avoid in decompensated heart failure. May increase edema. Extended/controlled/sustained-release forms: swallow whole; do not chew or crush. Avoid grapefruit juice.*

AMLODIPINE (*Norvasc*) HTN: Start 5 mg PO daily, max 10 mg/day. Elderly, small, frail, or with hepatic insufficiency: Start 2.5 PO daily. [Generic/Trade: Tabs, unscored 2.5, 5, 10 mg.] ▶L ♀C ▶– $

CLEVIDIPINE (*Cleviprex*) HTN: Start 1 to 2 mg/h IV, titrate q 1.5 to 10 min to BP response, usual maintenance dose 4 to 6 mg/h, max 32 mg/h IV. An increase of 1 to 2 mg/h will decrease SBP approximately 2 to 4 mmHg. ▶KL ♀C ▶? $$$$$

FELODIPINE (*Plendil, ✦Renedil*) HTN: Start 2.5 to 5 mg PO daily, max 10 mg/day. [Generic/Trade: Tabs, extended-release, unscored 2.5, 5, 10 mg.] ▶L ♀C ▶? $$

ISRADIPINE HTN: Start 2.5 mg PO two times per day, max 20 mg/day (max 10 mg/day in elderly). [Generic only: Immediate-release caps 2.5, 5 mg.] ▶L ♀C ▶? $$$$

NICARDIPINE (*Cardene, Cardene SR*) HTN emergency: Begin IV infusion at 5 mg/h, titrate to effect, max 15 mg/h. HTN: Start 20 mg PO three times per day, max 120 mg/day. Sustained-release: Start 30 mg PO two times per day, max 120 mg/day. Short-term management of HTN, patient receiving PO nicardipine: If using 20 mg PO q 8 h, give 0.5 mg/h IV; if using 30 mg PO q 8 h, give 1.2 mg/h IV; if using 40 mg PO q 8 h, give 2.2 mg/h. [Generic/Trade: Caps, immediate-release 20, 30 mg. Trade only: Caps, sustained-release 30, 45, 60 mg.] ▶L ♀C ▶? $$$

NIFEDIPINE (*Procardia, Adalat, Procardia XL, Adalat CC, Afeditab CR, ✦Adalat XL*) HTN/angina: Extended-release: 30 to 60 mg PO daily, max 120 mg/day. Angina: Immediate-release: Start 10 mg PO three times per day, max 120 mg/day. Avoid sublingual administration, may cause excessive hypotension, acute MI, CVA. Do not use immediate-release caps for treating HTN, hypertensive emergencies, or ST-elevation MI. Preterm labor: Loading dose: 10 mg PO q 20 to 30 min if contractions persist, up to 40 mg within the 1st h. Maintenance dose: 10 to 20 mg PO q 4 to 6 h or 60 to 160 mg extended-release PO daily. [Generic/Trade: Caps 10, 20 mg. Tabs, extended-release (Adalat CC, Afeditab CR, Procardia XL) 30, 60 mg. (Adalat CC, Procardia XL) 90 mg.] ▶L ♀C ▶– $$

NISOLDIPINE (*Sular*) HTN: Start 17 mg PO daily, max 34 mg/day. Take on an empty stomach. [Generic/Trade: Tabs, extended-release 8.5, 17, 25.5, 34 mg. These replace the former 10, 20, 30, 40 mg tabs. Generic only: Tabs, extended-release 20, 30, 40 mg.] ▶L ♀C ▶? $$$$$

Calcium Channel Blockers (CCBs)—Non-Dihydropyridines

NOTE: *See also Antihypertensive Combinations. Avoid in decompensated heart failure, 2nd/3rd degree heart block without pacemaker, acute MI and pulmonary congestion, or systolic blood pressure less than 90 mm Hg systolic.*

DILTIAZEM (*Cardizem, Cardizem LA, Cardizem CD, Cartia XT, Dilacor XR, Diltiazem CD, Diltzac, Diltia XT, Matzim LA, Tiazac, Taztia XT*) Atrial fibrillation/flutter, PSVT: Bolus 20 mg (0.25 mg/kg) IV over 2 min. Rebolus 15 min later (if

(cont.)

needed) 25 mg (0.35 mg/kg). Infusion 5 to 15 mg/h. HTN, once daily, extended-release: Start 120 to 240 mg PO daily, max 540 mg/day. HTN, once daily, graded extended-release (Cardizem LA): Start 180 to 240 mg PO daily, max 540 mg/day. HTN, twice daily, sustained-release: Start 60 to 120 mg PO two times per day, max 360 mg/day. Angina, immediate-release: Start 30 mg PO four times per day, max 360 mg/day divided three to four times per day. Angina, extended-release: Start 120 to 240 mg PO daily, max 540 mg/day. Angina, once daily, graded extended-release (Cardizem LA): Start 180 mg PO daily, doses more than 360 mg may provide no additional benefit. [Generic/Trade: Tabs, immediate-release, unscored (Cardizem) 30 mg, scored 60, 90, 120 mg. Caps, extended-release (Cardizem CD, Cartia XT daily) 120, 180, 240, 300, 360 mg, (Diltzac, Taztia XT, Tiazac daily) 120, 180, 240, 300, 360, 420 mg, (Dilacor XR, Diltia XT) 120, 180, 240 mg. Tabs, extended-release (Cardizem LA daily, Matzim LA) 180, 240, 300, 360, 420 mg. Generic only: Caps, extended release (twice daily) 60, 90, 120 mg. Trade only: Tabs, extended-release (Cardizem LA) 120 mg.] ▶L ♀C ▶+ $$

VERAPAMIL (*Isoptin SR, Calan, Calan SR, Verelan, Verelan PM*) SVT adults: 5 to 10 mg IV over 2 min. SVT peds (age 1 to 15 yo): 2 to 5 mg (0.1 to 0.3 mg/kg) IV, max dose 5 mg. Angina, immediate-release: start 40 to 80 mg PO three to four times per day, max 480 mg/day. Angina, sustained-release: Start 120 to 240 mg PO daily, max 480 mg/day (use twice daily dosing for doses greater than 240 mg/day with Isoptin SR and Calan SR). HTN: Same as angina, except (Verelan PM) 100 to 200 mg PO at bedtime, max 400 mg/day; immediate-release tabs should be avoided in treating HTN. Use cautiously with impaired renal/hepatic function. [Generic/Trade: Tabs, immediate-release, scored (Calan) 40, 80, 120 mg. Tabs, sustained-release, unscored (Isoptin SR, Calan SR) 120, scored 180, 240 mg. Caps, sustained-release (Verelan) 120, 180, 240, 360 mg. Caps, sustained-release (Verelan PM) 100, 200, 300 mg.] ▶L ♀C ▶– $$

Diuretics—Loop

NOTE: *Thiazides are preferred diuretics for HTN. With decreased renal function (CrCl less than 30 mL/min), loop diuretics may be more effective than thiazides for HTN. Rare hypersensitivity in patients allergic to sulfa-containing drugs, except ethacrynic acid. For diuretics given twice daily, give second dose in mid-afternoon to avoid nocturia.*

BUMETANIDE (*Bumex, ✦Burinex*) Edema: 0.5 to 1 mg IV/IM; 0.5 to 2 mg PO daily. 1 mg bumetanide is roughly equivalent to 40 mg furosemide. [Generic only: Tabs, scored 0.5, 1, 2 mg.] ▶K ♀C ▶? $

ETHACRYNIC ACID (*Edecrin*) Can be safely used in patients with true sulfa allergy. Edema: 0.5 to 1 mg/kg IV, max 100 mg/dose; 25 to 100 mg PO daily to two times per day. [Trade only: Tabs, scored 25 mg.] ▶K ♀B ▶? $$$$$

FUROSEMIDE (*Lasix*) HTN: Start 10 to 40 mg PO twice daily, max 600 mg daily. Edema: Start 20 to 80 mg IV/IM/PO, increase dose by 20 to 40 mg in 6 to 8 h until desired response is achieved, max 600 mg/day. Ascites: 40 mg PO daily in combination with spironolactone; may increase dose after 2 to 3 days if no

(cont.)

response. [Generic/Trade: Tabs, unscored 20, scored 40, 80 mg. Generic only: Oral soln 10 mg/mL, 40 mg/5 mL.] ▶K ♀C ▶? $

TORSEMIDE (*Demadex*) HTN: Start 5 mg PO daily, increase prn q 4 to 6 weeks, max 10 mg daily. Edema: 10 to 20 mg IV/PO daily, max 200 mg IV/PO daily. [Generic/Trade: Tabs, scored 5, 10, 20, 100 mg.] ▶LK ♀B ▶? $

Diuretics—Potassium Sparing

NOTE: *See also antihypertensive combinations and aldosterone antagonists. May cause hyperkalemia. Use cautiously with other agents that may cause hyperkalemia (ie, ACE inhibitors, ARBs, aliskiren, potassium containing salt substitutes).*

AMILORIDE (*Midamor*) Edema/HTN: Start 5 mg PO daily in combination with another diuretic, usually a thiazide for HTN, max 20 mg/day. [Generic only: Tabs, unscored 5 mg.] ▶LK ♀B ▶? $$$

TRIAMTERENE (*Dyrenium*) Edema (cirrhosis, nephrotic syndrome, heart failure): Start 100 mg PO two times per day, max 300 mg/day. [Trade only: Caps 50, 100 mg.] ▶LK ♀B ▶– $$$

Diuretics—Thiazide Type

NOTE: *See also Antihypertensive Combinations. Possible hypersensitivity in sulfa allergy. Should be used for most patients with HTN, alone or combined with other antihypertensive agents. Thiazides are not recommended for gestational HTN. Coadministration with NSAIDs, including selective COX-2 inhibitors, may reduce the antihypertensive, diuretic, and natriuretic effects of thiazides. Thiazide-induced hypokalemia is associated with increased fasting blood glucose and new onset DM; keep potassium 4.0 mg/dL or greater to minimize risk; may use thiazide in combination with oral potassium supplementation, ACE inhibitor, ARB, or potassium-sparing diuretic to maintain K^+ level. Lithium level may increase with concomitant use; monitor lithium level.*

CHLOROTHIAZIDE (*Diuril*) HTN: Start 125 to 250 mg PO daily or divided two times per day, max 1000 mg/day divided two times per day. [Trade only: Susp 250 mg/5 mL. Generic only: Tabs, scored 250, 500 mg.] ▶L ♀C, D if used in pregnancy-induced HTN ▶+ $

CHLORTHALIDONE HTN: 12.5 to 25 mg PO daily, max 50 mg/day. Edema: 50 to 100 mg PO daily, max 200 mg/day. Nephrolithiasis (unapproved use): 25 to 50 mg PO daily. [Generic only: Tabs, unscored 25, 50 mg.] ▶L ♀B, D if used in pregnancy-induced HTN ▶+ $

HYDROCHLOROTHIAZIDE (*HCTZ, Oretic, Microzide*) HTN: 12.5 to 25 mg PO daily, max 50 mg/day. Edema: 25 to 100 mg PO daily, max 200 mg/day. [Generic/Trade: Tabs, scored 25, 50 mg. Caps 12.5 mg.] ▶L ♀B, D if used in pregnancy-induced HTN ▶+ $

INDAPAMIDE (*✦Lozide*) HTN: 1.25 to 5 mg PO daily, max 5 mg/day. Edema: 2.5 to 5 mg PO q am. [Generic only: Tabs, unscored 1.25, 2.5 mg.] ▶L ♀B, D if used in pregnancy-induced HTN ▶? $

METHYCLOTHIAZIDE (*Enduron*) HTN: Start 2.5 mg PO daily, usual maintenance dose 2.5 to 5 mg/day. [Generic only: Tabs, scored, 5 mg.] ▶L ♀B, D if used in pregnancy-induced HTN ▶? $$$

METOLAZONE Edema: 5 to 10 mg PO daily, max 10 mg/day in heart failure, 20 mg/day in renal disease. If used with loop diuretic, start with 2.5 mg PO daily. [Generic: Tabs 2.5, 5, 10 mg.] ▶L ♀B, D if used in pregnancy-induced HTN ▶? $$$

Nitrates

NOTE: *Avoid if systolic BP below 90 mmHg, severe bradycardia, tachycardia, or right ventricular infarction. Avoid if patient takes PDE-5 inhibitor (e.g., avanafil, sildenafil, tadalafil, vardenafil) or guanylate cyclase stimulators (eg, riociguat).*

ISOSORBIDE DINITRATE (*Isordil, Dilatrate-SR*) Angina prophylaxis: 5 to 40 mg PO three times per day (7 am, noon, 5 pm), sustained-release: 40 to 80 mg PO two times per day (8 am, 2 pm). [Generic/Trade: Tabs, scored 5 mg. Trade only: Tabs, scored (Isordil) 40 mg. Caps, extended-release (Dilatrate-SR) 40 mg. Generic only: Tabs, scored 10, 20, 30 mg. Tabs, scored, sustained-release 40 mg.] ▶L ♀C ▶? $$$

ISOSORBIDE MONONITRATE Angina: 20 mg PO two times per day (8 am and 3 pm). Extended-release: Start 30 to 60 mg PO daily, max 240 mg/day. Do not use for acute angina. [Generic only: Tabs, 10, 20 mg. Tabs, extended-release, scored 30, 60; unscored 120 mg.] ▶L ♀C ▶? $

NITROGLYCERIN INTRAVENOUS INFUSION Perioperative HTN, acute MI/heart failure, acute angina: Mix 50 mg in 250 mL D5W (200 mcg/mL), start at 10 to 20 mcg/min (3 to 6 mL/h), then titrate upward by 10 to 20 mcg/min prn. ▶L ♀C ▶? $

NITROGLYCERIN OINTMENT (*Nitro-BID*) Angina prophylaxis: Start 0.5 inch q 8 h, maintenance 1 to 2 inch q 8 h, max 4 inch q 4 h; 15 mg/inch. Allow for a nitrate-free period of 10 to 14 h to avoid nitrate tolerance. 1 inch ointment contains about 15 mg. Do not use for acute angina attack. [Trade only: Oint, 2%, tubes 1, 30, 60 g (Nitro-BID).] ▶L ♀C ▶? $$

NITROGLYCERIN SPRAY (*Nitrolingual, NitroMist*) Acute angina: 1 to 2 sprays under the tongue prn, max 3 sprays in 15 min. [Generic/Trade: Nitrolingual soln, 4.9, 12 g. 0.4 mg/spray (60 or 200 sprays/canister). NitroMist aerosol, 4.1, 8.5 g; 0.4 mg/spray (90 or 200 sprays/canister).] ▶L ♀C ▶? $$$$$

NITROGLYCERIN SUBLINGUAL (*Nitrostat*) Acute angina: 0.4 mg SL, repeat dose q 5 min prn up to 3 doses in 15 min. [Trade only: Sublingual tabs, unscored 0.3, 0.4, 0.6 mg; in bottles of 100 or package of 4 bottles with 25 tabs each.] ▶L ♀B ▶? $

NITROGLYCERIN SUSTAINED RELEASE Angina prophylaxis: Start 2.5 mg PO two to three times per day, then titrate upward prn. [Generic only: Caps, extended-release 2.5, 6.5, 9 mg.] ▶L ♀C ▶? $$

NITROGLYCERIN TRANSDERMAL (*Minitran, Nitro-Dur, ✦Trinipatch, Transderm-Nitro*) Angina prophylaxis: 1 patch 12 to 14 h each day. Allow for a nitrate-free period of 10 to 14 h each day to avoid nitrate tolerance. Do not use for acute angina attack. [Generic/Trade: Transdermal system 0.1, 0.2, 0.4, 0.6 mg/h. Trade only: (Nitro-Dur) 0.3, 0.8 mg/h.] ▶L ♀C ▶? $$

CARDIOVASCULAR

Pressors/Inotropes

DOBUTAMINE Inotropic support: 2 to 20 mcg/kg/min. Dilute 250 mg in 250 mL D5W (1 mg/mL); a rate of 21 mL/h delivers 5 mcg/kg/min for a 70 kg patient. ▶plasma ♀D ▶− $

DOPAMINE Pressor: Start at 5 mcg/kg/min, increase prn by 5 to 10 mcg/kg/min increments at 10-min intervals, max 50 mcg/kg/min. Mix 400 mg in 250 mL D5W (1600 mcg/mL); a rate of 13 mL/h delivers 5 mcg/kg/min in a 70 kg patient. Doses in mcg/kg/min: 2 to 4 (traditional renal dose, apparently ineffective) dopaminergic receptors; 5 to 10 (cardiac dose) dopaminergic and beta-1 receptors; more than 10 dopaminergic, beta-1, and alpha-1 receptors. ▶plasma ♀C ▶− $ ■

EPHEDRINE Pressor: 10 to 25 mg IV slow injection, with repeat doses q 5 to 10 min prn, max 150 mg/day. Orthostatic hypotension: 25 mg PO daily to four times per day. Bronchospasm: 25 to 50 mg PO q 3 to 4 h prn. [Generic only: Caps, 50 mg.] ▶K ♀C ▶? $

EPINEPHRINE (*EpiPen, EpiPen Jr, Auvi-Q, Adrenalin*) Cardiac arrest: 1 mg IV q 3 to 5 min. Anaphylaxis: 0.1 to 0.5 mg SC/IM, may repeat SC dose q 10 to 15 min. Acute asthma and hypersensitivity reactions: Adults: 0.1 to 0.3 mg of 1:1000 soln SC or IM. Peds: 0.01 mg/kg (up to 0.3 mg) of 1:1000 soln SC or IM. [Soln for injection: 1:1000 (1 mg/mL in 1 mL amps or 1 mL vial-$). Trade only: EpiPen autoinjector delivers one 0.3 mg (1:1000, 0.3 mL) IM/SC dose. EpiPen Jr. autoinjector delivers one 0.15 mg (1:2000, 0.3 mL) IM/SC dose. Auvi-Q autoinjector delivers one 0.15 mg (1:1000, 0.15 mL) or 0.3 mg (1:1000, 0.3 mL) IM/SC dose. EpiPen and Auvi-Q only available in a 2-pack ($$$$$).] ▶plasma ♀C ▶− varies by therapy

MIDODRINE (*✦Amatine*) Orthostatic hypotension: 10 mg PO three times per day. The last daily dose should be no later than 6 pm to avoid supine HTN during sleep. [Generic: Tabs, scored 2.5, 5, 10 mg.] ▶LK ♀C ▶? $$$$$ ■

MILRINONE Systolic heart failure (NYHA class III, IV): Load 50 mcg/kg IV over 10 min, then begin IV infusion of 0.375 to 0.75 mcg/kg/min. ▶K ♀C ▶? $$

NOREPINEPHRINE (*Levophed*) Acute hypotension: Start 8 to 12 mcg/min, adjust to maintain BP, average maintenance rate 2 to 4 mcg/min. Mix 4 mg in 500 mL D5W (8 mcg/mL); a rate of 22.5 mL/h delivers 3 mcg/min. Ideally through central line. ▶plasma ♀C ▶? $ ■

PHENYLEPHRINE—INTRAVENOUS Severe hypotension: Infusion: 20 mg in 250 mL D5W (80 mcg/mL), start 100 to 180 mcg/min (75 to 135 mL/h), usual dose once BP is stabilized 40 to 60 mcg/min. ▶plasma ♀C ▶− $ ■

VASOPRESSIN (*Vasostrict, ADH, ✦Pressyn AR*) Diabetes insipidus: 5 to 10 units IM/SC two to four times per day prn. Cardiac arrest: 40 units IV; may repeat if no response after 3 min. Septic shock: 0.01 to 0.04 units/min. Variceal bleeding: 0.2 to 0.4 units/min initially (max 0.8 units/min). ▶LK ♀C ▶? $$$$$

Pulmonary Arterial Hypertension

AMBRISENTAN (*Letairis, ✦Volibris*) Pulmonary arterial hypertension: Start 5 mg PO daily; if tolerated, may increase to 10 mg/day. Contraindicated with idiopathic

(cont.)

pulmonary fibrosis or pregnancy. Monitor hemoglobin. If pulmonary edema occurs, consider veno-occlusive disease; if confirmed, discontinue therapy. Not recommended with moderate or severe hepatic impairment. Do not exceed 5 mg when given with cyclosporine. May reduce sperm count. Do not split, crush, or chew tablets. Only available through restricted program; prescribers, pharmacies, female patients must enroll. [Trade only: Tabs, unscored 5, 10 mg.] ▶L ♀X ▶– $$$$$ ■

BOSENTAN (*Tracleer*) Pulmonary arterial hypertension: Start 62.5 mg PO two times per day for 4 weeks, increase to 125 mg two times per day maintenance dose. Contraindicated in pregnancy. If pulmonary edema occurs, consider veno-occlusive disease; if confirmed, discontinue therapy. Monitor hemoglobin. Hepatotoxicity; monitor LFTs. May reduce sperm count. Many drug interactions; see prescribing information. Available only through access program. [Trade only: Tabs, unscored 62.5, 125 mg.] ▶L ♀X ▶–? $$$$$ ■

EPOPROSTENOL (*Flolan, Veletri*) Pulmonary arterial hypertension (PAH): Start 2 ng/kg/min IV infusion via central venous catheter. Adjust dose based on response. Avoid abrupt dose decreases or cessation. If pulmonary edema occurs, consider veno-occlusive disease; if confirmed, discontinue therapy. ▶plasma ♀B ▶? $$$$$

ILOPROST (*Ventavis*) Pulmonary arterial hypertension: Start 2.5 mcg/dose by inhalation (as delivered at mouthpiece); if well tolerated, increase to 5 mcg/dose by inhalation (as delivered at mouthpiece). Use 6 to 9 times a day (minimum of 2 h between doses) while awake. Only administer with I-neb AAD Systems. Avoid contact with skin/eyes or oral ingestion. Monitor vital signs when initiating therapy. Do not initiate therapy if SBP less than 85 mmHg. Discontinue therapy if pulmonary edema occurs; this may be sign of pulmonary venous hypertension. May reduce bronchospasm. ▶L ♀C ▶? $$$$$

MACITENTAN (*Opsumit*) Pulmonary arterial hypertension: 10 mg PO daily. Contraindicated with pregnancy. Only available through restricted program; prescribers, pharmacies, female patients must enroll. [Trade: Tabs 10 mg.] ▶L ♀X ▶– $$$$$ ■

RIOCIGUAT (*Adempas*) Pulmonary arterial hypotension: Start 1 mg PO three times daily; max 2.5 mg three times daily. Contraindicated with pregnancy, nitrates, nitric oxide donors, PDE-5 inhibitors (eg, sildenafil, tadalafil, vardenafil), nonspecific PDE inhibitors (eg, dipyridamole, theophylline). Only available through restricted program; prescribers, pharmacies, female patients must enroll. [Trade: Tabs 0.5, 1, 1.5, 2, 2.5 mg.] ▶LK ♀X ▶– $$$$$ ■

SILDENAFIL (*Revatio*) Pulmonary arterial hypertension: 5 mg or 20 mg PO three times per day, with doses 4 to 6 h apart; or 2.5 mg or 10 mg IV three times per day. Contraindicated with nitrates or guanylate cyclase stimulators (eg, riociguat). Coadministration is not recommended with ritonavir, potent CYP3A inhibitors, or other phosphodiesterase-5 inhibitors. Teach patients to seek medical attention for vision loss, hearing loss, or in men if erections last longer than 4 h. [Generic/Trade: Tabs 20 mg. Trade only: Susp 10 mg/mL.] ▶LK ♀B ▶– $$$$

TADALAFIL (*Adcirca*) Pulmonary arterial hypertension: 40 mg PO daily. Contraindicated with nitrates or guanylate cyclase stimulators (eg, riociguat). Coadministration is not recommended with potent CYP3A inhibitors (itraconazole, ketoconazole), potent CYP3A inducers (rifampin), other phosphodiesterase-5 inhibitors. Caution with ritonavir, see prescribing info for specific dose adjustments. Teach patients to seek medical attention for vision loss, hearing loss, or in men if erections last longer than 4 h. [Trade only (Adcirca): Tabs 20 mg.] ▶L ♀B ▶– $$$$

TREPROSTINIL SODIUM—INJECTABLE (*Remodulin*) Pulmonary arterial hypertension: Continuous SC (preferred) or central IV infusion. Start 1.25 ng/kg/min based on ideal body wt. Dose based on clinical response and tolerance. Avoid abruptly lowering the dose or cessation. Use cautiously in the elderly and those with liver or renal dysfunction. Initiate in setting with personnel and equipment for physiological monitoring and emergency care. Administer by continuous infusion using infusion pump. May potentiate bleeding risk for patients on anticoagulants. May potentiate hypotensive effects of other medications. ▶KL ♀B ▶? $$$$$

TREPROSTINIL—INHALED SOLUTION (*Tyvaso*) Pulmonary arterial hypertension: Start 3 breaths (18 mcg) per treatment session four times per day while awake; treatments should be at least 4 h apart; max 9 breaths (54 mcg) per treatment four times per day. Administer undiluted with the Tyvaso Inhalation System. Avoid contact with skin/eyes or oral ingestion. May need to adjust doses if CYP2C8 inducers or CYP2C8 inhibitors are added or withdrawn. Use cautiously in the elderly and those with liver or renal dysfunction. May potentiate bleeding risk of anticoagulants. May potentiate hypotensive effects of other medications. [1.74 mg in 2.9 mL inhalation soln.] ▶KL – ♀B ▶? $$$$$

TREPROSTINIL—ORAL (*Orenitram*) Pulmonary artery hypertension: Start 0.25 mg PO two times daily; increase by 0.25 to 0.5 mg two times daily or 0.125 mg three times daily q 3 to 4 days as tolerated. Use lower starting dose with mild hepatic impairment or with strong CYP2C8 inhibitor. Take with food. Swallow whole. Do not abruptly discontinue. Avoid use with moderate or severe hepatic impairment. Avoid alcohol. [Trade: Extended-release tabs 0.125, 0.25, 1, 2.5 mg.] ▶L ♀C ▶? $$$$$

Thrombolytics

ALTEPLASE (*TPA, tPA, Activase, Cathflo, ✦Activase rt-PA*) Acute MI: wt 67 kg or less, give 15 mg IV bolus, then 0.75 mg/kg (max 50 mg) over 30 min, then 0.5 mg/kg (max 35 mg) over the next 60 min; wt greater than 67 kg, give 15 mg IV bolus, then 50 mg over 30 min, then 35 mg over the next 60 min. Acute ischemic stroke with symptoms 3 h or less: 0.9 mg/kg (max 90 mg); give 10% of total dose as an IV bolus, and the remainder IV over 60 min. Multiple exclusion criteria. Acute pulmonary embolism: 100 mg IV over 2 h, then restart heparin when PTT twice normal or less. Occluded central venous access device: 2 mg/mL in catheter for 2 h. May use 2nd dose if needed. ▶L ♀C ▶? $$$$$

RETEPLASE (*Retavase*) Acute MI: 10 units IV over 2 min; repeat once in 30 min. ▶L ♀C ▶? $$$$$

STREPTOKINASE (*Streptase, Kabikinase*) Acute MI: 1.5 million units IV over 60 min. ▶L ♀C ▷? $$$$$

TENECTEPLASE (*TNKase*) Acute MI: Single IV bolus dose over 5 sec based on body wt: Wt less than 60 kg: 30 mg; wt 60 kg to 69 kg: 35 mg; wt 70 to 79 kg: 40 mg; wt 80 to 89 kg: 45 mg; wt 90 kg or more: 50 mg. ▶L ♀C ▷? $$$$$

Volume Expanders

ALBUMIN (*Albuminar, Buminate, Albumarc, ✦Plasbumin*) Shock, burns: 500 mL of 5% soln IV infusion as rapidly as tolerated, repeat in 30 min if needed. ▶L ♀C ▷? $$$$

DEXTRAN (*Rheomacrodex, Gentran, Macrodex*) Shock/hypovolemia: up to 20 mL/kg in 1st 24 h, then up to 10 mL/kg for 4 days. ▶K ♀C ▷? $$

HETASTARCH (*Hespan, Hextend, Voluven*) Shock/hypovolemia: 500 to 1000 mL IV infusion. Hespan, Hextend: usually should not exceed 20 mL/kg/day. Voluven: Do not exceed 50 mL/kg/day. ▶K ♀C ▷? $$ ∎

PLASMA PROTEIN FRACTION (*Plasmanate, Protenate, Plasmatein*) Shock/hypovolemia: 5% soln 250 to 500 mL IV prn. ▶L ♀C ▷? $$$$

Other

BiDil (hydralazine + isosorbide dinitrate) Heart failure (adjunct to standard therapy in black patients): Start 1 tab PO three times per day, increase as tolerated to max 2 tabs three times per day. May decrease to ½ tab three times per day with intolerable side effects. [Trade only: Tabs, scored 37.5/20 mg.] ▶LK ♀C ▷? $$$$$

CILOSTAZOL (*Pletal*) Intermittent claudication: 100 mg PO two times per day on empty stomach. 50 mg PO two times per day with CYP3A4 inhibitors (eg, ketoconazole, itraconazole, erythromycin, diltiazem) or CYP2C19 inhibitors (eg, omeprazole). Contraindicated in heart failure of any severity due to decreased survival. [Generic/Trade: Tabs 50, 100 mg.] ▶L ♀C ▷? $$$$ ∎

IVABRADINE (*Corlanor*) Stable, symptomatic heart failure with ejection fraction less than or equal to 35%, sinus rhythm with heart rate of at least 70 beats per minute, and either maximally tolerated beta-blocker dose or intolerant to beta-blocker: Start 5 mg PO two times per day, max 15 mg/day. With conduction defect or if bradycardia could lead to hemodynamic compromise, start 2.5 mg PO two times daily. Fetal toxicity; females should use effective contraception. Contraindicated with strong CYP3A4 inhibitors (eg, azole antifungals, macrolide antibiotics, HIV protease inhibitors, nefazodone); acute decompensated heart failure; BP less than 90/50 mmHg; sick sinus syndrome, sinoatrial block, or 3rd degree AV block without functioning pacemaker; resting heart rate less than 60 bpm prior to treatment; severe hepatic impairment; or pacemaker dependent. Monitor for atrial fibrillation, bradycardia. Not recommended with 2nd degree heart block or with demand pacemakers set to at least 60 beats per minute. Avoid concomitant CYP3A4 inhibitors or CYP3A4 inducers. Negative chronotropes increase risk of bradycardia; monitor heart rate. [Trade only: Tabs, unscored 5, 7.5 mg.] ▶L ♀? ▷– $$$$$

NESIRITIDE (*Natrecor*) Hospitalized patients with decompensated heart failure with dyspnea at rest: 2 mcg/kg IV bolus over 1 min, then 0.01 mcg/kg/min IV infusion for up to 48 h. Do not initiate at higher doses. Limited experience with increased doses. Mix 1.5 mg vial in 250 mL D5W (6 mcg/mL); a bolus of 23.3 mL is 2 mcg/kg for a 70 kg patient; infusion set at rate 7 mL/h delivers a 0.01 mcg/kg/min for a 70 kg patient. Contraindicated with cardiogenic shock or SBP less than 100 mmHg. Symptomatic hypotension. May increase mortality. Not indicated for outpatient infusion, for scheduled repetitive use, to improve renal function, or to enhance diuresis. May worsen renal impairment. ▶K, plasma ♀C ▶? $$$$$

PENTOXIFYLLINE Intermittent claudication: 400 mg PO three times per day with meals. Contraindicated with recent cerebral/retinal bleed. [Generic: Tabs, extended-release 400 mg.] ▶L ♀C ▶? $$$

RANOLAZINE (*Ranexa*) Chronic angina: 500 mg PO two times per day, max 1000 mg two times per day. Max 500 mg two times per day, if used with diltiazem, verapamil, or moderate CYP3A inhibitors. Baseline and follow-up ECGs; may prolong QT interval. If CrCl is less than 60 mL/min at baseline, monitor renal function; discontinue ranolazine if acute renal failure occurs. Contraindicated with hepatic cirrhosis, potent CYP3A4 inhibitors, CYP3A inducers. Increases level of cyclosporine, digoxin, lovastatin, simvastatin, sirolimus, tacrolimus, antipsychotics, TCA(s). Swallow whole; do not crush, break, or chew. Teach patients to report palpitations or fainting spells. [Trade only: Tabs, extended-release 500, 1000 mg.] ▶LK ♀C ▶? $$$$$

CONTRAST MEDIA

MRI Contrast—Gadolinium-Based

NOTE: *Avoid gadolinium-based contrast agents if severe renal insufficiency (GFR less than 30 mL/min/1.73 m²) due to risk of nephrogenic systemic fibrosis/nephrogenic fibrosing dermopathy. Similarly avoid in acute renal insufficiency of any severity due to hepatorenal syndrome or during the perioperative phase of liver transplant.*

GADOBENATE (*MultiHance*) ▶K ♀C ▶? $$$$ ■
GADOBUTROL (*Gadavist, ✦Gadavist*) ▶K – ♀C ▶? ⊙V $$$$ ■
GADODIAMIDE (*Omniscan*) ▶K ♀C ▶? $$$$ ■
GADOPENTETATE (*Magnevist*) ▶K ♀C ▶? $$$ ■
GADOTERIDOL (*ProHance*) ▶K ♀C ▶? $$$$ ■
GADOVERSETAMIDE (*OptiMARK*) ▶K ♀C ▶– $$$$ ■

MRI Contrast—Other

FERUMOXSIL (*GastroMARK*) Non-iodinated, nonionic, iron-based, oral GI contrast for MRI: 600 mL (105 mg Fe) administered orally at a rate of about 300 mL over 15 minutes (max 900 mL or 157.5 mg Fe). Take after fasting at least 4 hours. Shake bottles for vigorously for one minute before use. [300 mL bottles] ▶L ♀B ▶? $$$$
MANGAFODIPIR (*Teslascan*) Non-iodinated manganese-based IV contrast for MRI. ▶L ♀– ▶– $$$$

Radiography Contrast

NOTE: *Beware of allergic or anaphylactoid reactions. Avoid IV contrast in renal insufficiency or dehydration. Hold metformin (Glucophage) prior to or at the time of iodinated contrast dye use and for 48 h after procedure. Restart after procedure only if renal function is normal.*

BARIUM SULFATE Noniodinated GI (oral, rectal) contrast: Dosage depends on indication and form, see package insert. ▶Not absorbed ♀? ▶+ $
DIATRIZOATE (*Cystografin, Gastrografin, Hypaque, MD-Gastroview, RenoCal, Reno-DIP, Reno-60, Renografin*) Iodinated, ionic, high osmolality IV or GI contrast: Dosage varies based on study and form, see package insert. Oral contrast for abdominal CT: typical dose is 250 mL of solution made by mixing 25 mL of GI formulation (Gastrografin, MD-Gastroview) in one liter of water. Have patient complete drinking 30 minutes prior to study. Avoid use if there is a risk of aspiration. ▶K ♀C ▶? $
IODIXANOL (*Visipaque*) Iodinated, nonionic, iso-osmolar IV contrast. ▶K ♀B ▶? $$$
IOHEXOL (*Omnipaque*) Iodinated, nonionic, low osmolality for IV, intrathecal, and oral/body cavity contrast. Dosages vary depending on forms and type of study, see package insert. Oral pass-thru examination of the GI tract: Dosages

(cont.)

vary depending on forms, however one example dose would be to mix 50 mL of Omnipaque 350 into one liter of water and have patient drink 500 mL one hour prior to study and remainder 30 min prior to study. [Omnipaque 140, 180, 240, 300, 350] ▶K ♀B ▶? $$$

IOPAMIDOL (*Isovue*) Iodinated, nonionic, low-osmolality IV contrast. ▶K ♀? ▶? $$

IOPROMIDE (*Ultravist*) Iodinated, nonionic, low-osmolality IV contrast. ▶K ♀B ▶? $$$

IOTHALAMATE (*Conray*, ✦*Vascoray*) Iodinated, ionic, high-osmolality IV contrast. ▶K ♀B ▶— $

IOVERSOL (*Optiray*) Iodinated, nonionic, low-osmolality IV contrast. ▶K ♀B ▶? $$

IOXAGLATE (*Hexabrix*) Iodinated, ionic, low-osmolality IV contrast. ▶K ♀B ▶— $$$

IOXILAN (*Oxilan*) Iodinated, nonionic, low-osmolality IV contrast. ▶K ♀B ▶— $$$

DERMATOLOGY

CORTICOSTEROIDS: TOPICAL

Potency*	Generic	Trade Name**	Forms	Frequency
Low	alclometasone dipropionate	Aclovate	0.05% C/O	bid-tid
Low	clocortolone pivalate	Cloderm	0.1% C	tid
Low	desonide	DesOwen, Tridesilon	0.05% C/L/O	bid-tid
Low	hydrocortisone	Hytone, others	0.5% C/L/O; 1% C/L/O; 2.5% C/L/O	bid-qid
Low	hydrocortisone acetate	Cortaid, Corticaine	0.5% C/O; 1% C/O/Sp	bid-qid
Medium	betamethasone valerate	Luxiq	0.1% C/L/O; 0.12% F (Luxiq)	qd-bid
Medium	desoximetasone‡	Topicort	0.05% C	bid
Medium	fluocinolone	Synalar	0.01% C/S; 0.025% C/O	bid-qid
Medium	flurandrenolide	Cordran	0.025% C/O; 0.05% C/L/O/T	bid-qid
Medium	fluticasone propionate	Cutivate	0.005% O; 0.05% C/L	daily-bid
Medium	hydrocortisone butyrate	Locoid	0.1% C/O/S	bid-tid
Medium	hydrocortisone valerate	Westcort	0.2% C/O	bid-tid
Medium	mometasone furoate	Elocon	0.1% C/L/O	qd
Medium	triamcinolone‡	Aristocort, Kenalog	0.025% C/L/O; 0.1% C/L/O/S	bid-tid
High	amcinonide	Cyclocort	0.1% C/L/O	bid-tid
High	betamethasone dipropionate‡	Maxivate, others	0.05% C/L/O (non-Diprolene)	qd-bid
High	desoximetasone‡	Topicort	0.05% G; 0.25% C/O	bid

(cont.)

CORTICOSTEROIDS: TOPICAL (*continued*)

High	diflorasone diacetate‡	Maxiflor	0.05% C/O	bid
High	fluocinonide	Lidex	0.05% C/G/O/S	bid-qid
High	halcinonide	Halog	0.1% C/O/S	bid-tid
High	triamcinolone‡	Aristocort, Kenalog	0.5% C/O	bid-tid
Very high	betamethasone dipropionate‡	Diprolene, Diprolene AF	0.05% C/G/L/O	qd-bid
Very high	clobetasol	Temovate, Cormax, Olux	0.05% C/G/O/L /S/Sp/F (Olux)	bid
Very high	diflorasone diacetate‡	Psorcon	0.05% C/O	qd-tid
Very high	halobetasol propionate	Ultravate	0.05% C/O	qd-bid

bid=two times per day; tid=three times per day; qid=four times per day.

* Potency based on vasoconstrictive assays, which may not correlate with efficacy. Not all available.

** Not all brand name products are commercially available, but generic versions are marketed. products are listed, including those lacking potency ratings.

‡These drugs have formulations in more than once potency category.

C, cream; O, ointment; L, lotion; T, tape; F, foam; S, solution; G, gel; Sp, spray

Acne Preparations

ACANYA (clindamycin—topical + benzoyl peroxide) Apply daily. [Trade only: Gel (clindamycin 1.2% + benzoyl peroxide 2.5%) 50 g.] ▶K ♀C ▶+ $$$$$

ADAPALENE (*Differin*) Apply at bedtime. [Generic/Trade: Gel 0.1%. Cream 0.1% (45 g). Gel 0.3% (45 g). Trade only: Soln 0.1% (59 mL).] ▶bile ♀C ▶? $$$$

AZELAIC ACID (*Azelex, Finacea, Finevin*) Apply two times per day. [Trade only: Cream 20%, 30, 50 g (Azelex). Gel 15% 50 g (Finacea).] ▶K ♀B ▶? $$$$$

BENZACLIN (clindamycin—topical + benzoyl peroxide) Apply two times per day. [Generic/Trade: Gel (clindamycin 1% + benzoyl peroxide 5%) 25, 50 g (jar). Trade only: 35 g (pump) and 50 g (pump).] ▶K ♀C ▶? $$$$$

BENZAMYCIN (erythromycin base—topical + benzoyl peroxide) Apply two times per day. [Generic/Trade: Gel (erythromycin 3% + benzoyl peroxide 5%) 23.3, 46.6 g. Trade only: Benzamycin Pak, #60 gel pouches.] ▶LK ♀C ▶? $$$

BENZOYL PEROXIDE (*Benzac, Benzagel 10%, Desquam, Clearasil, ✦Solugel*) Apply once daily; increase to two to three times per day if needed. [OTC and Rx generic: Liquid 2.5, 5, 10%. Bar 5, 10%. Mask 5%. Lotion 4, 5, 8, 10%. Cream 5, 10%. Gel 2.5, 4, 5, 6, 10, 20%. Pad 3, 4, 6, 8, 9%. Other strengths available.] ▶LK ♀C ▶? $

CLINDAMYCIN—TOPICAL (*Cleocin T, Clindagel, Evoclin, ✦Dalacin T*) Apply daily (Evoclin, Clindagel, ClindaMax) or two times per day (Cleocin T). [Generic/Trade: Gel 1% 30, 60 g. Lotion 1% 60 mL. Soln 1% 30, 60 mL. Foam 1% 50, 100 g. Pads 1% 60 ct.] ▶L ♀B ▶– $$$

DIANE-35 (cyproterone + ethinyl estradiol) Canada only. 1 tab PO daily for 21 consecutive days, stop for 7 days, repeat cycle. [Canada Generic/Trade: Blister pack of 21 tabs 2 mg cyproterone acetate/0.035 mg ethinyl estradiol.] ▶L ♀X ▶– $$

DUAC (clindamycin—topical + benzoyl peroxide, ✦*Clindoxyl*) Apply at bedtime. [Generic/Trade: Gel (clindamycin 1% + benzoyl peroxide 5%) 45 g.] ▶K ♀C ▶+ $$$$$

EPIDUO, EPIDUO FORTE (adapalene + benzoyl peroxide, ✦*Tactuo*) Apply daily. [Trade only: Epiduo, Tactuo Gel (0.1% adapalene + benzoyl peroxide 2.5%) 45 g. Epiduo Forte (0.3% adapalene + benzoyl peroxide 2.5%) 15, 30, 45, 60, 70 g.] ▶Bile, K ♀C ▶ $$$$$

ERYTHROMYCIN—TOPICAL (*Eryderm, Erycette, Erygel, A/T/S, ✦Sans-Acne, Ery-Sol*) Apply two times per day. [Generic/Trade: Soln 2% 60 mL. Pads 2%. Gel 2% 30, 60 g.] ▶L ♀B ▶? $$

ISOTRETINOIN (*Amnesteem, Claravis, Sotret, Absorica, Myorisan, Zenatane, ✦Accutane Roche, Clarus*) 0.5 to 2 mg/kg/day PO divided two times per day for 15 to 20 weeks. Typical target dose is 1 mg/kg/day. Potent teratogen; use extreme caution. Can only be prescribed by healthcare professionals who are registered with the iPLEDGE program. May cause depression. Not for long-term use. [Generic: Caps 10, 20, 40 mg. Generic only: Caps (Absorica) 25, 35 mg. Caps (Sotret, Absorica, Claravis, and Zenatane) 30 mg.] ▶LK ♀X ▶– $$$$$

ONEXTON (clindamycin—topical + benzoyl peroxide) Apply once daily to the face. [Trade only: Gel (clindamycin 1.2% + benzoyl peroxide 3.75%) 50 g.] ▶K ♀C ▶+ $$$$

SALICYLIC ACID (*Akurza, Clearasil Cleanser, Stridex Pads*) Apply/wash area up to three times per day. [OTC Generic/Trade: Pads, Gel, Lotion, Liquid, Mask scrub, 0.5%, 1%, 2%. Rx Trade only (Akurza): Cream 6% 340 g. Lotion 6%, 355 mL.] ▶not absorbed ♀? ▶? $

SULFACET-R (sulfacetamide—topical + sulfur) Apply one to three times per day. [Generic/Trade: Lotions, cleansers, washes.] ▶K ♀C ▶? $$$

SULFACETAMIDE—TOPICAL (*Klaron*) Apply two times per day. [Generic/Trade: Lotion 10% 118 mL.] ▶K ♀C ▶? $$$$

TAZAROTENE (*Tazorac, Avage, Fabior*) Acne: Apply 0.1% cream (Tazorac) or foam (Fabior) at bedtime. Psoriasis: Apply 0.05% cream at bedtime, increase to 0.1% prn. Wrinkles: Apply 0.1% cream (Avage) once daily. [Trade only: Cream (Tazorac) 0.05% and 0.1% 30, 60 g. Foam (Fabior) 0.1% 50, 100 g. Gel 0.05% and 0.1% 30, 100 g. Cream only: Cream (Avage) 0.1% 15, 30 g.] ▶L ♀X ▶? $$$$

TRETINOIN—TOPICAL (*Retin-A, Retin-A Micro, Renova, Retisol-A, Atralin, ✦Stieva-A, Rejuva-A, Vitamin A Acid Cream*) Acne, wrinkles: Apply at bedtime. [Generic/Trade: Cream 0.025% 20, 45 g; 0.05% 20, 45 g; 0.1% 20, 45 g. Gel 0.01% 15, 45 g; 0.025% 15, 45 g; 0.05% 45 g. Micro gel 0.04%, 0.1% 20, 45 g, and 50 g pump 0.08% 50 g pump. Trade only: Renova cream 0.02% 40, 60 g.] ▶LK ♀C ▶? $$$

VELTIN (**clindamycin—topical + tretinoin**) Apply at bedtime. [Trade: Gel clindamycin 1.2% + tretinoin 0.025%, 30, 60 g.] ▶LK ♀C ▶? $$$$$

ZIANA (**clindamycin—topical + tretinoin**) Apply at bedtime. [Trade only: Gel clindamycin 1.2% + tretinoin 0.025% 30, 60 g.] ▶LK ♀C ▶? $$$$$

Actinic Keratosis Preparations

DICLOFENAC—TOPICAL (*Solaraze, Voltaren, Pennsaid*) Actinic/solar keratoses: Apply two times per day to lesions for 60 to 90 days (Solaraze). Osteoarthritis of areas amenable to topical therapy: 2 g (upper extremities) to 4 g (lower extremities) four times per day (Voltaren). 40 gtts to knee(s) four times daily (Pennsaid). [Generic/Trade: Gel 3% (Solaraze) 100 g. Soln 1.5% (Pennsaid) 150 mL. Trade only: Gel 1% (Voltaren) 100 g. Soln 2.0% Pump (Pennsaid) 112 g.] ▶L ♀B ▶? $$$

FLUOROURACIL—TOPICAL (*5-FU, Carac, Efudex, Fluoroplex*) Actinic keratoses: Apply two times per day for 2 to 6 weeks. Superficial basal cell carcinomas: Apply 5% cream/soln two times per day. [Trade only: Cream 1% 30 g (Fluoroplex). Generic/Trade: Cream 0.5% 30 g (Carac); Soln 2%, 5% 10 mL (Efudex). Cream 5% 40 g.] ▶L ♀X ▶— $$$

INGENOL (*Picato*) Apply 0.015% gel to affected area on face and scalp once daily for 3 days or 0.05% gel on affected areas of trunk and extremities once daily for 2 days. [Trade: Gel 0.015% 0.25 g, 0.05% 0.25 g.] ▶not absorbed ♀C ▶? $$$$$

METHYLAMINOLEVULINATE (*Metvix, Metvixia*) Actinic keratosis: Apply cream to non-hyperkeratotic actinic keratoses lesion and surrounding area on face or scalp; cover with dressing for 3 h; remove dressing and cream and perform illumination therapy. Repeat in 7 days. [Trade only: Cream 16.8%, 2 g tube.] ▶not absorbed ♀C ▶?

Antibacterials (Topical)

BACITRACIN—TOPICAL Apply daily to three times per day. [OTC Generic/Trade: Oint 500 units/g 1, 15, 30 g.] ▶not absorbed ♀C ▶? $

FUSIDIC ACID—TOPICAL (*✦Fucidin*) Canada only. Apply three to four times per day. [Canada trade only: Cream 2% fusidic acid 5, 15, 30 g. Oint 2% sodium fusidate 5, 15, 30 g.] ▶L ♀? ▶? $

GENTAMICIN—TOPICAL Apply three to four times per day. [Generic only: Oint 0.1% 15, 30 g. Cream 0.1% 15, 30 g.] ▶K ♀D ▶? $$$

MAFENIDE (*Sulfamylon*) Apply one to two times per day. [Trade Only: Topical Soln 50 g packets. Cream 5% 57, 114, 454 g.] ▶LK ♀C ▶? $$$

METRONIDAZOLE—TOPICAL (*Noritate, MetroCream, MetroGel, MetroLotion, ✦Rosasol*) Rosacea: Apply daily (1%) or two times per day (0.75%). [Trade only: Cream (Noritate) 1% 60 g. Generic/Trade: Gel (MetroGel) 1% 45, 60 g. Gel 0.75% 45 g. Cream 0.75% 45 g. Lotion (MetroLotion) 0.75% 59 mL.] ▶KL ♀B (– in 1st trimester) ▶— $$$$

MUPIROCIN (*Bactroban, Centany*) Impetigo/infected wounds: Apply three times per day. Nasal MRSA eradication: 0.5 g of nasal formulation only in each nostril

(cont.)

two times per day for 5 days. [Generic/Trade: Oint 2% 22 g. Nasal oint 2% 1 g single-use tubes (for MRSA eradication). Trade only: Cream 2% 15, 30 g.] ▶not absorbed ♀B ▶? $$

NEOSPORIN CREAM **(neomycin—topical + polymyxin—topical + bacitracin—topical)** Apply one to three times per day. [OTC Trade only: neomycin 3.5 mg/g + polymyxin 10,000 units/g; 15 g and unit dose 0.94 g.] ▶K ♀C ▶? $

NEOSPORIN OINTMENT **(bacitracin—topical + neomycin—topical + polymyxin—topical)** Apply one to three times per day. [OTC Generic/Trade: bacitracin 400 units/g + neomycin 3.5 mg/g + polymyxin 5000 units/g 15, 30 g and "to go" 0.9 g packets.] ▶K ♀C ▶? $

POLYSPORIN **(bacitracin—topical + polymyxin—topical, ✦*Polytopic*)** Apply one to three times per day. [OTC Trade only: Oint 15, 30 g and unit dose 0.9 g. Powder 10 g.] ▶K ♀C ▶? $

RETAPAMULIN (*Altabax*) Impetigo: Apply thin layer two times per day for 5 days. [Trade only: Oint 1% 15, 30 g.] ▶not absorbed ♀B ▶? $$$$

SILVER SULFADIAZINE (*Silvadene*, ✦*Flamazine*) Apply one to two times per day. [Generic/Trade: Cream 1% 20, 50, 85, 400, 1000 g.] ▶LK ♀B ▶– $$

Antifungals (Topical)

BUTENAFINE (*Lotrimin Ultra, Mentax*) Treatment of tinea pedis: Apply daily for 4 weeks or two times per day for 7 days. Tinea corporis, tinea versicolor, or tinea cruris: Apply daily for 2 weeks. [Rx Trade only: Cream 1% 15, 30 g (Mentax). OTC Trade only: Cream 1% 12, 24 g (Lotrimin Ultra).] ▶L ♀B ▶? $

CICLOPIROX (*Loprox, Loprox TS, Penlac, ✦Stieprox shampoo*) Tinea pedis, tinea cruris, tinea corporis, tinea versicolor, and candidiasis (cream, lotion): Apply two times per day. Fungal nail infection (Penlac): Apply daily to affected nails; apply over previous coat; remove with alcohol every 7 days. Seborrheic dermatitis (Loprox shampoo): Shampoo two times per week for 4 weeks. [Generic/Trade: Shampoo (Loprox) 1% 120 mL. Nail soln (Penlac) 8% 6.6 mL. Generic only: Gel 0.77% 30, 45, 100 g. Cream (Loprox) 0.77% 15, 30, 90 g. Lotion (Loprox TS) 0.77% 30, 60 mL.] ▶K ♀B ▶? $$$$

CLOTRIMAZOLE—TOPICAL (*Lotrimin AF, Mycelex, ✦Canesten, Clotrimaderm*) Treatment of tinea pedis, tinea cruris, tinea corporis, tinea versicolor, and cutaneous candidiasis: Apply two times per day. [Note that Lotrimin brand cream and soln are clotrimazole, while Lotrimin powders and liquid spray are miconazole. Rx Generic only: Cream 1% 15, 30, 45 g. Soln 1% 10, 30 mL. OTC Generic/Trade (Lotrimin AF): Cream 1% 12, 24 g.] ▶L ♀B ▶? $

ECONAZOLE (*Ecoza*) Tinea pedis, tinea cruris, tinea corporis, tinea versicolor: Apply daily. Cutaneous candidiasis: Apply two times per day. [Generic only: Cream 1% 15, 30, 85 g. Trade only: Foam 1% 70 g (Ecoza-$$$$$)] ▶not absorbed ♀C ▶? $$

EFINACONAZOLE (*Jublia*) Onychomycosis of toenail: Apply once daily to affected toenail for 48 weeks. [Trade: Soln 1% 4, 8 mL brush applicator.] ▶minimal absorption ♀C ▶? $$$$$

KETOCONAZOLE—TOPICAL (*Extina, Nizoral, Nizoral AD, Xolegel, ✦Ketoderm*) Tinea/candidal infections: Apply daily. Seborrheic dermatitis: Apply cream one

(cont.)

to two times per day for 4 weeks or gel daily for 2 weeks or foam two times per day for 4 weeks. Dandruff (Nizoral AD): Apply shampoo twice a week. Tinea versicolor: Apply shampoo to affected area, leave on for 5 min, rinse. [Generic/Trade: Shampoo 2% 120 mL. Generic only: Cream 2% 15, 30, 60 g. Trade only: Shampoo 1% 125, 200 mL (OTC Nizoral AD). Gel 2% 45 g (Xolegel). Foam 2% 50, 100 g (Extina).] ▶L ♀C ▶? $$

LULICONAZOLE (*Luzu*) Tinea pedis: Apply once daily for 2 weeks. Tinea cruris, tinea corporis: Apply once daily for 1 week. [Trade: 1% cream, 60g.] ▶minimal absorption ♀C ▶? $$$$$

MICONAZOLE—TOPICAL (*Micatin, Lotrimin AF, ZeaSorb AF*) Tinea, candida: Apply two times per day. [Note that Lotrimin brand cream and soln are clotrimazole, while Lotrimin powders and liquid spray are miconazole. OTC Generic only: Cream 2% 15, 45 g. OTC Trade only: Powder 2% 70, 160 g. Spray powder 2% 90, 100, 140 g. Spray liquid 2% 90, 105 mL. Gel 2% 24 g.] ▶L ♀+ ▶? $

NAFTIFINE (*Naftin*) Tinea: Apply daily (cream) or two times per day (gel). [Generic/Trade: Cream 1% 60, 90 g. Trade only: Cream 1% Pump 90 g. Gel 1% 40, 60, 90 g. Gel 2% 45, 60 g. Cream 2% 45, 60 g.] ▶LK ♀B ▶? $$$$$

NYSTATIN—TOPICAL (*Mycostatin, Nyamyc, ✦Nyaderm*) Candidiasis: Apply two to three times per day. [Generic only: Cream, Oint 100,000 units/g 15, 30 g. Generic/Trade: Powder 100,000 units/g 15, 30, 60 g.] ▶not absorbed ♀C ▶? $$

OXICONAZOLE (*Oxistat, Oxizole*) Tinea pedis, tinea cruris, and tinea corporis: Apply one to two times per day. Tinea versicolor (cream only): Apply daily. [Trade only: Cream 1% 30, 60, 90 g. Lotion 1% 30, 60 mL.] ▶minimal absorption ♀B ▶? $$$$$

SERTACONAZOLE (*Ertaczo*) Tinea pedis: Apply two times per day. [Trade only: Cream 2% 60 g.] ▶minimal absorption ♀C ▶? $$$$$

TERBINAFINE—TOPICAL (*Lamisil, Lamisil AT*) Tinea: Apply one to two times per day. [OTC Generic/Trade: (Lamisil AT): Cream 1% 12, 24 g. OTC Trade only: Spray pump soln 1% 30 mL. Gel 1% 6, 12 g.] ▶L ♀B ▶? $

TOLNAFTATE (*Tinactin*) Apply two times per day. [OTC Generic/Trade: Cream 1% 15, 30 g. Soln 1% 10 mL. Powder 1% 45 g. OTC Trade only: Gel 1% 15 g. Powder 1% 90 g. Spray powder 1% 100, 133, 150 g. Spray liquid 1% 100, 113 mL.] ▶? ♀? ▶? $

Antiparasitics (Topical)

BENZYL ALCOHOL (*Ulesfia*) Lice: Apply to dry hair to saturate scalp and hair. Rinse after 10 minutes. Reapply in 7 to 10 days. Flammable. [Trade only: Lotion 5% 60 mL and in 2-pack with nit comb.] ▶not absorbed ♀B ▶? $$$$

CROTAMITON (*Eurax*) Scabies: Apply cream/lotion topically from chin to feet, repeat in 24 h, bathe 48 h later. Pruritus: Massage prn. [Trade only: Cream 10% 60 g. Lotion 10% 60, 480 mL.] ▶? ♀C ▶? $$$$$

LINDANE Other drugs preferred. Scabies: Apply 30 to 60 mL of lotion, wash after 8 to 12 h. Lice: 30 to 60 mL of shampoo, wash off after 4 min. Can cause seizures in epileptics or if overused/misused in children. Not for infants. [Generic only: Lotion 1% 60 mL. Shampoo 1% 60 mL.] ▶L ♀B ▶? $$$$

MALATHION (*Ovide*) Lice: Apply to dry hair, let dry naturally, wash off in 8 to 12 h. Repeat in 7 to 10 days, if lice present. Flammable. [Generic/Trade only: Lotion 0.5% 59 mL.] ▶? ♀B ▶? $$$$

PERMETHRIN (*Elimite, Acticin, Nix, ✝Kwellada-P*) Scabies: Apply cream from head (avoid mouth/nose/eyes) to soles of feet and wash after 8 to 14 h. 30 g is typical adult dose. Repeat in 7 days. Lice: Saturate hair and scalp with 1% rinse, wash after 10 min. Do not use in age younger than 2 mo. May repeat therapy in 7 days, as necessary. [Generic/Trade: Cream (Elimite, Acticin) 5% 60 g. OTC Generic/Trade: Liquid creme rinse (Nix) 1% 60 mL.] ▶L ♀B ▶? $$

PYRETHRINS + PIPERONYL BUTOXIDE (*✝R&C*) Lice: Apply shampoo, wash after 10 min. Reapply in 5 to 10 days. A-200 brand name no longer available. [OTC Generic/Trade: Shampoo (0.33% pyrethrins, 4% piperonyl butoxide) 60, 120 mL.] ▶L♀C ▶? $

RID (pyrethrins + piperonyl butoxide) Lice: Apply shampoo/mousse, wash after 10 min. Reapply in 5 to 10 days prn. [OTC Generic/Trade: Shampoo 60, 120, 240 mL. OTC Trade only: Mousse 5.5 oz.] ▶L ♀C ▶? $

SPINOSAD (*Natroba*) Lice: Apply to dry hair/scalp to cover. Leave on 10 min then rinse. Retreat if live lice seen after 7 days. [Generic/Trade: Topical susp, 0.9%, 120 mL.] ▶not absorbed – ♀B ▶? $$$$$

Antipsoriatics

ACITRETIN (*Soriatane*) 25 to 50 mg PO daily. Avoid pregnancy during therapy and for 3 years after discontinuation. [Generic/Trade: Caps 10, 17.5, 25 mg.] ▶L ♀X ▶– $$$$$

ANTHRALIN (*Zithranol*) Scalp psoriasis: Apply shampoo to scalp 3 to 4 times a week. Lather and leave on for 3 to 5 min. Rinse. Psoriasis of skin or scalp: Apply cream once a day. Initially use short contact times (5 to 15 min) and gradually increase to 30 min. Wash off. [Trade: Shampoo 1% (Zithranol shampoo) 85 g. Cream 1.2% (Zithranol RR cream) 15, 45 g.] ▶minimal absorption ♀C ▶? $$$$$

ANTHRALIN (*Drithocreme*) Apply daily. Short contact periods (ie, 15 to 20 min) followed by removal may be preferred. [Trade only: Cream 0.5, 1% 50 g.] ▶? ♀C ▶– $$$

CALCIPOTRIENE (*Dovonex, Sorilux*) Apply two times per day. [Trade only: Oint 0.005% 30, 60, 100 g (Dovonex). Cream 0.005% 30, 60, 100 g (Dovonex). Foam for scalp 0.005% 60, 120 g (Sorilux). Generic/Trade: Scalp soln 0.005% 60 mL.] ▶L ♀C ▶? $$$$

CALCIPOTRIOL + BETAMETHASONE (*✝Dovobet*) Canada only. Apply once daily for up to 4 weeks (severe scalp psoriasis) or up to 8 weeks (mild to moderate plaque psoriasis of body). [Rx: Trade: Gel (50 mcg/g calcipotriol and 0.5 mg/g betamethasone) 30g, 60g.] ▶L ♀D ▶? $$$$$

TACLONEX (calcipotriene + betamethasone—topical) Apply daily for up to 4 weeks. [Calcipotriene 0.005% + betamethasone dipropionate 0.064%. Generic/Trade: Oint 60, 100 g. Trade only: Topical susp (Taclonex) 60, 120 g.] ▶L ♀C ▶? $$$$$

USTEKINUMAB (*Stelara*) Severe plaque psoriasis, active psoriatic arthritis, wt less than or equal to 100 kg: 45 mg SC initially and again 4 weeks later, followed by

(cont.)

45 mg SC q 12 weeks. For wt greater than 100 kg and psoriatic arthritis with moderate to severe plaque psoriasis: 90 mg SC initially and again 4 weeks later, followed by 90 mg SC q 12 weeks. [Trade only: 45 and 90 mg prefilled syringe and vial.] ▶L ♀B ▶? $$$$$

Antivirals (Topical)

ACYCLOVIR—TOPICAL (*Zovirax*) Herpes genitalis: Apply ointment q 3 h (6 times per day) for 7 days. Recurrent herpes labialis: Apply cream 5 times per day for 4 days. [Generic/Trade: Oint 5% 5, 15, 30 g. Trade only: Cream 5% 5 g.] ▶K ♀C ▶? $$$$$

DOCOSANOL (*Abreva*) Oral-facial herpes (cold sores): Apply 5 times per day until healed. [OTC Trade only: Cream 10% 2 g.] ▶not absorbed ♀B ▶? $

IMIQUIMOD (*Aldara, Zyclara, ✦Vyloma*) Genital/perianal warts: Apply once daily for up to 8 weeks. Wash off after 8 h. Non-hyperkeratotic, non-hypertrophic actinic keratoses on face/scalp in immunocompetent adults: Apply two times per week overnight for 16 weeks (Aldara) or once daily for two 2-week periods separated by a 2-week break (Zyclara). Wash off after 8 h. Primary superficial basal cell carcinoma: Apply 5 times a week for 6 weeks (Aldara). Wash off after 8 h. [Generic/Trade: Cream 5% (Aldara) single-use packets. Trade only: Cream 3.75% (Zyclara-$$$$$) single-use packets, box of 28 and 7.5 g pump. Cream 2.5% 7.5 g pump.] ▶not absorbed ♀C ▶? $$$

PENCICLOVIR (*Denavir*) Herpes labialis (cold sores): Apply cream q 2 h while awake for 4 days. [Trade only: Cream 1% tube 5 g.] ▶not absorbed ♀B ▶? $$$$$

PODOFILOX (*Condylox, ✦Condyline, Wartec*) External genital warts (gel and soln) and perianal warts (gel only): Apply two times per day for 3 consecutive days of the week and repeat for up to 4 weeks. [Generic/Trade: Soln 0.5% 3.5 mL. Trade only: Gel 0.5% 3.5 g.] ▶? ♀C ▶? $$$

PODOPHYLLIN (*Podocon-25, Podofin, Podofilm*) Warts: Apply by physician. [Not to be dispensed to patients. For hospital/clinic use, not intended for outpatient prescribing. Trade only: Liquid 25% 15 mL.] ▶? ♀− ▶− $$$

SINECATECHINS (*Veregen*) Apply three times per day to external genital and perianal warts for up to 16 weeks. [Trade only: Oint 15% 30 g.] ▶minimal absorption ♀C ▶? $$$$$

Atopic Dermatitis Preparations

NOTE: *Potential risk of cancer. Should only be used as second-line agent for short-term and intermittent treatment of atopic dermatitis in those unresponsive to or intolerant of other treatments.*

PIMECROLIMUS (*Elidel*) Atopic dermatitis: Apply two times per day. [Trade only: Cream 1% 30, 60, 100 g.] ▶L ♀C ▶? $$$$$ ■

TACROLIMUS—TOPICAL (*Protopic*) Atopic dermatitis: Apply two times per day. [Generic/Trade: Oint 0.03%, 0.1% 30, 60, 100 g.] ▶minimal absorption ♀C ▶? $$$$$ ■

Corticosteroid/Antimicrobial Combinations

CORTISPORIN (neomycin—topical + polymyxin—topical + hydrocortisone—topical) Apply two to four times per day. [Trade only: Cream 7.5 g. Oint (also contains bacitracin) 15 g.] ▶LK ♀C ▶? $$$$

FUSIDIC ACID—TOPICAL + HYDROCORTISONE—TOPICAL (✦*Fucidin-H*) Canada only. Apply three times per day. [Canada Trade only: Cream (2% fusidic acid, 1% hydrocortisone acetate) 30 g.] ▶L ♀? ▶? $$

LOTRISONE (clotrimazole—topical + betamethasone—topical, ✦*Lotriderm*) Apply two times per day. Do not use for diaper rash. [Generic/Trade: Cream (clotrimazole 1% + betamethasone 0.05%) 15, 45 g. Lotion (clotrimazole 1% + betamethasone 0.05%) 30 mL.] ▶L ♀C ▶? $$$

MYCOLOG II (nystatin—topical + triamcinolone—topical) Apply two times per day. [Generic only: Cream, Oint 15, 30, 60 g.] ▶L ♀C ▶? $$$$$

Hemorrhoid Care

DIBUCAINE (*Nupercainal*) Apply three to four times per day prn. [OTC Generic/Trade: Oint 1% 30, 60 g.] ▶L ♀? ▶? $

HYDROCORTISONE—TOPICAL + PRAMOXINE—TOPICAL (*Analpram-HC, Epifoam, Proctofoam HC, Pramosone*) [Generic/Trade: Cream (Analpram-HC 1% hydrocortisone + 1% pramoxine, 2.5% hydrocortisone + 1% pramoxine) 4 g, 30 g. Trade only: Topical aerosol foam (Proctofoam HC, Epifoam 1% hydrocortisone + 1% pramoxine) 10 g. Lotion (Analpram-HC, Pramosone 2.5% hydrocortisone + 1% pramoxine) 60, 120 mL. Lotion (Pramosone 1% hydrocortisone + 1% pramoxine) 60, 120, 240 mL. Oint (Pramosone 1% hydrocortisone + 1% pramoxine, 2.5% hydrocortisone + 1% pramoxine) 28 g.] ▶L ♀C ▶? $$$

PRAMOXINE (*Tucks Hemorrhoidal Ointment, Fleet Pain Relief, ProctoFoam NS*) Apply up to 5 times per day prn. [OTC Trade only: Oint (Tucks Hemorrhoidal Ointment) 30 g. Pads (Fleet Pain Relief) 100 each. Aerosol foam (ProctoFoam NS) 15 g.] ▶not absorbed ♀+ ▶+ $

STARCH (*Tucks Suppositories*) 1 suppository up to 6 times per day prn. [OTC Trade only: Supp (51% topical starch; vegetable oil, tocopheryl acetate) 12, 24 each.] ▶not absorbed ♀+ ▶+ $

WITCH HAZEL (*Tucks*) Apply to anus/perineum up to 6 times per day prn. [OTC Generic/Trade: Pads 50% 12, 40, 100 ea, generically available in various quantities.] ▶? ♀+ ▶+ $

Other Dermatologic Agents

ALITRETINOIN (*Panretin, ✦Toctino*) Apply two times per day to four times per day to cutaneous Kaposi's lesions. [Trade only: Gel 0.1% 60 g.] ▶not absorbed ♀D ▶− $$$$$

ALUMINUM CHLORIDE (*Drysol, Certain Dri*) Apply at bedtime. [Rx Trade only: Soln 20% 37.5 mL bottle, 35, 60 mL bottle with applicator. OTC Trade only (Certain Dri): Soln 12.5% 36 mL bottle.] ▶K ♀? ▶? $

BECAPLERMIN (*Regranex*) Diabetic ulcers: Apply daily. [Trade only: Gel 0.01%, 15 g.] ▶minimal absorption ♀C ▷? $$$$$ ■

BRIMONIDINE (*Mirvaso*) Persistent erythema associated with rosacea: Apply once daily to chin, forehead, nose, and each cheek. [0.33% gel, 30, 45 g.] ▶L ♀B ▷− $$$$$

CALAMINE Apply three to four times per day prn for poison ivy/oak or insect bite itching. [OTC Generic only: Lotion 120, 240, 480 mL.] ▶? ♀? ▷? $

CAPSAICIN (*Zostrix, Zostrix-HP, Qutenza*) Arthritis, post-herpetic or diabetic neuralgia: Apply three to four times per day. Post-herpetic neuralgia: 1 patch (Qutenza) applied for 1 hour in medical office, may repeat q 3 months. [Rx: Patch 8% (Qutenza). OTC Generic/Trade: Cream 0.025% 60 g, 0.075% (HP) 60 g. OTC Generic only: Lotion 0.025% 59 mL, 0.075% 59 mL.] ▶? ♀? ▷? $

COAL TAR (*Polytar, Tegrin, Cutar, Tarsum*) Seborrheic dermatitis: Apply shampoo at least twice a week. Psoriasis: Apply one to four times per day. [OTC Generic/Trade: Shampoo, cream, ointment, gel, lotion, liquid, oil, soap.] ▶? ♀? ▷? $

DEET (*Off, Cutter, Repel, Ultrathon, n,n-diethyl-m-toluamide*) Mosquito repellant: 10% to 50% every 2 to 6 h. Higher concentration products do not work better, but have a longer duration of action. [OTC Generic/Trade: Spray, lotion, towelette 4.75% to 100%.] ▶? ♀? ▷? $

DEOXYCHOLIC ACID (*Kybella*) Reduction of chin (submental) fullness: 0.2 mL injections 1 cm apart until all of planned treatment area have been injected. [Injectable solution.] ▶not absorbed ♀? ▷? $$$$$

DOXEPIN—TOPICAL (*Prudoxin, Zonalon*) Pruritus: Apply four times per day for up to 8 days. [Trade only: Cream 5% 30, 45 g.] ▶L ♀B ▷− $$$$$

EFLORNITHINE (*Vaniqa*) Reduction of facial hair: Apply to face two times per day. [Trade only: Cream 13.9% 30, 45 g.] ▶K ♀C ▷? $$$

HYALURONIC ACID (*Bionect, Restylane, Perlane*) Moderate to severe facial wrinkles: Inject into wrinkle/fold (Restylane, Perlane). Protection of dermal ulcers: Apply gel/cream/spray two or three times per day (Bionect). [OTC Trade only: Cream 2% 15, 30 g. Rx Generic/Trade: Soln 3% 30 mL. Gel 4% 30 g. Cream 4% 15, 30, 60 g. Injectable gel 2%.] ▶? ♀? ▷? $$$$$

HYDROQUINONE (*Eldopaque, Eldoquin, Eldoquin Forte, EpiQuin Micro, Esoterica, Glyquin, Lustra, Melanex, Solaquin, Claripel, ✦Ultraquin*) Hyperpigmentation: Apply two times per day. [OTC Generic/Trade: Cream 2% 15, 30 g. Rx Generic/Trade: Soln 3% 30 mL. Gel 4% 30 g. Cream 4% 15, 30, 60 g.] ▶? ♀C ▷?

IVERMECTIN—TOPICAL (*Sklice, Soolantra*) Lice (Sklice): Apply lotion to dry hair and scalp. Rinse after 10 min. Single application only. Rosacea (Soolantra): Apply cream to affected area once daily. [Trade: Lotion (Sklice) 0.5%, 120 mL. Cream (Soolantra) 1% 30, 45, 60 g.] ▶minimal absorption —♀C ▷? $$$$$

LACTIC ACID (*Lac-Hydrin, AmLactin, ✦Dermalac*) Apply two times per day. [Trade only: Lotion 12% 150, 360 mL. OTC: Cream 12% 140, 385 g. AmLactin AP is lactic acid (12%) with pramoxine (1%).] ▶? ♀? ▷? $$

LIDOCAINE—TOPICAL (*Xylocaine, Lidoderm, Numby Stuff, LMX, Zingo, ✦Maxilene*) Apply prn. Dose varies with anesthetic procedure, degree of anesthesia required, and individual patient response. Postherpetic neuralgia:

(cont.)

Apply up to 3 patches to affected area at once for up to 12 h within a 24-h period. Apply 30 min prior to painful procedure (ELA-Max 4%). Discomfort with anorectal disorders: Apply prn (ELA-Max 5%). Intradermal powder injection for venipuncture/IV cannulation, 3 to 18 yo (Zingo): 0.5 mg to site 1 to 10 min prior. [For membranes of mouth and pharynx: Spray 10%, Oint 5%, Liquid 5%, Soln 2%, 4%, Dental patch. For urethral use: Jelly 2%. Patch (Lidoderm $$$$$) 5%. Intradermal powder injection system: 0.5 mg (Zingo). OTC Trade only: Liposomal lidocaine 4% (ELA-Max).] ▶LK ♀B ▶+ $ - varies by therapy

MINOXIDIL—TOPICAL (*Rogaine, Women's Rogaine, Rogaine Extra Strength, Minoxidil for Men*) Androgenetic alopecia in men or women: 1 mL to dry scalp two times per day. [OTC Generic/Trade: Soln 2% 60 mL (Rogaine, Women's Rogaine). Soln 5% 60 mL (Rogaine Extra Strength, Theroxidil Extra Strength—for men only). Foam 5% 60 g (Rogaine Extra Strength).] ▶K ♀C ▶- $

OATMEAL (*Aveeno*) Pruritus from poison ivy/oak, varicella: Apply lotion four times per day prn. Also bath packets for tub. [OTC Generic/Trade: Lotion. Bath packets.] ▶not absorbed ♀? ▶? $

PLIAGLIS (tetracaine—topical + lidocaine—topical) Superficial dermatological procedures: Apply 20 to 30 min prior procedure. Tattoo removal: Apply 60 min prior procedure. [Generic/Trade: Cream lidocaine 7% + tetracaine 7%.] ▶minimal absorption ♀B ▶? $$

PRAMOSONE (pramoxine—topical + hydrocortisone—topical, *Pramox HC*) Inflammatory and pruritic manifestations of corticosteroid-responsive dermatoses: Apply three to four times per day. [Generic/Trade: 1% pramoxine/1% hydrocortisone: Cream 30, 60 g. 1% pramoxine/2.5% hydrocortisone acetate: Cream 30, 60 g. Trade only: 1% pramoxine/1% hydrocortisone: Oint 30 g. Lotion 60, 120, 240 mL. 1% pramoxine/2.5% hydrocortisone acetate: Oint 30 g. Lotion 60, 120 mL.] ▶not absorbed ♀C ▶? $$$

SELENIUM SULFIDE (*Selsun, Exsel, Versel, Tersi*) Dandruff, seborrheic dermatitis: Apply 5 to 10 mL two times per week for 2 weeks then less frequently, thereafter. Tinea versicolor: Apply 2.5% to affected area daily for 7 days. [OTC Generic/Trade: Lotion/Shampoo 1% 120, 210, 240, 325 mL, 2.5% 120 mL. Rx Generic/Trade: Lotion/Shampoo 2.5% 120 mL. Trade only: Foam 2.25% 70 g] ▶? ♀C ▶? $

SUNSCREEN Apply according to manufacturer's directions. [Many formulations available.] ▶minimal absorption ♀? ▶+ $

SYNERA (tetracaine—topical + lidocaine—topical) Superficial dermatologic procedures: Apply 20 to 30 min prior to procedure. [Trade only: Topical patch (lidocaine 70 mg + tetracaine 70 mg).] ▶minimal absorption ♀B ▶? $$

TRI-LUMA (fluocinolone—topical + hydroquinone + tretinoin) Melasma of the face: Apply at bedtime for 4 to 8 weeks. [Trade only: Cream 30 g (fluocinolone 0.01% + hydroquinone 4% + tretinoin 0.05%).] ▶minimal absorption ♀C ▶? $$$$

VUSION (miconazole—topical + zinc oxide + white petrolatum) Diaper rash: Apply to affected area with each change for 7 days. [Trade only: Oint 50 g.] ▶minimal absorption ♀C ▶? $$$$$

XERESE (acyclovir + hydrocortisone) Recurrent herpes labialis: Apply 5 times a day, starting at the 1st signs and symptoms. ▶minimal absorption ♀B ▶? $$$$$

ENDOCRINE AND METABOLIC

A1C REDUCTION IN TYPE 2 DIABETES

Intervention	Expected A1C Reduction with Monotherapy
Alpha-glucosidase inhibitors	0.5–0.8%
Canagliflozin	0.7–1%
DPP-4 Inhibitors (gliptins)	0.5–0.8%
GLP-1 agonists	0.5–1%
Insulin	1.5–3.5%
Lifestyle modifications	1–2%
Meglitinides	0.5–1.5%
Metformin	1–2%
Pramlintide	0.5–1%
Sulfonylureas	1–2%
Thiazolidinediones	0.5–1.4%

References: *Diabetes Care* 2009; 32:195. *Diabetes Obes Metab* 2013;15:372–82.

IV SOLUTIONS

Solution	Dextrose	Calories/ Liter	Na*	Ca*	Lactate*	Osm*
0.9 NS	0 g/L	0	154	0	0	310
LR	0 g/L	9	130	3	28	273
D5 W	50 g/L	170	0	0	0	253
D5 0.2 NS	50 g/L	170	34	0	0	320
D5 0.45 NS	50 g/L	170	77	0	0	405
D5 0.9 NS	50 g/L	170	154	0	0	560
D5 LR	50 g/L	170	130	2.7	28	527

* All given in mEq/L

CORTICOSTEROIDS

CORTICOSTEROIDS	Approximate Equivalent Dose (mg)	Relative Anti-inflammatory Potency	Relative Mineralocorti-coid Potency	Biological Half-life (h)
betamethasone	0.6–0.75	20–30	0	36–54
cortisone	25	0.8	2	8–12
dexamethasone	0.75	20–30	0	36–54
fludrocortisone	n.a.	10	125	18–36
hydrocortisone	20	1	2	8–12
methylprednisolone	4	5	0	18–36
prednisolone	5	4	1	18–36
prednisone	5	4	1	18–36
triamcinolone	4	5	0	12–36

n.a., not available.

DIABETES NUMBERS*

Criteria for diagnosis Pre-diabetes: Fasting glucose 100–125 mg/dL A1C 5.7–6.4% 2 h after 75 g oral glucose load: 140–199 mg/dL **Diabetes**:[†] A1C ≥ 6.5% Fasting glucose ≥ 126 mg/dL Random glucose with symptoms ≥ 200 mg/dL 2 h after 75 g oral glucose load ≥ 200 mg/dL	**Self-monitoring glucose goals** Preprandial: 80–130 mg/dL Postprandial: < 180 mg/dL **A1C goal**: < 7% for most non-pregnant adults, individualize based on age, comorbid conditions, microvascular complications, known cardiovascular disease, hypoglycemia, and other patient specific factors. A1C goal < 7.5% for pediatric Type 1 Diabetes.

(cont.)

DIABETES NUMBERS* (*continued*)

Hospitalized patients: may consider more stringent goal if safely achievable without hypoglycemia	**Mean gluose levels by A1C:**

A1C (%)	Glucose (mg/dL)
6	126
7	154
8	183
9	212
10	240

Critically ill glucose goal: 140–180 mg/dL

Non-critically ill glucose goal (hospitalized patients): premeal blood glucose < 140 mg/dL, random < 180 mg/dL

Estimated average glucose (eAG):
eAG (mg/dL) = $(28.7 \times A1C) - 46.7$

Complications prevention and management:

ASA[‡] (75–162 mg/day) in Type 1 & 2 adults for primary prevention if 10-year cardiovascular risk > 10% (includes most men older than 50 yo or women older than 60 yo with at least one other major risk factor of hypertension, smoking dyslipidemia, albuminuria or family history of cardiovascular disease) and secondary prevention (those with vascular disease)

ACE inhibitor or ARB if hypertensive or albuminuria

Statin: high intensity therapy in those with overt cardiovascular disease (CVD) or as below in other risk groups.

Statin Recommendations for those without overt CVD

Age	CVD Risk Factors (hypertension, overweight/obesity, smoking, LDL ≥ 100 mg/dL)	Statin Intensity Recommendation
Less than 40 yo	No	None
	Yes	Moderate or high
40 yo or older	No	Moderate
	Yes	High, if 40–75 yo Moderate or high, if older than 75 yo

(cont.)

ENDOCRINE AND METABOLIC

DIABETES NUMBERS* (continued)

> **Immunizations:** annual flu vaccine; hepatitis B vaccine if previously unvaccinated and 19 to 59 yo, consider if age 60 yo or older; pneumococcal vaccine: PPSV23 to all age 2 or older, if age 65 or older and unvaccinated give PCV13 then PPSV23 6–12 months later, if age 65 yo or older and previously vaccinated with PPSV23, give PCV13 ≥ 12 months later.
>
> **Every visit:** Measure wt & BP (goal < 140/90 mm Hg§); visual foot exam; review self-monitoring glucose record; review/adjust meds; review self-mgmt skills, dietary needs, and physical activity; smoking cessation counseling.
>
> **Twice a year:** A1C in those meeting treatment goals with stable glycemia (quarterly if not); dental exam.
>
> **Annually:** Screening fasting lipid profile (or q 2 years with low-risk lipid values)**; creatinine; albumin to creatinine ratio spot collection; dilated eye exam (q2 years if no evidence of retinopathy).

*See recommendations at: care.diabetesjournals.org. References: Diabetes Care 2015; 38(Suppl 1):S1-93.

Glucose values are plasma.

†In the absence of symptoms, confirm diagnosis with glucose testing on subsequent day.

‡Avoid ASA if younger than 21 yo due to Reye's Syndrome risk; use if younger than 30 yo has not been studied.

§Lower systolic targets (i.e. < 130 mm Hg) may be considered on a patient-specific basis if treatment goals can be met without excessive treatment burden.

**In those on statin therapy, check a fasting lipid panel as needed to monitor for adherence.

Androgens/Anabolic Steroids

NOTE: *See OB/GYN section for other hormones.*

TESTOSTERONE (*Androderm, AndroGel, Axiron, Aveed, Delatestryl, Depo-Testosterone, Striant, Testim, Testopel, Testro AQ, Vogelxo, Natesto, ✦Andriol*) Hypogonadism: Injectable enanthate or cypionate: 50 to 400 mg IM q 2 to 4 weeks. Injectable undecanoate (Aveed): 750 mg IM, repeat in 4 weeks then q 10 weeks thereafter. Testopel: 2 to 6 (150 to 450 mg testosterone) pellets SC q 3 to 6 months. Transdermal: Androderm: Start 4 mg patch to nonscrotal skin at bedtime. AndroGel 1%: Apply 5 g from gel pack or 4 pumps (5 g gel; 50 mg testosterone) from dispenser daily to shoulders/upper arms/abdomen. Androgel 1.62%: Apply 2 pumps (40.5 mg testosterone) from dispenser daily to shoulders or upper arms. Adjust based on serum testosterone concentration q14 to 28 days. Dose range 1 to 4 pumps daily. Axiron: 60 mg (1 pump of 30 mg to each axilla) once daily. Testim: 1 tube (5 g) daily to shoulders/upper arms. Vogelxo: 50 mg (1 tube, 1 packet, or 4 pumps) once daily. Buccal: Striant: 30 mg q 12 h on upper gum above the incisor tooth; alternate sides for each

(cont.)

application.   [Generic/Trade: Gel 1% 2.5, 5 g packet, 75 g multidose pump (AndroGel 1% 1.25 g gel containing 12.5 mg testosterone per actuation). Gel (Fortesta) 10 mg/actuation. Injection 100, 200 mg/mL (cypionate), 200 mg/mL (ethanate). Trade only: Patch 2, 4 mg/24 h (Androderm). Gel 1.62%, (AndroGel 1.62%) 1.25, 2.5 g (package of 30), 75 g multidose pump (AndroGel 1.62% 20.25 mg testosterone/actuation). Gel 1%, 5 g tube (Testim). Gel (Vogelxo): 50 mg tube, 50 mg packet or multi-dose pump: 12.5 mg/actuation. Soln 90 mL multidose pump (Axiron, 30 mg/actuation). Nasal Gel (Natesto 5.5 mg/ actuation pump) 7.32 g. Pellet 75 mg (Testopel). Buccal: Blister packs: 30 mg (Striant). IM injection (Aveed): 750 mg/3 mL through restricted access program.] ▶L ♀X ▷? ⊚lll varies by therapy ■

Bisphosphonates

ALENDRONATE (*Fosamax, Fosamax Plus D, Binosto, ✦Fosavance*) Prevention of postmenopausal osteoporosis (Fosamax): 5 mg PO daily or 35 mg PO weekly. Treatment of postmenopausal osteoporosis (Fosamax, Fosamax Plus D, Binosto): 10 mg daily, 70 mg PO weekly, 70 mg/vitamin D3 2800 international units PO weekly, or 70 mg/vitamin D3 5600 international units PO weekly. Treatment of glucocorticoid-induced osteoporosis (Fosamax): 5 mg PO daily in men and women or 10 mg PO daily in postmenopausal women not taking estrogen. Treatment of osteoporosis in men (Fosamax, Fosamax Plus D, Binosto): 10 mg PO daily, 70 mg PO weekly, or 70 mg/vitamin D3 2800 international units PO weekly, or 70 mg/vit D3 5600 international units PO weekly. Paget's disease (Fosamax): 40 mg PO daily for 6 months. [Generic/Trade (Fosamax): Tabs 10, 70 mg. Oral Soln 70 mg/75 mL. Generic only: Tabs 5, 35, 40 mg. Trade only: Fosamax Plus D: 70 mg + either 2800 or 5600 units of vitamin D3. Binosto: 70 mg effervescent tab.] ▶K ♀C ▷− $

ETIDRONATE (*Didronel*) Paget's disease:–5 to 10 mg/kg PO daily for 6 months or 11 to 20 mg/kg daily for 3 months. [Generic only: Tabs 200, 400 mg.] ▶K ♀C ▷? $$$$$

IBANDRONATE (*Boniva*) Prevention and treatment of postmenopausal osteoporosis: Oral: 150 mg PO once a month. IV: 3 mg IV q 3 months. [Generic/Trade: Tab 150 mg. IV: 3 mg.] ▶K ♀C ▷? $$$$

PAMIDRONATE (*Aredia*) Hypercalcemia of malignancy: 60 to 90 mg IV over 2 to 24 h. Wait at least 7 days before considering retreatment. ▶K ♀D ▷? $$$$

RISEDRONATE (*Actonel, Atelvia*) Prevention and treatment of postmenopausal osteoporosis: 5 mg PO daily, 35 mg PO weekly, or 150 mg once a month. Treatment of osteoporosis in men: 35 mg PO weekly. Prevention and treatment of glucocorticoid-induced osteoporosis: 5 mg PO daily. Paget's disease: 30 mg PO daily for 2 months. [Generic/Trade: Tabs 5, 30, 35, 150 mg. Delayed-release tab (Atelvia): 35 mg.] ▶K ♀C ▷? $$$$$

ZOLEDRONIC ACID (*Reclast, Zometa, ✦Aclasta*) Treatment of osteoporosis (Reclast): 5 mg once yearly IV infusion over 15 min or longer. Prevention of postmenopausal osteoporosis: (Reclast) 5 mg IV infusion q 2 years. Prevention

(cont.)

and treatment of glucocorticoid-induced osteoporosis (Reclast): 5 mg once a year IV infusion over 15 min or longer. Hypercalcemia (Zometa): 4 mg IV infusion over 15 min or longer. Wait at least 7 days before considering retreatment. Paget's disease (Reclast): 5 mg IV single dose infused over 15 min or longer. Multiple myeloma and metastatic bone lesions from solid tumors (Zometa): 4 mg IV infusion over 15 min or longer q 3 to 4 weeks. [Generic/Trade: 4 mg/5 mL IV (Zometa), 5 mg/100 mL IV (Reclast)] ▶K ♀D ▶? $$$$$

Corticosteroids

NOTE: See also Dermatology, Ophthalmology.

BETAMETHASONE (*Celestone, Celestone Soluspan, ✦Betaject*) Anti-inflammatory/immunosuppressive: 0.6 to 7.2 mg/day PO divided two to four times per day; up to 9 mg/day IM. Fetal lung maturation, maternal antepartum: 12 mg IM q 24 h for 2 doses. [Trade only: Syrup 0.6 mg/5 mL.] ▶L ♀C ▶– $$$$$

CORTISONE (*Cortone*) 25 to 300 mg PO daily. [Generic only: Tabs 25 mg.] ▶L ♀D ▶– $$$$$

DEXAMETHASONE (*Decadron, DexPak, ✦Dexasone*) Anti-inflammatory/immunosuppressive: 0.5 to 9 mg/day PO/IV/IM, divided two to four times per day. Cerebral edema: 10 to 20 mg IV load, then 4 mg IM q 6 h (off-label IV use common) or 1 to 3 mg PO three times per day. Bronchopulmonary dysplasia in preterm infants: 0.5 mg/kg PO/IV divided q 12 h for 3 days, then taper. Croup: 0.6 mg/kg PO or IM for 1 dose. Acute asthma: age older than 2 yo: 0.6 mg/kg to max 16 mg PO daily for 2 days. Fetal lung maturation, maternal antepartum: 6 mg IM q 12 h for 4 doses. Antiemetic, prophylaxis: 8 mg IV or 12 mg PO prior to chemotherapy; 8 mg PO daily for 2 to 4 days. Antiemetic, treatment: 10 to 20 mg PO/IV q 4 to 6 h. [Generic only: Tabs 0.5, 0.75, 1.0, 1.5, 2, 4, 6 mg; elixir 0.5 mg/5 mL; Soln 0.5 mg/5 mL, 1 mg/1 mL (concentrate). Trade only: DexPak 13 day (51 total 1.5 mg tabs for a 13-day taper), DexPak 10 day (35 total 1.5 mg tabs for 10-day taper), DexPak 6 days (21 total 1.5 mg tabs for 6-day taper).] ▶L ♀C ▶– $

FLUDROCORTISONE (*Florinef*) Mineralocorticoid activity: 0.1 mg PO three times per week to 0.2 mg PO daily. Postural hypotension: 0.05 to 0.4 mg PO daily. [Generic only: Tabs 0.1 mg.] ▶L ♀C ▶? $

HYDROCORTISONE (*Cortef, Cortenema, Solu-Cortef*) Adrenocortical insufficiency: 100 to 500 mg IV/IM q 2 to 6 h prn (sodium succinate) or 20 to 240 mg/day PO divided three to four times per day. Ulcerative colitis: 100 mg retention enema at bedtime (laying on side for 1 h or longer) for 21 days. [Generic/Trade: Tabs 5, 10, 20 mg; Enema 100 mg/60 mL.] ▶L ♀C ▶– $$$

METHYLPREDNISOLONE (*Solu-Medrol, Medrol, Depo-Medrol*) Anti-inflammatory/immunosuppressive: Oral (Medrol): Dose varies, 4 to 48 mg PO daily. Medrol Dosepak tapers 24 to 0 mg PO over 7 days. IM/Joints (Depo-Medrol): Dose varies, 4 to 120 mg IM q 1 to 2 weeks. Parenteral (Solu-Medrol): Dose varies, 10 to 250 mg IV/IM. Peds: 0.5 to 1.7 mg/kg PO/IV/IM divided q 6 to 12 h. [Trade only: Tabs 2 mg. Generic/Trade: Tabs 4, 8, 16, 32 mg. Medrol Dosepak (4 mg, 21 tabs).] ▶L ♀C ▶– $$

PREDNISOLONE (*Flo-Pred, Prelone, Pediapred, Orapred, Orapred ODT, Millipred*) 5 to 60 mg PO daily. [Generic/Trade: Tabs 5 mg. Soln 5 mg/5 mL (Pediapred, raspberry flavor). Orally disintegrating tabs 10, 15, 30 mg (Orapred ODT). Trade only: Soln 10 mg/5 mL (Millipred, grape), 20mg/5 mL (Veripred). Susp 15 mg/5 mL (Flo-Pred; cherry flavor). Generic only: Syrup 5 mg/5 mL, 15 mg/5 mL (cherry flavor). Soln 15 mg/5 mL (grape flavor).] ▶L ♀C ▶+ $$$

PREDNISONE (*Rayos, Prednisone Intensol, ✦Winpred*) 1 to 2 mg/kg or 5 to 60 mg PO daily. [Generic only: Tabs 1, 2.5, 5, 10, 20, 50 mg. Soln 5 mg/5 mL, 5 mg/mL (Prednisone Intensol). Dosepacks (5 mg tabs: Tapers 30 to 5 mg PO over 6 days or 30 to 10 mg over 12 days), Dosepacks Double Strength (10 mg tabs: Tapers 60 to 10 mg over 6 days, or 60 to 20 mg PO over 12 days) taper packs. Trade only: Delayed-release tabs 1, 2, 5 mg.] ▶L ♀C ▶+ $

TRIAMCINOLONE (*Aristospan, Kenalog, Triesence*) 4 to 48 mg PO/IM daily. Intra-articular 2.5 to 40 mg (Kenalog, Trivaris), 2 to 20 mg (Aristospan). [Trade only: Injection 10 mg/mL, 40 mg/mL, 5 mg/mL, 20 mg/mL (Aristospan).] ▶L ♀C ▶– $

Diabetes-Related—Alpha-Glucosidase Inhibitors

ACARBOSE (*Precose, ✦Glucobay*) DM, Type 2: Start 25 mg PO three times per day with meals, and gradually increase as tolerated to maintenance, 50 to 100 mg three times per day. [Generic/Trade: Tabs 25, 50, 100 mg.] ▶Gut/K ♀B ▶– $$$

MIGLITOL (*Glyset*) DM, Type 2: Start 25 mg PO three times per day with meals, maintenance 50 to 100 mg three times per day. [Trade only: Tabs 25, 50, 100 mg.] ▶K ♀B ▶– $$$

Diabetes-Related—Combinations

ACTOPLUS MET, ACTOPLUS MET XR (**pioglitazone + metformin**) DM, Type 2: 1 tab PO daily or two times per day. If inadequate control with metformin monotherapy, start 15/500 or 15/850 mg PO one to two times per day. If inadequate control with pioglitazone monotherapy, start 15/500 mg two times per day or 15/850 mg daily. Max 45/2550 mg/day. Extended-release, start 1 tab (15/100 mg or 30/1000 mg) daily with evening meal. Max: 45/2000 mg/day. Obtain LFTs before therapy and periodically thereafter. [Generic/Trade: Tabs 15/500, 15/850 mg. Trade only: Extended-release (Actoplus Met XR) tabs: 15/1000, 30/1000 mg.] ▶KL ♀C ▶? $$$$$ ∎

AVANDAMET (**rosiglitazone + metformin**) DM, Type 2, initial therapy (drug-naive): Start 2/500 mg PO one or two times per day. If inadequate control with metformin alone, select tab strength based on adding 4 mg/day rosiglitazone to existing metformin dose. If inadequate control with rosiglitazone alone, select tab strength based on adding 1000 mg/day metformin to existing rosiglitazone dose. Max 8/2000 mg/day. Obtain LFTs before therapy and periodically thereafter. ▶KL ♀C ▶? $$$$$ ∎

AVANDARYL (**rosiglitazone + glimepiride**) DM, Type 2, initial therapy (drug-naive): Start 4/1 mg PO daily. If switching from monotherapy with a sulfonylurea or glitazone, consider 4/2 mg PO daily. Max 8/4 mg/day. Obtain LFTs before

(cont.)

therapy and periodically thereafter. [Trade only: Tabs 4/1, 4/2, 4/4, 8/2, 8/4 mg rosiglitazone/glimepiride.] ▶LK ♀C ▶? $$$$ ■

DUETACT (pioglitazone + glimepiride) DM, Type 2: Start 30/2 mg PO daily. Start up to 30/4 mg PO daily if prior glimepiride therapy, or 30/2 mg PO daily if prior pioglitazone therapy; max 30/4 mg/day. Obtain LFTs before therapy and periodically thereafter. [Generic/Trade: Tabs 30/2, 30/4 mg pioglitazone/ glimepiride.] ▶LK ♀C ▶? $$$$ ■

GLUCOVANCE (glyburide + metformin) DM, Type 2, Initial therapy (drug-naive): Start 1.25/250 mg PO daily or two times per day with meals; max 10/2000 mg daily. Inadequate control with a sulfonylurea or metformin alone: Start 2.5/500 or 5/500 mg PO two times per day with meals; max 20/2000 mg daily. [Generic/ Trade: Tabs 1.25/250, 2.5/500, 5/500 mg.] ▶KL ♀B ▶? $$$ ■

GLYXAMBI (empagliflozin + linagliptin) DM, Type 2: 1 tab (10 mg empagliflozin/5 mg linagliptin) PO daily in morning. May increase to 25 mg empagliflozin/5 mg linagliptin PO daily. [Trade only: 10/5, 25/5 mg empagliflozin/linagliptin tablets.] ▶LK ♀C ▶? $$$$$

INVOKAMET (canagliflozin + metformin) DM, Type 2: 1 tablet PO twice daily. In patients not taking metformin, start with low dose of 500 mg metformin with gradual dose titration for GI tolerance. In patients not taking canagliflozin, start 50 mg canagliflozin. [Trade only: 50/500, 50/1000, 150/500, 150/1000 canagliflozin/metformin tablets.] ▶KL ♀C ▶? $$$$$ ■

JANUMET, JANUMET XR (sitagliptin + metformin) DM, Type 2: Individualize based on patient's current therapy. Immediate-release: 1 tab PO two times per day. Extended-release: 1 tab PO daily. If inadequate control with metformin monotherapy: Immediate-release: Start 50/500 or 50/1000 mg two times per day based on current metformin dose. Extended-release: Start 100 mg sitagliptin daily plus current daily metformin. If inadequate control on sitagliptin: Immediate-release: Start 50/500 two times per day. Extended-release: Start 100/1000 daily. Max 100/2000 mg/day. Give with meals. [Trade only: Immediate-release tabs 50/500, 50/1000 mg, extended-release tabs 100/1000, 50/500, 50/1000 mg sitagliptin/metformin.] ▶K ♀B ▶? $$$$ ■

JENTADUETO (linagliptin + metformin) DM, Type 2: If prior metformin, start 2.5 mg linagliptin and current metformin dose two times per day. If no prior metformin, start 2.5/5 mg PO two times per day. If current linagliptin/metformin, start at current doses. Max 2.5/1000 mg. [Trade only: 2.5/500, 2.5/850, 2.5/1000 mg.] ▶KL – ♀B ▶? $$$$$ ■

KAZANO (alogliptin + metformin) DM, Type 2: Individualize based on patient's current therapy. 1 tab PO two times per day. Max 25/2000 mg/day. Give with meals. [Trade only: 12.5/500, 12.5/1000 mg alogliptin/metformin.] ▶K – ♀B ▶? $$$$$

KOMBIGLYZE XR (saxagliptin + metformin, ✦Komboglyze) DM, Type 2: If inadequately controlled on metformin alone, start 2.5 to 5 mg of saxagliptin plus current dose of metformin; give once daily with evening meal. If inadequately controlled on saxagliptin, start 5/500 mg once daily with evening meal. Max: 5/2000 mg/day. [Trade only: Tabs 5/500, 2.5/1000, 5/1000 mg.] ▶ ♀B ▶? $$$$$ ■

METAGLIP (glipizide + metformin) DM, Type 2, Initial therapy (drug-naive): Start 2.5/250 mg PO daily to 2.5/500 mg PO two times per day with meals; max 10/2000 mg daily. Inadequate control with a sulfonylurea or metformin alone: Start 2.5/500 or 5/500 mg PO two times per day with meals; max 20/2000 mg daily. [Generic/Trade: Tabs 2.5/250, 2.5/500, 5/500 mg.] ▶KL ♀C ▶? $$$ ■

OSENI (alogliptin + pioglitazone) DM, Type 2: Individualize based on patient's current therapy. 1 tab PO daily. Max 25/45 mg/day. Obtain LFTs before therapy and periodically thereafter. [Trade only: Tabs 12.5/15, 12.5/30, 12.5/45, 25/15, 25/30, 25/45 mg alogliptin/pioglitazone.] ▶KL – ♀C ▶? $$$$$ ■

PRANDIMET (repaglinide + metformin) DM, Type 2, initial therapy (drug-naive): Start 1/500 mg PO daily before meals; max 10/2500 mg daily or 4/1000 mg/meal. May start higher if already taking coadministered doses of repaglinide and metformin. [Trade: Tabs 1/500, 2/500 mg.] ▶KL ♀C ▶? $$$ ■

XIGDUO XR (dapagliflozin + metformin) DM, Type 2: 1 tablet PO once daily in the morning with food. Individualize starting dose based on current treatment. [Trade only: 5/500, 5/1000, 10/500, 10/1000 mg dapagliflozin/metformin extended-release tabs.] ▶KL ♀C ▶? $$$$$ ■

Diabetes-Related—DPP-4 inhibitors

ALOGLIPTIN (*Nesina*) DM, Type 2: 25 mg PO daily. [Trade only: Tabs 6.25, 12.5, 25 mg.] ▶K – ♀B ▶? $$$$$

LINAGLIPTIN (*Tradjenta*, *✦Trajenta*) DM, Type 2: 5 mg PO once daily. [Trade only: Tab 5 mg.] ▶L – ♀B ▶? $$$$$

SAXAGLIPTIN (*Onglyza*) DM, Type 2: 2.5 or 5 mg PO daily. [Trade only: Tabs 2.5, 5 mg.] ▶LK ♀B ▶? $$$$$

SITAGLIPTIN (*Januvia*) DM, Type 2: 100 mg PO daily. [Trade only: Tabs 25, 50, 100 mg.] ▶K ♀B ▶? $$$$$

Diabetes-Related—GLP-1 agonists

ALBIGLUTIDE (*Tanzeum*) DM, Type 2, adjunctive therapy: 30 mg SC once weekly. May increase to 50 mg SC once weekly. [Trade only: 30, 50 mg single-dose pen.] ▶proteolysis ♀C ▶? $$$$$ ■

DULAGLUTIDE (*Trulicity*) DM, Type 2: Start 0.75 mg SC once weekly. May increase to 1.5 mg SC once weekly. [Trade only: 0.75, 1.5 mg single-dose pen; 0.75, 1.5 mg single-dose prefilled syringe.] ▶proteolysis ♀C ▶? $$$$$ ■

EXENATIDE (*Byetta, Bydureon*) DM, Type 2, adjunctive therapy: Immediate-release: 5 mcg SC two times per day (within 1 h before the morning and evening meals, or 1 h before the two main meals of the day at least 6 h apart). May increase to 10 mcg SC two times per day after 1 month. Extended-release: 2 mg SC once weekly given any time of day without regard to meals. [Trade only: Byetta, prefilled pen (60 doses each) 5 mcg/dose, 1.2 mL; 10 mcg/dose, 2.4 mL. Bydureon (extended-release): 2 mg/vial; 2 mg/prefilled pen (single-use).] ▶K/proteolysis ♀C ▶? $$$$$ ■

LIRAGLUTIDE (*Victoza, Saxenda*) DM, Type 2 (Victoza): Start 0.6 mg SC daily for 1 week, then increase to 1.2 mg SC daily. May increase to 1.8 mg SC daily. Chronic weight management (Saxenda): Start 0.6 mg SC daily for 1 week, then increase at weekly intervals to effective dose of 3 mg SC daily. [Trade only (Victoza): Multidose pen (18 mg/3 mL) delivers doses of 0.6, 1.2, or 1.8 mg. Trade only (Saxenda): Multidose pen (18 mg/3 mL) delivers doses of 0.6, 1.2, 1.8, 2.4, or 3 mg.] ▶proteolysis ♀C (Victoza), X (Saxenda) ▶? $$$$$ ■

INJECTABLE INSULINS*

		Onset (h)	Peak (h)	Duration (h)
Rapid-/short-acting	Insulin aspart (NovoLog)	< 0.2	1–3	3–5
	Insulin glulisine (Apidra)	0.30–0.4	1	4–5
	Insulin lispro (Humalog)	0.25–0.5	0.5–2.5	≤5
	Regular (Novolin R, Humulin R)	0.5–1	2–3	3–6
Intermediate-/long-acting	NPH (Novolin N, Humulin N)	2–4	4–10	10–16
	Insulin detemir (Levemir)	n.a.	flat action profile	up to 23
	Insulin glargine (Lantus, Toujeo)	2–4	peakless	24
	Insulin degludec (Tresiba)	1	peakless	>42
Mixtures	Insulin aspart protamine susp/aspart (NovoLog Mix 70/30)	0.25	1–4 (biphasic)	up to 24
	Insulin lispro protamine susp/insulin lispro (Humalog Mix 75/25, Humalog Mix 50/50)	< 0.25	1–3 (biphasic)	10–20
	NPH/Reg (Humulin 70/30, Novolin 70/30)	0.5–1	2–10 (biphasic)	10–20
	Insulin degludec/aspart (Ryzodeg 70/30)	0.25	2–3	>24

*These are general guidelines, as onset, peak, and duration of activity are affected by the site of injection, physical activity, body temperature, and blood supply.

†Dose-dependent duration of action, range from 6 to 23 h.

n.a. = not available.

Diabetes-Related—Insulins

INSULIN—INHALED SHORT-ACTING (*Afrezza*) Diabetes: Insulin naïve: Start 4 units inhaled at each meal. Switching from prandial insulin: 4 to 24 units inhaled per meal depending on prior insulin dose; round up to the nearest 4 units. Switching from premixed insulin: Estimate the mealtime dose by dividing half of the total daily injected premixed dose equally among three meals. Administer 4 to 24 units inhaled per meal depending on prior mealtime insulin dose; round up to the nearest 4 units. [Trade only: 4, 8, 12 unit cartridges.] ▶K ♀C ▶? $$$$$ ■

INSULIN—INJECTABLE COMBINATIONS (*Humalog Mix 75/25, Humalog Mix 50/50, Humulin 70/30, Novolin 70/30, NovoLog Mix 70/30, ReliOn Novolin 70/30, Ryzodeg 70/30*) Diabetes: Doses vary, but typically total insulin 0.3 to 1 unit/kg/day SC in divided doses (Type 1), and 0.5 to 1.5 unit/kg/day SC in divided doses (Type 2). Administer Humalog, Novolog within 15 min before or immediately after a meal. Administer Ryzodeg with a meal. Administer regular insulin mixtures 30 min before meals. [Trade only: Insulin lispro protamine susp/insulin lispro (Humalog Mix 75/25, Humalog Mix 50/50). Insulin aspart protamine/insulin aspart (NovoLog Mix 70/30,). NPH and regular mixtures (Humulin 70/30, Novolin 70/30, ReliOn Novolin 70/30). Insulin degludec/insulin aspart mixture (Ryzodeg 70/30). Insulin available in pen form: Novolin 70/30 InnoLet, NovoLog Mix 70/30 FlexPen, Humulin 70/30, Humalog Mix 75/25 KwikPen, Humalog Mix 50/50 KwikPen, Ryzodeg 70/30 FlexTouch.] ▶LK ♀B/C ▶+ $$$$

INSULIN—INJECTABLE INTERMEDIATE (*Novolin N, Humulin N, ReliOn Novolin N*) Diabetes: Doses vary, but typically total insulin 0.3 to 0.5 unit/kg/day SC in divided doses (Type 1), and 1 to 1.5 unit/kg/day SC in divided doses (Type 2). Generally, 50 to 70% of insulin requirements are provided by rapid- or short-acting insulin and the remainder from intermediate- or long-acting insulin. [Trade only: Injection NPH (Novolin N, Humulin N, ReliOn Novolin N). Insulin available in pen form: Humulin N KwikPen. Premixed preparations of NPH and regular insulin also available.] ▶LK ♀B/C ▶+ $$$$

INSULIN—INJECTABLE SHORT-/RAPID-ACTING (*Apidra, Novolin R, NovoLog, Humulin R, Humalog, ✦NovoRapid*) Diabetes: Doses vary, but typically total insulin 0.3 to 0.5 unit/kg/day SC in divided doses (Type 1), and 1 to 1.5 unit/kg/day SC in divided doses (Type 2). Generally, 50 to 70% of insulin requirements are provided by rapid- or short-acting insulin and the remainder from intermediate- or long-acting insulin. Administer rapid-acting insulin (Humalog, NovoLog, Apidra) within 15 min before or immediately after a meal. Administer regular insulin 30 min before meals. Severe hyperkalemia: 5 to 10 units regular insulin plus concurrent dextrose IV. Profound hyperglycemia (eg, DKA): 0.1 unit regular/kg IV bolus, then initial infusion 100 units regular in 100 mL NS (1 unit/mL), at 0.1 units/kg/h. [Trade only: Injection regular 100 units/mL (Novolin R, Humulin R). Injection regular 500 units/mL (Humulin U-500, concentrated). Insulin glulisine (Apidra). Insulin lispro 100 units/mL (Humalog). Insulin aspart (NovoLog). Insulin available in pen form (100 units/mL): Novolin R InnoLet, Humulin R, Apidra SoloSTAR, Humalog KwikPen, NovoLog FlexPen. Insulin lispro 200 units/mL (Humalog U-200 KwikPen).] ▶LK ♀B/C ▶+ $$$$

INSULIN—INJECTABLE, LONG-ACTING (*Lantus, Levemir, Toujeo, Tresiba*) Diabetes: Doses vary, but typically total insulin 0.3 to 0.5 units/kg/day SC in divided doses (Type 1), and 1 to 1.5 units/kg/day SC in divided doses (Type 2). Generally, 50 to 70% of insulin requirements are provided by rapid- or short-acting insulin and the remainder from intermediate- or long-acting insulin. Lantus, Type 2 DM: Start 10 units or 0.2 units/kg SC daily (same time every day) in insulin-naive patients. Levemir, Type 2 DM: Start 10 units or 0.1 to 0.2 units/kg SC daily in the evening or divided twice daily in insulin-naive patients. DM, Type 1 (Lantus/Levemir):

(cont.)

Start with $1/3$ of total daily insulin dose; remainder of requirements from rapid- or short-acting insulin. [Trade only: Lantus (insulin glargine), Levemir (insulin detemir) 100 units/mL (U-100), 10 ml vial. Insulin available in pen form: Lantus SoloSTAR (glargine, U-100, 3 mL), Toujeo SoloSTAR (glargine, U-300, 1.5 mL), Levemir FlexTouch (detemir, U-100, 3 mL) Tresiba FlexTouch (degludec, U-100, U-200, 3 mL).] ▶LK ♀B/C ▶+

Diabetes-Related—Meglitinides

NATEGLINIDE (*Starlix*) DM, Type 2: 120 mg PO three times per day within 30 min before meals; use 60 mg PO three times per day in patients who are near goal A1C. [Generic/Trade: Tabs 60, 120 mg.] ▶L ♀C ▶? $$$

REPAGLINIDE (*Prandin*, *GlucoNorm*) DM, Type 2: Start 0.5 to 2 mg PO three times per day before meals, maintenance 0.5 to 4 mg three to four times per day, max 16 mg/day. [Generic/Trade: Tabs 0.5, 1, 2 mg.] ▶L ♀C ▶? $$$

Diabetes-Related—SGLT2 Inhibitors

CANAGLIFLOZIN (*Invokana*) DM, Type 2: 100 mg PO daily before 1st meal of the day. If tolerated and needed for glycemic control, may increase to 300 mg PO daily if CrCl greater than 60 mL/min. [Trade only: Tabs 100, 300 mg.] ▶LK – ♀C ▶? $$$$$

DAPAGLIFLOZIN (*Farxiga*, *Forxiga*) DM, Type 2: 5 mg PO daily in the morning, with or without food. If tolerated and needed for glycemic control, may increase to 10 mg PO daily. [Trade only: Tabs 5, 10 mg] ▶LK ♀C ▶– $$$$$

EMPAGLIFLOZIN (*Jardiance*) DM, Type 2: Start 10 mg PO daily in morning, with or without food. May increase up to 25 mg PO daily in morning, with or without food. [Trade only: 10, 25 mg.] ▶LK ♀C ▶? $$$$$

Diabetes-Related—Sulfonylureas—2nd Generation

GLICLAZIDE (*Diamicron, Diamicron MR*) Canada only. DM, Type 2, immediate-release: Start 80 to 160 mg PO daily, max 320 mg PO daily (160 mg or more per day should be in divided doses. Modified-release: Start 30 mg PO daily, max 120 mg PO daily. [Generic/Trade: Tabs 80 mg (Diamicron). Trade only: Tabs, modified-release 30 mg (Diamicron MR).] ▶KL ♀C ▶? $

GLIMEPIRIDE (*Amaryl*) DM, Type 2: Start 1 to 2 mg PO daily, usual 1 to 4 mg/day, max 8 mg/day. [Generic/Trade: Tabs 1, 2, 4 mg. Generic only: Tabs 3, 6, 8 mg.] ▶LK ♀C ▶– $$

GLIPIZIDE (*Glucotrol, Glucotrol XL*) DM, Type 2: Start 5 mg PO daily, usual 10 to 20 mg/day, max 40 mg/day (divide two times per day if more than 15 mg/day). Extended-release: Start 5 mg PO daily, usual 5 to 10 mg/day, max 20 mg/day. [Generic/Trade: Tabs 5, 10 mg. Extended-release tabs 2.5, 5, 10 mg.] ▶LK ♀C ▶? $

GLYBURIDE (*DiaBeta, Glynase PresTab*, *Euglucon*) DM, Type 2: Start 1.25 to 5 mg PO daily, usual 1.25 to 20 mg daily or divided two times per day, max 20 mg/day. Micronized tabs: Start 1.5 to 3 mg PO daily, usual 0.75 to 12 mg/day divided

(cont.)

two times per day, max 12 mg/day. [Generic/Trade: Tabs (scored) 1.25, 2.5, 5 mg. Micronized Tabs (scored) 1.5, 3, 4.5, 6 mg.] ▶LK ♀B ▷? $

Diabetes-Related—Thiazolidinediones

PIOGLITAZONE (Actos) DM, Type 2: Start 15 to 30 mg PO daily, max 45 mg/day. Monitor LFTs. [Generic/Trade: Tabs 15, 30, 45 mg.] ▶L ♀C ▷– $ ■

ROSIGLITAZONE (Avandia) DM, Type 2 monotherapy or in combination with metformin or sulfonylurea: Start 4 mg PO daily or divided two times per day, max 8 mg/day. Obtain LFTs before therapy and periodically thereafter. [Trade only: Tabs 2, 4, 8 mg.] ▶L ♀C ▷– $$$$ ■

Diabetes-Related—Other

DEXTROSE (Glutose, B-D Glucose, Insta-Glucose, Dex-4) Hypoglycemia: 15 to 20 g PO once, repeat in 15 minutes if continued hypoglycemia per self-monitoring, or 0.5 to 1 g/kg (1 to 2 mL/kg) up to 25 g (50 mL) of 50% soln IV. Dilute to 25% for pediatric administration. [OTC Generic/Trade: Chewable tabs 4 g (Dex-4), 5 g (Glutose). Trade only: Oral gel 40%.] ▶L ♀C ▷? $

GLUCAGON (GlucaGen) Hypoglycemia: 1 mg IV/IM/SC, onset 5 to 20 min. Diagnostic aid: 1 mg IV/IM/SC. [Trade only: Injection 1 mg.] ▶LK ♀B ▷? $$$

METFORMIN (Glucophage, Glucophage XR, Glumetza, Fortamet, Riomet) DM, Type 2: Immediate-release: Start 500 mg PO one to two times per day or 850 mg PO daily with meals, may gradually increase to max 2550 mg/day. Extended-release: Glucophage XR: 500 mg PO daily with evening meal; increase by 500 mg once a week to max 2000 mg/day (may divide two times per day). Glumetza: 1000 mg PO daily with evening meal; increase by 500 mg once a week to max 2000 mg/day (may divide two times per day). Fortamet: 500 to 1000 mg daily with evening meal; increase by 500 mg once a week to max 2500 mg/day. Polycystic ovary syndrome (unapproved, immediate-release): 500 mg PO three times per day. DM prevention, Type 2 (with lifestyle modifications, unapproved): 850 mg PO daily for 1 month, then increase to 850 mg PO two times per day. All products started at low doses to improve GI tolerability, gradually increase as tolerated. [Generic/Trade: Tabs 500, 850, 1000 mg, extended-release 500, 750 mg. Trade only, extended-release (Fortamet, Glumetza): 500, 1000 mg. Trade only (Riomet): Oral soln 500 mg/5 mL.] ▶K ♀B ▷? $ ■

PRAMLINTIDE (Symlin, SymlinPen) DM, Type 1 with mealtime insulin therapy: Initiate 15 mcg SC immediately before major meals and titrate by 15 mcg increments (if significant nausea has not occurred for at least 3 days) to maintenance 30 to 60 mcg as tolerated. DM, Type 2 with mealtime insulin therapy: Initiate 60 mcg SC immediately before major meals and increase to 120 mcg as tolerated (if significant nausea has not occurred for 3 to 7 days). Decrease initial premeal short-acting insulin doses by 50% including fixed-mix insulin (ie, 70/30). [Trade only: 600 mcg/mL in 5 mL vials, 1000 mcg/mL pen injector (SymlinPen) 1.5, 2.7 mL.] ▶K ♀C ▷? $$$$ ■

ENDOCRINE AND METABOLIC

Diagnostic Agents

COSYNTROPIN (*Cortrosyn, ✦Synacthen*) Rapid screen for adrenocortical insufficiency: 0.25 mg IM/IV over 2 min; measure serum cortisol before and 30 to 60 min after. ▶L ♀C ▷? $

Minerals

CALCIUM ACETATE (*PhosLo, Eliphos, Phoslyra*) Phosphate binder to reduce serum phosphorous in end-stage renal disease: Initially 2 tabs/caps or 10 mL of soln PO with each meal. [Generic/Trade: Gelcaps 667 mg (169 mg elem Ca). Tabs 667 mg (169 mg elem Ca). Trade only: Soln (Phoslyra): 667 mg (169 mg elemental calcium)/5 mL.] ▶K ♀C ▷? $

CALCIUM CARBONATE (*Caltrate, Mylanta Children's, Os-Cal, Oyst-Cal, Tums, Surpass, Viactiv, ✦Calsan*) Supplement: 1 to 2 g elemental Ca/day or more PO with meals divided two to four times per day. Antacid: 1000 to 3000 mg PO q 2 h prn or 1 to 2 pieces gum chewed prn, max 7000 mg/day. [OTC Generic/Trade: Tabs 500, 650, 750, 1000, 1250, 1500 mg. Chewable tabs 400, 500, 750, 850, 1000, 1177, 1250 mg. Caps 1250 mg. Gum 300, 450 mg. Susp 1250 mg/5 mL. Calcium carbonate is 40% elem Ca and contains 20 mEq of elem Ca/g calcium carbonate. Not more than 500 to 600 mg elem Ca/dose. Available in combination with sodium fluoride, vitamin D, and/or vitamin K. Trade examples: Caltrate 600 + vitamin D = 600 mg elemental Ca/200 units vitamin D, Os-Cal 500 + D = 500 mg elemental Ca/200 units vitamin D, Os-Cal Extra D = 500 mg elemental Ca/400 units vitamin D, Tums (regular strength) = 200 mg elemental Ca, Tums (ultra) = 400 mg elemental Ca, Viactiv (chewable) 500 mg elemental Ca + 100 units vitamin D + 40 mcg vitamin K.] ▶K ♀+ (? 1st trimester) ▷? $

CALCIUM CHLORIDE 500 to 1000 mg slow IV q 1 to 3 days via central line or deep vein. [Generic only: Injectable 10% (1000 mg/10 mL) 10 mL ampules, vials, syringes.] ▶K ♀+ ▷+ $

CALCIUM CITRATE (*Citracal*) 1 to 2 g elemental Ca/day or more PO with meals divided two to four times per day. [OTC Trade/generic (mg elem Ca/units vitamin D): 200/250, 250/200, 315/250, 600/500 (slow release); some products available with magnesium and/or phosphorus. Chewable gummies: 250 mg with 250 units vitamin D.] ▶K ♀+ ▷+ $

CALCIUM GLUCONATE 2.25 to 14 mEq slow IV. 500 to 2000 mg PO two to four times per day. [Generic only: Injectable 10% (1000 mg/10 mL, 4.65 mEq/10 mL) 1, 10, 50, 100, 200 mL. OTC Generic only: Tabs 50, 500, 650, 975, 1000 mg. Chewable tabs 650 mg.] ▶K ♀+ ▷+ $

FERRIC CARBOXYMALTOSE (*Injectafer*) Iron deficiency anemia (unsatisfactory response to oral iron; non-dialysis dependent): If less than 50 kg: 15 mg/kg elemental iron IV for 2 doses, separated by at least 7 days. If 50 kg or greater: 750 mg elemental iron IV for 2 doses, separated by at least 7 days. Max: 1500 mg per course. [Trade only: 750 mg iron/15 mL vial.] ▶NA ♀C ▷? $$$$$

FERRIC GLUCONATE COMPLEX (*Ferrlecit*) 125 mg elemental iron IV over 10 min or diluted in 100 mL NS IV over 1 h. Peds age 6 yo or older: 1.5 mg/kg

(cont.)

(max 125 mg) elemental iron diluted in 25 mL NS and administered IV over 1 h. ▶KL ♀B ▷? $$$$$

FERROUS GLUCONATE (*Fergon*) 800 to 1600 mg ferrous gluconate PO divided three times per day. [OTC Generic/Trade: Tabs (ferrous gluconate) 240 mg (27 mg elemental iron). Generic only: Tabs 324, 325 mg.] ▶K ♀+ ▷+ $

FERROUS SULFATE (*Fer-in-Sol, Feosol, Slow FE, ✦Ferodan, Slow-Fe*) 500 to 1000 mg ferrous sulfate (100 to 200 mg elemental iron) PO divided three times per day. [OTC Generic/Trade (mg ferrous sulfate): Tabs, extended-release 160 mg. Tabs 200, 324, 325 mg. OTC Generic only (mg ferrous sulfate): Soln 75 mg/0.6 mL. Elixir 220 mg/5 mL.] ▶K ♀+ ▷+ $

FERUMOXYTOL (*Feraheme*) Iron deficiency in chronic kidney disease: Give 510 mg IV infusion, followed by 510 mg IV infusion once given 3 to 8 days after initial injection. ▶KL ♀C ▷? $$$$$ ■

FLUORIDE SUPPLEMENTATION

Age	<0.3 ppm in drinking water	0.3–0.6 ppm in drinking water	>0.6 ppm in drinking water
0–6 mo	none	none	none
6 mo–3 yo	0.25 mg PO daily	none	none
3–6 yo	0.5 mg PO daily	0.25 mg PO daily	none
6–16 yo	1 mg PO daily	0.5 mg PO daily	none

JADA 2010;141:1480–1489

FLUORIDE (*Luride, ✦Fluor-A-Day*) Adult dose: 10 mL of topical rinse, swish and spit daily. Peds daily dose based on fluoride content of drinking water (table). [Generic only: Chewable tabs 0.5, 1 mg. Tabs 1 mg. Gtts 0.125, 0.25, 0.5 mg/dropperful. Lozenges 1 mg. Soln 0.2 mg/mL. Gel 0.1, 0.5, 1.23%. Rinse (sodium fluoride) 0.05, 0.1, 0.2%.] ▶K ♀? ▷? $

IRON DEXTRAN (*InFeD, DexFerrum, ✦Dexiron, Infufer*) 25 to 100 mg IM daily prn. Equations available to calculate IV dose based on wt and Hb. ▶KL ♀C ▷? $$$$ ■

IRON POLYSACCHARIDE (*Niferex, Niferex-150, Nu-Iron 150, Ferrex 150*) 50 to 200 mg PO divided one to three times per day. [OTC Trade only: Caps 60 mg (Niferex). OTC Generic/Trade: Caps 150 mg (Niferex-150, Nu-Iron 150, Ferrex 150), Elixir 100 mg/5 mL (Niferex). 1 mg iron polysaccharide = 1 mg elemental iron.] ▶K ♀+ ▷+ $$ ■

IRON SUCROSE (*Venofer*) Iron deficiency with hemodialysis: 5 mL (100 mg elemental iron) IV over 5 min or diluted in 100 mL NS IV over 15 min or longer. Iron deficiency in nondialysis-dependent chronic kidney disease: 10 mL (200 mg elemental iron) IV over 5 min. ▶KL ♀B ▷? $$$$$

MAGNESIUM CHLORIDE (*Slow-Mag*) 2 tabs PO daily. [OTC Trade only: Enteric-coated tab 64 mg. 64 mg tab Slow-Mag = 64 mg elemental magnesium.] ▶K ♀A ▷+ $

MAGNESIUM GLUCONATE (*Almora, Magtrate,* manganate, *♦Maglucate*) 500 to 1000 mg PO divided three times per day. [OTC Generic only: Tabs 500 mg (27 mg elemental Mg), liquid 54 mg elemental Mg/5 mL.] ▶K ♀A ▶+ $

MAGNESIUM OXIDE (*Mag-200, Mag-Ox 400*) 400 to 800 mg PO daily. [OTC Generic/Trade: Caps: 140 (84.5 mg elemental Mg), 250 (elemental), 400 (240 mg elemental Mg), 420 (253 mg elemental Mg), 500 mg (elemental).] ▶K ♀A ▶+ $

MAGNESIUM SULFATE Hypomagnesemia: 1 g of 20% soln IM q 6 h for 4 doses, or 2 g IV over 1 h (monitor for hypotension). Peds: 25 to 50 mg/kg IV/IM q 4 to 6 h for 3 to 4 doses, max single dose 2 g. Eclampsia: 4 to 6 g IV over 30 min, then 1 to 2 g/h. Drip: 5 g in 250 mL D5W (20 mg/mL), 2 g/h is a rate of 100 mL/h. Preterm labor: 6 g IV over 20 min, then 1 to 3 g/h titrated to decrease contractions. Monitor respirations and reflexes. If needed, may reverse toxic effects with calcium gluconate 1 g IV. Torsades de pointes: 1 to 2 g IV in D5W over 5 to 60 min. ▶K ♀D C/D ▶+ $

PHOSPHORUS (*Neutra-Phos, K-Phos*) 1 cap/packet PO four times per day. 1 to 2 tabs PO four times per day. Severe hypophosphatemia (eg, less than 1 mg/dL): 0.08 to 0.16 mmol/kg IV over 6 h. [OTC Trade only: (Neutra-Phos, Neutra-Phos K) tab/cap/packet 250 mg (8 mmol) phosphorus. Rx: Trade only: (K-Phos) tab 250 mg (8 mmol) phosphorus.] ▶K ♀C ▶? $

POTASSIUM (ORAL FORMS)*

Effervescent Granules	
20 mEq	Klorvess Effervescent, K-vescent
Effervescent Tabs	
10 mEq	Effer-K
20 mEq	Effer-K
25 mEq	Effer-K, K+Care ET, K-Lyte, K-Lyte/Cl, Klor-Con/EF
50 mEq	K-Lyte DS, K-Lyte/Cl 50
Liquids	
20 mEq/15 mL	Cena-K, Kaochlor S-F, K-G Elixir, Kaochlor 10%, Kay Ciel, Kaon, Kaylixir, Kolyum, Potasalan, Twin-K
30 mEq/15 mL	Rum-K
40 mEq/15 mL	Cena-K, Kaon-Cl 20%
45 mEq/15 mL	Tri-K

(cont.)

POTASSIUM (ORAL FORMS)* (*continued*)

Powders	
15 mEq/pack	K+Care
20 mEq/pack	Gen-K, K+Care, Kay Ciel, K-Lor, Klor-Con
25 mEq/pack	K+Care, Klor-Con 25
Tabs/Caps	
8 mEq	K+8, Klor-Con 8, Slow-K, Micro-K
10 mEq	K+10, K-Norm, Kaon-Cl 10, Klor-Con M10 Klotrix, K-Tab, K-Dur 10, Micro-K 10
20 mEq	Klor-Con M20, K-Dur 20

* Table provides examples and is not intended to be all inclusive.

POTASSIUM (*Cena-K*) IV infusion 10 mEq/h (diluted). 20 to 40 mEq PO one or two times per day. Use IV or immediate-release PO if rapid replacement needed. [Injectable, many different products in a variety of salt forms (ie, chloride, bicarbonate, citrate, acetate, gluconate), available in tabs, caps, liquids, effervescent tabs, packets. Potassium gluconate is available OTC. See table.] ▶K ♀C ▷? $

ZINC ACETATE (*Galzin*) Dietary supplement: 8 to 12 mg (elemental) daily. Zinc deficiency: 25 to 50 mg (elemental) daily. Wilson's disease: 25 to 50 mg (elemental) PO three times per day. [Trade only: Caps 25, 50 mg elemental zinc.] ▶Minimal absorption ♀A ▷– $$$

ZINC SULFATE (*Orazinc, Zincate*) Dietary supplement: 8 to 12 mg (elemental) daily, Zinc deficiency: 25 to 50 mg (elemental) PO daily. [OTC Generic/Trade: Tabs 66, 110, 200 mg. Rx Generic/Trade: Caps 220 mg.] ▶Minimal absorption ♀A ▷– $

Nutritionals

BANANA BAG Alcoholic malnutrition (example formula): Add thiamine 100 mg + folic acid 1 mg + IV multivitamins to 1 liter NS and infuse over 4 h. Magnesium sulfate 2 g may be added. "Banana bag" and "rally pack" are jargon and not valid drug orders. Specify individual components. ▶KL ♀+ ▷+ $

FAT EMULSION (*Intralipid, Liposyn*) Dosage varies. ▶L ♀C ▷? $$$$$

LEVOCARNITINE (*Carnitor*) 10 to 20 mg/kg IV at each dialysis session. [Generic/Trade: Tabs 330 mg, Oral soln 1 g/10 mL.] ▶KL ♀B ▷? $$$$$

Phosphate Binders

FERRIC CITRATE (*Auryxia*) Treatment of hyperphosphatemia in end stage renal disease on dialysis: Start 2 tab PO three times daily with meals. Titrate by 1 to

(cont.)

ENDOCRINE AND METABOLIC

2 tabs q week to achieve target serum phosphorous levels. Max 12 tabs/day. [Trade only (Tabs): 210 mg ferric iron (equivalent to 1 g ferric citrate).] ▶KL ♀? $$$$$

LANTHANUM CARBONATE (*Fosrenol*) Hyperphosphatemia in end-stage renal disease: Start 1500 mg/day PO in divided doses with meals. Titrate dose q 2 to 3 weeks in increments of 750 mg/day until acceptable serum phosphate is reached. Most will require 1500 to 3000 mg/day to reduce phosphate to less than 6.0 mg/dL. Chew or crush tabs completely before swallowing; not to be swallowed whole. [Trade only: Chewable tabs 500, 750, 1000 mg.] ▶Not absorbed ♀C ▶? $$$$$

SEVELAMER (*Renagel, Renvela*) Hyperphosphatemia: 800 to 1600 mg PO three times per day with meals. [Trade only (Renagel—sevelamer hydrochloride): Tabs 400, 800 mg. (Renvela—sevelamer carbonate): Tabs 800 mg. Powder: 800, 2400 mg packets.] ▶Not absorbed ♀C ▶? $$$$$

SUCROFERRIC OXYHYDROXIDE (*Velphoro*) Hyperphosphatemia in kidney disease on dialysis: Start 1 tab (500 mg) PO three times daily with meals, adjust weekly according to serum phosphorus concentrations. Tablets must be chewed. [Trade only: Tabs 500 mg.] ▶not absorbed ♀B ▶+ $$$$$

Thyroid Agents

LEVOTHYROXINE (*Synthroid, Tirosint, Unithroid, T4, ✦Eltroxin, Euthyrox*) Start 100 to 200 mcg PO daily (healthy adults) or 12.5 to 50 mcg PO daily (elderly or cardiovascular disease), increase by 12.5 to 25 mcg/day at 3- to 8-week intervals. Usual maintenance dose 100 to 200 mcg/day, max 300 mcg/day. [Generic/Trade: Tabs 25, 50, 75, 88, 100, 112, 125, 137, 150, 175, 200, 300 mcg. Trade only: Caps (Tirosint) 13, 25, 50, 75, 88, 100, 112, 125, 137, 150 mcg.] ▶L ♀A ▶+ $ ■

LIOTHYRONINE (*T3, Cytomel, Triostat*) Start 25 mcg PO daily, max 100 mcg/day. [Generic/Trade: Tabs 5, 25, 50 mcg.] ▶L ♀A ▶? $$ ■

METHIMAZOLE (*Tapazole*) Start 5 to 20 mg PO three times per day or 10 to 30 mg PO daily, then adjust. [Generic/Trade: Tabs 5, 10 mg. Generic only: Tabs 15, 20 mg.] ▶L ♀D ▶+ $$$

PROPYLTHIOURACIL (*PTU, ✦Propyl Thyracil*) Hyperthyroidism: Start 100 mg PO three times per day, then adjust. Thyroid storm: 200 to 300 mg PO four times per day, then adjust. [Generic only: Tabs 50 mg.] ▶L ♀D (but preferred over methimazole in 1st trimester) ▶+ $ ■

Vitamins

ASCORBIC ACID (*vitamin C, ✦Redoxon*) 70 to 1000 mg PO daily. [OTC Generic only: Tabs 25, 50, 100, 250, 500, 1000 mg. Chewable tabs 100, 250, 500 mg. Timed-release tabs 500, 1000, 1500 mg. Timed-release caps 500 mg. Lozenges 60 mg. Liquid 35 mg/0.6 mL. Oral soln 100 mg/mL. Syrup 500 mg/5 mL.] ▶K ♀C ▶? $

CALCITRIOL (*Rocaltrol, Calcijex*) 0.25 to 2 mcg PO daily. Hypocalcemia and/or secondary hyperparathyroidism in chronic renal dialysis IV: 1 to 2 mcg, three times a week; increase dose by 0.5 to 1 mcg q 2 to 4 weeks. Adjust based on PTH. [Generic/Trade: Caps 0.25, 0.5 mcg. Oral soln 1 mcg/mL. Injection 1, 2 mcg/mL.] ▶L ♀C ▶? $$

CYANOCOBALAMIN (**vitamin B12**, *CaloMist, Nascobal*) Deficiency states: 100 to 200 mcg IM once a month or 1000 to 2000 mcg PO daily for 1 to 2 weeks followed by 1000 mcg PO daily, 500 mcg intranasal weekly (Nascobal: 1 spray 1 nostril once a week), or 50 to 100 mcg intranasal daily (CaloMist: 1 to 2 sprays each nostril daily). [OTC Generic only: Tabs 100, 500, 1000, 5000 mcg. Lozenges 100, 250, 500 mcg. Rx Trade only: Nasal spray 500 mcg/spray (Nascobal 2.3 mL), 25 mcg/spray (CaloMist, 18 mL).] ▶K ♀C ▶+ $

DOXERCALCIFEROL (*Hectorol*) Secondary hyperparathyroidism on dialysis: Oral: 10 mcg PO three times a week. May increase q 8 weeks by 2.5 mcg/dose; max 60 mcg/week. IV: 4 mcg IV three times a week. May increase dose q 8 weeks by 1 to 2 mcg/dose; max 18 mcg/week. Secondary hyperparathyroidism not on dialysis: Start 1 mcg PO daily, may increase by 0.5 mcg/dose q 2 weeks. Max 3.5 mcg/day. [Generic/Trade: Caps 0.5, 1, 2.5 mcg.] ▶L ♀B ▶? $$$$$

ERGOCALCIFEROL (**vitamin D2**, *Calciferol, Drisdol, ✦Osteoforte*) Osteoporosis prevention and treatment (age 50 yo or older): 800 to 1000 units daily. Familial hypophosphatemia (vitamin D–resistant Rickets): 12,000 to 500,000 units PO daily. Hypoparathyroidism: 50,000 to 200,000 units PO daily. Vitamin D deficiency: 50,000 units PO weekly or biweekly for 8 to 12 weeks. Adequate daily intake: 1 to 70 yo: 600 units (15 mcg); older than 70 yo: 800 units (20 mcg). [OTC Generic only: Caps 400, 1000, 5000 units. Soln 8000 units/mL (Calciferol). Rx Generic/Trade: Caps 50,000 units. Rx Generic only: Caps 25,000 units.] ▶L ♀A (C if exceed RDA) ▶+ $

FOLIC ACID (**folate**, *Folvite*) 0.4 to 1 mg IV/IM/PO/SC daily. [OTC Generic only: Tabs 0.4, 0.8 mg. Rx Generic: Tabs 1 mg.] ▶K ♀A ▶+ $

MULTIVITAMINS (*MVI*) Dose varies with product. Tabs come with and without iron. [OTC and Rx: Many different brands and forms available with and without iron (tabs, caps, chewable tabs, gtts, liquid).] ▶LK ♀+ ▶+ $

NEPHRO-VITE (**ascorbic acid + folic acid + niacin + thiamine + riboflavin + pyridoxine + pantothenic acid + biotin + cyanocobalamin**) 1 tab PO daily. If on dialysis, take after treatment. [Generic/Trade: Vitamin C 60 mg/folic acid 1 mg/niacin 20 mg/thiamine 1.5 mg/riboflavin 1.7 mg/pyridoxine 10 mg/pantothenic acid 10 mg/biotin 300 mcg/cyanocobalamin 6 mcg.] ▶K ♀? ▶? $

NEPHROCAP (**ascorbic acid + folic acid + niacin + thiamine + riboflavin + pyridoxine + pantothenic acid + biotin + cyanocobalamin**) 1 cap PO daily. If on dialysis, take after treatment. [Generic/Trade: Vitamin C 100 mg/folic acid 1 mg/niacin 20 mg/thiamine 1.5 mg/riboflavin 1.7 mg/pyridoxine 10 mg/pantothenic acid 5 mg/biotin 150 mcg/cyanocobalamin 6 mcg.] ▶K ♀? ▶? $

NIACIN (**vitamin B3, nicotinic acid,** *Niacor, Nicolar, Slo-Niacin, Niaspan*) Niacin deficiency: 10 to 500 mg PO daily. Hyperlipidemia: Start 50 to 100 mg PO two to three times per day with meals, increase slowly, usual maintenance range 1.5

(cont.)

ENDOCRINE AND METABOLIC

to 3 g/day, max 6 g/day. Extended-release (Niaspan): Start 500 mg at bedtime, increase monthly up to max 2000 mg. Extended-release formulations not listed here may have greater hepatotoxicity. Start with low doses and increase slowly to minimize flushing; 325 mg aspirin (non-EC) 30 to 60 min prior to niacin ingestion will minimize flush. [OTC Generic only: Tabs 50, 100, 250, 500 mg. Timed-release caps 125, 250, 400 mg. Timed-release tabs 250, 500 mg. Liquid 50 mg/5 mL. Trade only: 250, 500, 750 mg (Slo-Niacin). Rx: Generic/Trade: Timed-release tabs 500, 750, 1000 mg (Niaspan, $$$$). Trade only: Tabs 500 mg (Niacor).] ▶K ♀C ▶? $

PARICALCITOL (*Zemplar*) Prevention/treatment of secondary hyperparathyroidism with renal insufficiency: 1 to 2 mcg PO daily or 2 to 4 mcg PO three times per week; increase dose by 1 mcg/day or 2 mcg/week until desired PTH level is achieved. Prevention/treatment of secondary hyperparathyroidism with renal failure (CrCl less than 15 mL/min): PO: To calculate initial dose divide baseline iPTH by 80 and then administer this dose in mcg three times per week. To titrate dose based on response, divide recent iPTH by 80 then administer this dose in mcg three times per week. IV: 0.04 to 0.1 mcg/kg (2.8 to 7 mcg) IV three times per week at dialysis; increase dose by 2 to 4 mcg q 2 to 4 weeks until desired PTH level is achieved. Max dose 0.24 mcg/kg (16.8 mcg). [Generic/Trade: Caps 1, 2, 4 mcg.] ▶L ♀C ▶? $$$$$

PHYTONADIONE (vitamin K, *Mephyton, AquaMephyton*) Single dose of 0.5 to 1 mg IM within 1 h after birth. Excessive oral anticoagulation: Dose varies based on INR. INR 4.5 to 10: 2012 CHEST guidelines recommend AGAINST routine vitamin K administration; INR greater than 10 with no bleeding: 2012 CHEST guidelines recommend giving vitamin K, but do not specify a dose, 2008 guidelines previously recommended 5 to 10 mg PO; serious bleeding and elevated INR: 5 to 10 mg slow IV infusion. Adequate daily intake: 120 mcg (males) and 90 mcg (females). [Trade only: Tabs 5 mg.] ▶L ♀C ▶+ ■

PYRIDOXINE (vitamin B6) 10 to 200 mg PO daily. Prevention of deficiency due to isoniazid in high-risk patients: 10 to 25 mg PO daily. Treatment of neuropathies due to isoniazid: 50 to 200 mg PO daily. Hyperemesis of pregnancy: 10 to 50 mg PO q 8 h. [OTC Generic only: Tabs 25, 50, 100 mg; Timed-release tab 100 mg.] ▶K ♀A ▶+ $

RIBOFLAVIN (vitamin B2) 5 to 25 mg PO daily. [OTC Generic only: Tabs 25, 50, 100 mg.] ▶K ♀A ▶+ $

THIAMINE (vitamin B1) 10 to 100 mg IV/IM/PO daily. [OTC Generic only: Tabs 50, 100, 250, 500 mg. Enteric-coated tab 20 mg.] ▶K ♀A ▶+ $

VITAMIN A RDA: 900 mcg retinol equivalents (RE) (males), 700 mcg RE (females). Treatment of deficiency: 100,000 units IM daily for 3 days, then 50,000 units IM daily for 2 weeks. 1 RE is equivalent to 1 mcg retinol or 6 mcg beta-carotene. Max recommended daily dose 3000 mcg. [OTC Generic only: Caps 10,000, 15,000 units. Trade only: Tabs 5000 units. Rx: Generic: 25,000 units. Trade only: Soln 50,000 units/mL.] ▶L ♀A (C if exceed RDA, X in high doses) ▶+ $

VITAMIN D3 (cholecalciferol, *DDrops*) Osteoporosis prevention and treatment (age 50 or older): 800 to 1000 units daily. Familial hypophosphatemia (Vitamin D–resistant Rickets): 12,000 to 500,000 units PO daily. Hypoparathyroidism:

(cont.)

50,000 to 200,000 units PO daily. Adequate daily intake: 1 to 70 yo: 600 units; older than 70 yo: 800 units. [OTC Generic: 200, 400, 800, 1000, 2000 units (caps/tabs). Trade only: Soln 400, 1000, 2000 units/drop.] ▶L −♀D+ $

VITAMIN E (tocopherol, ✦Aquasol E) RDA: 22 units (natural, d-alpha-tocopherol) or 33 units (synthetic, d,l-alpha-tocopherol) or 15 mg (alpha-tocopherol). Max recommended 1000 mg alpha-tocopherol (1500 units) daily. [OTC Generic only: Tabs 200, 400 units. Caps 73.5, 100, 147, 165, 200, 330, 400, 500, 600, 1000 units. Gtts 50 mg/mL.] ▶L ♀A D? $

Other

BROMOCRIPTINE (Cycloset, Parlodel) Type 2 DM: 0.8 mg PO q am (within 2 h of waking), may increase weekly by 0.8 mg to max tolerated dose of 1.6 to 4.8 mg. Hyperprolactinemia: Start 1.25 to 2.5 mg PO at bedtime, then increase q 3 to 7 days to usual effective dose of 2.5 to 15 mg/day, max 40 mg/day. Acromegaly: Usual effective dose is 20 to 30 mg/day, max 100 mg/day. Doses greater than 20 mg/day can be divided two times per day. Also approved for Parkinson's disease, but rarely used. Take with food to minimize dizziness and nausea. [Generic: Tabs 2.5 mg. Generic/Trade: Caps 5 mg. Trade only: Tabs 0.8 mg (Cycloset).] ▶L ♀B D− $$$$$

CABERGOLINE (Dostinex) Hyperprolactinemia: 0.25 to 1 mg PO two times per week. [Generic/Trade: Tabs 0.5 mg.] ▶L ♀B D− $$$$$

CALCITONIN (Miacalcin, Fortical, ✦Calcimar, Caltine) Osteoporosis: 100 units SC/IM every other day or 200 units (1 spray) intranasal daily (alternate nostrils). Paget's disease: 50 to 100 units SC/IM daily. Hypercalcemia: 4 units/kg SC/IM q 12 h. May increase after 2 days to max of 8 units/kg q 6 h. Skin test before using injectable product: 1 unit intradermally and observe for local reaction. Acute osteoporotic vertebral fracture pain (unapproved use): 100 units SC/IM daily or 200 units intranasal daily (alternate nostrils). [Generic/Trade: Nasal spray 200 units/activation in 3.7 mL bottle (minimum of 30 doses/bottle).] ▶plasma ♀C D? $$$$

DENOSUMAB (Prolia) Postmenopausal osteoporosis: 60 mg SC q 6 months. Osteoporosis in men: 60 mg SC q6 months. Increase bone mass in men receiving androgen deprivation therapy for nonmetastatic prostate cancer: 60 mg SC q 6 months. Increase bone mass in women receiving adjuvant aromatase inhibitor therapy for breast cancer at high risk of fracture: 60 mg SC q 6 months. [Trade only: 60 mg/1 mL vial (Prolia), prefilled syringe.] ▶? ♀X D? $$$$

DESMOPRESSIN (DDAVP, Stimate, ✦Minirin, Octostim) Diabetes insipidus: 10 to 40 mcg intranasally daily or divided two to three times per day, 0.05 to 1.2 mg/day PO or divided two to three times per day, or 0.5 to 1 mL/day SC/IV in 2 divided doses. Hemophilia A, von Willebrand's disease: 0.3 mcg/kg IV over 15 to 30 min, or 150 to 300 mcg intranasally. Enuresis: 0.2 to 0.6 mg PO at bedtime. Not for children younger than 6 yo. [Trade only: Stimate nasal spray 150 mcg/0.1 mL (1 spray), 2.5 mL bottle (25 sprays). Generic/Trade (DDAVP nasal spray): 10 mcg/0.1 mL (1 spray), 5 mL bottle (50 sprays). Note difference in concentration of nasal soln. Rhinal Tube: 2.5 mL bottle with 2 flexible plastic tube applicators with graduation marks for dosing. Generic only: Tabs 0.1, 0.2 mg.] ▶LK ♀B D? $$$$

PARATHYROID HORMONE (*Natpara*) Hypocalcemia in hypoparathyroidism: Start 50 mcg SC once daily in thigh (alternate thigh every other day). Adjust dose by 25 mcg q 4 weeks to max of 100 mcg to achieve serum calcium 8 to 9 mg/dL. [Trade only: 25, 50, 75, 100 mcg dose strength cartridges. Available through restricted access program (NATPARA REMS).] ▶LK ♀C ▶? $$$$$ ■

SODIUM POLYSTYRENE SULFONATE (*Kayexalate*) Hyperkalemia: 15 g PO one to four times per day or 30 to 50 g retention enema (in sorbitol) q 6 h prn. Retain for 30 min to several hours. Irrigate with tap water after enema to prevent necrosis. [Generic only: Susp 15 g/60 mL. Powdered resin.] ▶Fecal excretion ♀C ▶? $$$$

SOMATROPIN (human growth hormone, *Genotropin, Humatrope, Norditropin, Norditropin NordiFlex, Norditropin FlexPro, Nutropin AQ, Nutropin Depot, Omnitrope, Protropin, Serostim, Serostim LQ, Saizen, Valtropin, Zorbtive, Zomacton*) Dosages vary by indication and product. [Single-dose vials (powder for injection with diluent): Omnitrope: 1.5, 5.8 mg vial. Zomacton: 5 mg vial. Zorbtive: 8.8 mg vial. Cartridges: Genotropin: 1.5, 5.8, 13.8 mg cartridges. Humatrope: 6, 12, 24 mg pen cartridges; 5 mg vial (powder for injection with diluent). Nutropin AQ: 10 mg multidose vial, 5, 10, 20 mg/pen cartridges. Pens: Norditropin FlexPro: 5, 10, 15 mg prefilled pen. Norditropin NordiFlex: 30 mg prefilled pens. Saizen: Preassembled reconstitution device with autoinjector pen. Multiple forms: Serostim: 4, 5, 6 mg single-dose vials; 4, 8.8 mg multidose vials; and 8.8 mg cartridges for autoinjector. Valtropin: 5 mg single-dose vials, 5 mg prefilled syringe.] ▶LK ♀B/C ▶? $$$$$

TERIPARATIDE (*Forteo*) Treatment of postmenopausal osteoporosis, treatment of men and women with glucocorticoid-induced osteoporosis or to increase bone mass in men with primary or hypogonadal osteoporosis and high risk for fracture: 20 mcg SC daily in thigh or abdomen for no longer than 2 years. [Trade only: 28 dose pen injector (20 mcg/dose).] ▶LK ♀C ▶– $$$$$ ■

ENT

ENT COMBINATIONS (SELECTED)

	Decongestant	Antihistamine	Antitussive	Typical Adult Doses
OTC				
Actifed Cold & Allergy	phenylephrine	chlorpheniramine	-	1 tab q 4–6 h
Actifed Cold & Sinus‡	pseudoephedrine	chlorpheniramine	-	2 tabs q 6 h
Allerfrim, Aprodine	pseudoephedrine	triprolidine	-	1 tab or 10 mL q 4–6 h
Benadryl Allergy/Cold‡	phenylephrine	diphenhydramine	-	2 tabs q 4 h
Benadryl-D Allergy/Sinus Tablets	phenylephrine	diphenhydramine	-	1 tab q 4 h
Claritin-D 12-h, Alavert D-12	pseudoephedrine	loratadine	-	1 tab q 12 h
Claritin-D 24-h	pseudoephedrine	loratadine	-	1 tab daily
Dimetapp Cold & Allergy Elixir	phenylephrine	brompheniramine	-	20 mL q 4 h
Dimetapp DM Cold & Cough	phenylephrine	brompheniramine	dextromethorphan	20 mL q 4 h
Drixoral Cold & Allergy	pseudoephedrine	dexbrompheniramine	-	1 tab q 12 h
Mucinex-DM Extended-Release	-	-	guaifenesin, dextromethorphan	1-2 tabs q 12 h
Robitussin CF	phenylephrine	-	guaifenesin, dextromethorphan	10 mL q 4 h*
Robitussin DM, Mytussin DM	-	-	guaifenesin, dextromethorphan	10 mL q 4 h*
Robitussin PE, GuaitussPE	phenylephrine	-	guaifenesin	10 mL q 4 h*
Triaminic Cold & Allergy	phenylephrine	chlorpheniramine	-	10 mL q 4 h*
Rx Only				
Allegra-D 12-h	pseudoephedrine	fexofenadine	-	1 tab q 12 h
Allegra-D 24-h	pseudoephedrine	fexofenadine	-	1 tab daily
Bromfenex	pseudoephedrine	brompheniramine	-	1 cap q 12 h
Clarinex-D 24-h	pseudoephedrine-desloratadine	desloratadine	-	1 tab daily
Deconamine	pseudoephedrine	chlorpheniramine	-	1 tab or 10 mL tid-qid
Deconamine SR, Chlordrine SR	pseudoephedrine chlor-pheniramine	chlorpheniramine	-	1 tab q 12 h
Deconsal I	phenylephrine	-	guaifenesin	1-2 tabs q 12 h
Dimetane-DX	pseudoephedrine	brompheniramine	dextromethorphan	10 mL PO q 4 h
Duratuss	phenylephrine	-	guaifenesin	1 tab q 12 h

ENT COMBINATIONS (SELECTED) (*continued*)

Duratuss HD ©*II*	phenylephrine	-	guaifenesin, hydrocodone	5-10 mL q 4–6 h
Entex PSE, Guaifenex PSE 120	pseudoephedrine	-	guaifenesin	1 tab q 12 h
Histussin D ©*II*	pseudoephedrine	-	hydrocodone	5 mL qid
Histussin HC ©*II*	phenylephrine	chlorpheniramine	hydrocodone	10 mL q 4 h
Humibid DM	-	-	guaifenesin, dextromethorphan	1 tab q 12 h
Hycotuss ©*II*	-	-	guaifenesin, hydrocodone	5 mL after meals & at bedtime
Phenergan/Dextromethorphan	promethazine	promethazine	dextromethorphan	5 mL q 4–6 h
Phenergan VC	phenylephrine	promethazine	-	5 mL q 4–6 h
Phenergan VC w/codeine ©*V*	phenylephrine	promethazine	codeine	5 mL q 4–6 h
Robitussin AC ©*V (generic only)*	-	-	guaifenesin, codeine	10 mL q 4 h*
Robitussin DAC ©*V (generic only)*	pseudoephedrine	-	guaifenesin, codeine	10 mL q 4 h*
Rondec Syrup	phenylephrine	chlorpheniramine	-	5 mL qid†
Rondec DM Syrup	phenylephrine	chlorpheniramine	dextromethorphan	5 mL qid†
Rondec Oral Drops	phenylephrine	chlorpheniramine	-	0.75 to 1 mL qid
Rondec DM Oral Drops	phenylephrine	chlorpheniramine	dextromethorphan	0.75 to 1 mL qid
Rynatan	phenylephrine	chlorpheniramine	-	1-2 tabs q 12 h
Rynatan-P Pediatric	phenylephrine	chlorpheniramine	-	2.5-5 mL q 12 h*
Semprex-D	pseudoephedrine	acrivastine	-	1 c ap q 4-6 h
Tanafed (generic only)	pseudoephedrine	chlorpheniramine	-	10-20 mL q 12 h*
Tussionex ©*II*	-	chlorpheniramine	hydrocodone	5 mL q 12 h

tid=three times per day; qid=four times per day
*5 mL/dose if 6–11 yo. 2.5 mL if 2–5 yo.
†2.5 mL/dose if 6–11 yo. 1.25 mL if 2–5 yo.
‡Also contains acetaminophen.

Antihistamines—Non-Sedating

DESLORATADINE (*Clarinex, ✦Aerius*) 5 mg PO daily for age older than 12 yo. Peds: 2 mL (1 mg) PO daily for age 6 to 11 mo, ½ teaspoonful (1.25 mg) PO daily for age 12 mo to 5 yo, 1 teaspoonful (2.5 mg) PO daily for age 6 to 11 yo. [Generic/Trade: Tabs 5 mg. Orally disintegrating tabs 2.5, 5 mg. Trade only: Syrup 0.5 mg/mL.] ▶LK ♀C ▶+ $$$$

FEXOFENADINE (*Allegra*) 60 mg PO two times per day or 180 mg daily. Peds: 30 mg PO two times per day for age 2 to 11 yo. [OTC Generic/Trade: Tabs 30, 60, 180 mg. Susp 30 mg/5 mL. Trade only: Orally disintegrating tab 30 mg.] ▶LK ♀C▶+ $$

LORATADINE (*Claritin, Claritin Hives Relief, Claritin RediTabs, Alavert, Tavist ND*) 10 mg PO daily for age older than 6 yo, 5 mg PO daily for age 2 to 5 yo. [OTC Generic/Trade: Tabs 10 mg. Fast-dissolve tabs (Alavert, Claritin RediTabs) 5, 10 mg. Syrup 1 mg/mL. Rx Trade only (Claritin): Chewable tabs 5 mg, Liqui-gel caps 10 mg.] ▶LK ♀B▶+ $

Antihistamines—Other

NOTE: *Antihistamines ineffective when treating the common cold. Contraindicated in narrow-angle glaucoma, BPH, stenosing peptic ulcer disease, and bladder obstruction. Use half the normal dose in the elderly. May cause drowsiness and/or sedation, which may be enhanced with alcohol, sedatives, and other CNS depressants. Deaths have occurred in children younger than 2 yo attributed to toxicity from cough and cold medications; the FDA does not recommend their use in this age group.*

CETIRIZINE (*Zyrtec, ✦Reactine, Aller-Relief*) 5 to 10 mg PO daily for age older than 6 yo. Peds: Give 2.5 mg PO daily for age 6 to 23 mo, give 2.5 mg PO daily to two times per day for age 2 to 5 yo. [OTC Generic/Trade: Tabs 5, 10 mg. Syrup 5 mg/5 mL. Chewable tabs, grape flavored 5, 10 mg.] ▶LK ♀B▶– $$$

CHLORPHENIRAMINE (*Chlor-Trimeton, Aller-Chlor*) 4 mg PO q 4 to 6 h. Max 24 mg/day. Peds: Give 2 mg PO q 4 to 6 h for age 6 to 11 yo. Max 12 mg/day. [OTC Trade only: Tabs, extended-release 12 mg. Generic/Trade: Tabs 4 mg. Syrup 2 mg/5 mL. Tabs extended-release 8 mg.] ▶LK ♀B▶– $

CLEMASTINE (*Tavist-1*) 1.34 mg PO two times per day. Max 8.04 mg/day. [OTC Generic/Trade: Tabs 1.34 mg. Rx: Generic/Trade: Tabs 2.68 mg. Syrup 0.67 mg/5 mL. Rx: Generic only: Syrup 0.5 mg/5 mL.] ▶LK ♀B▶– $

CYPROHEPTADINE (*Periactin*) Start 4 mg PO three times per day. Max 32 mg/day. [Generic only: Tabs 4 mg. Syrup 2 mg/5 mL.] ▶LK ♀B▶– $

DEXCHLORPHENIRAMINE (*Polaramine*) 2 mg PO q 4 to 6 h. Timed-release tabs: 4 or 6 mg PO at bedtime or q 8 to 10 h. [Generic only: Tabs, immediate-release 2 mg; timed-release 4, 6 mg. Syrup 2 mg/5 mL.] ▶LK ♀? ▶– $$

DIPHENHYDRAMINE (*Benadryl, Banophen, Aller-Max, Diphen, Diphenhist, Dytan, Siladryl, Sominex, ✦Allerdryl, Nytol*) Allergic rhinitis, urticaria, hypersensitivity reactions: 25 to 50 mg IV/IM/PO q 4 to 6 h. Peds: 5 mg/kg/day divided q 4 to 6 h. EPS: 25 to 50 mg PO three to four times per day or 10 to 50 mg IV/IM three to four times per day. Insomnia: 25 to 50 mg PO at bedtime. [OTC Trade only: Tabs 25, 50 mg. Chewable tabs 12.5 mg. OTC and Rx: Generic only: Caps 25, 50 mg. Softgel cap 25 mg. OTC Generic/Trade: Soln 6.25 or 12.5 mg per 5 mL. Rx: Trade only: (Dytan) Susp 25 mg/mL. Chewable tabs 25 mg.] ▶LK ♀B▶– $

HYDROXYZINE (*Atarax, Vistaril*) 25 to 100 mg IM/PO one to four times per day or prn. [Generic only: Tabs 10, 25, 50, 100 mg. Caps 100 mg. Syrup 10 mg/5 mL. Generic/Trade: Caps 25, 50 mg. Susp 25 mg/5 mL (Vistaril). Caps = Vistaril; Tabs = Atarax.] ▶L ♀C▶– $$

LEVOCETIRIZINE (*Xyzal*) 5 mg PO daily for age 12 yo or older. Peds: Give 2.5 mg PO daily for age 6 to 11 yo. [Generic/Trade: Tabs, scored 5 mg. Oral soln 2.5 mg/5 mL (148 mL).] ▶K ♀B ▶– $$$

MECLIZINE (*Antivert, Bonine, Medivert, Meclicot, Meni-D*) Motion sickness: 25 to 50 mg PO 1 h prior to travel, then 25 to 50 mg PO daily. Vertigo: 25 mg PO q 6 h prn. [Rx/OTC/Generic/Trade: Tabs 12.5, 25 mg. Chewable tabs 25 mg. Rx/Trade only: Tabs 50 mg.] ▶L ♀B ▶? $

Antitussives/Expectorants

BENZONATATE (*Tessalon, Tessalon Perles, Zonatuss*) 100 to 200 mg PO three times per day. Swallow whole. Do not chew. Numbs mouth; possible choking hazard. [Generic/Trade: Softgel caps 100, 200 mg. Trade only: Caps 150 mg (Zonatuss).] ▶L ♀C ▶? $$

DEXTROMETHORPHAN (*Benylin, Delsym, DexAlone, Robitussin Cough, Vick's 44 Cough*) 10 to 20 mg PO q 4 h or 30 mg PO q 6 to 8 h. Sustained action liquid 60 mg PO q 12 h. [OTC Trade only: Caps 15 mg (Robitussin), 30 mg (DexAlone). Susp, extended-release 30 mg/5 mL (Delsym). Generic/Trade: Syrup 5, 7.5, 10, 15 mg/5 mL. Generic only: Lozenges 5, 10 mg.] ▶L ♀+ ▶+ $

GUAIFENESIN (*Robitussin, Hytuss, Guiatuss, Mucinex*) 100 to 400 mg PO q 4 h. 600 to 1200 mg PO q 12 h (extended-release). Peds: 50 to 100 mg/dose for age 2 to 5 yo, give 100 to 200 mg/dose for age 6 to 11 yo. [Rx Generic/Trade: Extended-release tabs 600, 1200 mg. OTC Generic/Trade: Liquid, Syrup 100 mg/5 mL. OTC Trade only: Caps 200 mg (Hytuss). Extended-release tabs 600 mg (Mucinex). OTC Generic only: Tabs 100, 200, 400 mg.] ▶L ♀C ▶+ $

Combination Products—Rx Only

NOTE: *Decongestants in some ENT combination products can increase BP, aggravate anxiety, or cause insomnia (use caution). Some contain sedating antihistamines. Sedation can be enhanced by alcohol and other CNS depressants. Deaths have occurred in children younger than 2 yo attributed to toxicity from cough and cold medications; the FDA does not recommend their use in this age group.*

REZIRA (hydrocodone + pseudoephedrine) [Trade: Syrup 5 mg hydrocodone/60 mg pseudoephedrine/5 mL.] ▶LK – ♀C ▶– ⊚II

ZUTRIPRO (hydrocodone + chlorpheniramine + pseudoephedrine) [Trade: Syrup 5 mg hydrocodone/4 mg chlorpheniramine/60 mg pseudoephedrine/5 mL.] ▶LK – ♀C ▶– ⊚II

Decongestants

NOTE: *See ENT—Nasal Preparations for nasal spray decongestants (oxymetazoline, phenylephrine). Deaths have occurred in children younger than 2 yo attributed to toxicity from cough and cold medications; the FDA does not recommend their use in this age group.*

PHENYLEPHRINE (*Sudafed PE*) 10 mg PO q 4 h. [OTC Trade only: Tabs 10 mg.] ▶L ♀C ▶+ $

PSEUDOEPHEDRINE (*Sudafed, Sudafed 12 Hour, Efidac/24, Dimetapp Decongestant Infant Drops, PediaCare Infants' Decongestant Drops, Triaminic Oral Infant Drops*) Adult: 60 mg PO q 4 to 6 h. Extended-release tabs: 120 mg PO two times per day or 240 mg PO daily. Peds: Give 15 mg PO q 4 to 6 h for age 2 to 5 yo, give 30 mg PO q 4 to 6 h for age 6 to 12 yo. [OTC Generic/Trade: Tabs 30, 60 mg. Tabs, extended-release 120 mg (12 h). Soln 15, 30 mg/5 mL. Trade only: Chewable tabs 15 mg. Tabs, extended-release 240 mg (24 h). Rx only in some states.] ▶L ♀C ▶+ $

Ear Preparations

AURALGAN (benzocaine—**otic** + antipyrine) 2 to 4 gtts in ear(s) three to four times per day prn. [Generic/Trade: Otic soln 10, 15 mL.] ▶Not absorbed ♀C ▶? $

CARBAMIDE PEROXIDE (*Debrox, Murine Ear*) 5 to 10 gtts in ear(s) two times per day for 4 days. [OTC Generic/Trade: Otic soln 6.5%, 15, 30 mL.] ▶Not absorbed ♀? ▶? $

CIPRO HC OTIC (ciprofloxacin—**otic** + hydrocortisone—**otic**) 3 gtts in ear(s) two times per day for 7 days for age 1 yo to adult. [Trade only: Otic susp 10 mL.] ▶Not absorbed ♀C ▶− $$$$

CIPRODEX OTIC (ciprofloxacin—**otic** + dexamethasone—**otic**) 4 gtts in ear(s) two times per day for 7 days for age 6 mo to adult. [Trade only: Otic susp 5, 7.5 mL.] ▶Not absorbed ♀C ▶− $$$$

CIPROFLOXACIN—OTIC (*Cetraxal*) 1 single-use container in ear(s) two times per day for 7 days for age 1 yo to adult. [Trade only: 0.25 mL single-use containers with 0.2% ciprofloxacin soln, #14.] ▶Not absorbed ♀C ▶? $$$$

CORTISPORIN OTIC (hydrocortisone—**otic** + polymyxin—**otic** + neomycin—**otic**) 4 gtts in ear(s) three to four times per day up to 10 days of soln or susp. Peds: 3 gtts in ear(s) three to four times per day up to 10 days. Caution in perforated TMs or tympanostomy tubes as this increases the risk of neomycin ototoxicity, especially if use prolonged or repeated. Use susp rather than acidic soln. [Generic only: Otic soln or susp 7.5, 10 mL.] ▶Not absorbed ♀? ▶? $

CORTISPORIN TC OTIC (hydrocortisone—**otic** + neomycin—**otic** + thonzonium + colistin) 4 to 5 gtts in ear(s) three to four times per day up to 10 days. [Trade only: Otic susp, 10 mL.] ▶Not absorbed ♀? ▶? $$$

DOMEBORO OTIC (acetic acid + aluminum acetate) 4 to 6 gtts in ear(s) q 2 to 3 h. Peds: 2 to 3 gtts in ear(s) q 3 to 4 h. [Generic only: Otic soln 60 mL.] ▶Not absorbed ♀? ▶? $

FLUOCINOLONE—OTIC (*DermOtic*) 5 gtts in affected ear(s) two times per day for 7 to 14 days for age 2 yo to adult. [Trade only: Otic oil 0.01% 20 mL.] ▶L ♀C ▶? $$

OFLOXACIN—OTIC (*Floxin Otic*) Otitis externa: 5 gtts in ear(s) daily for age 1 to 12 yo, 10 gtts in ear(s) daily for age 12 yo or older. [Generic/Trade: Otic soln 0.3% 5, 10 mL. Trade only: "Singles": Single-dispensing containers 0.25 mL (5 gtts), 2 per foil pouch.] ▶Not absorbed ♀C ▶− $$$

SWIM-EAR (isopropyl alcohol + anhydrous glycerins) 4 to 5 gtts in ears after swimming. [OTC Trade only: Otic soln 30 mL.] ▶Not absorbed ♀? ▶? $

VOSOL HC (*acetic acid + propylene glycol + hydrocortisone*) 5 gtts in ear(s) three to four times per day. Peds age older than 3 yo: 3 to 4 gtts in ear(s) three to four times per day. [Generic/Trade: Otic soln 2%/3%/1% 10 mL.] ▶Not absorbed ♀? ▶? $

Mouth and Lip Preparations

AMLEXANOX (*Aphthasol, OraDisc A*) Aphthous ulcers: Apply ¼ inch paste or mucoadhesive patch to affected area four times per day after oral hygiene for up to 10 days. Up to 3 patches may be applied at one time. [Trade only: Oral paste 5% (Aphthasol), 3, 5 g tube. Mucoadhesive patch (OraDisc) 2 mg, #20.] ▶LK ♀B ▶? $

CEVIMELINE (*Evoxac*) Dry mouth due to Sjögren's syndrome: 30 mg PO three times per day. [Generic/Trade: Caps 30 mg.] ▶L ♀C ▶– $$$$$

CHLORHEXIDINE GLUCONATE (*Peridex, Periogard*) Rinse with 15 mL of undiluted soln for 30 sec two times per day. Do not swallow. Spit after rinsing. [Generic/Trade: Oral rinse 0.12% 473 to 480 mL bottles.] ▶Fecal excretion ♀B ▶? $

DEBACTEROL (*sulfuric acid + sulfonated phenolics*) Aphthous stomatitis, mucositis: Apply to dry ulcer. Rinse with water. [Trade only: 1 mL prefilled, single-use applicator.] ▶Not absorbed ♀C ▶+ $$

GELCLAIR (*maltodextrin + propylene glycol*) Aphthous ulcers, mucositis, stomatitis: Rinse mouth with 1 packet three times per day or prn. Do not eat or drink for 1 h after treatment. [Trade only: 21 packets/box.] ▶Not absorbed ♀+ ▶+ $$$

LIDOCAINE—VISCOUS (*Xylocaine*) Mouth or lip pain in adults only: 15 to 20 mL topically or swish and spit q 3 h. [Generic/Trade: Soln 2%, 20 mL unit dose, 100 mL bottle.] ▶LK ♀B ▶+ $

MAGIC MOUTHWASH (*diphenhydramine + Mylanta + sucralfate*) 5 mL PO swish and spit or swish and swallow three times per day before meals and prn. [Compounded susp. A standard mixture is 30 mL diphenhydramine liquid (12.5 mg/5 mL)/60 mL Mylanta or Maalox/4 g Carafate.] ▶LK ♀– $$$

PILOCARPINE (*Salagen*) Dry mouth due to radiation of head and neck or Sjögren's syndrome: 5 mg PO three to four times per day. [Generic/Trade: Tabs 5, 7.5 mg.] ▶L ♀C ▶– $$$$

Nasal Preparations—Corticosteroids

BECLOMETHASONE—NASAL (*Beconase AQ, Qnasl*) Beconase AQ: 1 to 2 spray(s) per nostril two times per day. Qnasl: 1 to 2 spray(s) per nostril daily. [Trade only: Beconase AQ 42 mcg/spray, 200 sprays/bottle. Qnasl: 80 mcg/spray, 120 sprays/bottle.] ▶L ♀C ▶? $$$$

BUDESONIDE—NASAL (*Rhinocort Allergy Spray, Rhinocort Aqua*) 1 to 4 sprays per nostril daily. [Generic/Trade: Nasal inhaler 120 sprays/bottle. Rhinocort Allergy Spray available OTC.] ▶L ♀B ▶? $$$$

CICLESONIDE—NASAL (*Omnaris, Zetonna*) Omnaris: 2 sprays per nostril daily. Zetonna: 1 actuation per nostril daily. [Trade only: Nasal spray, 50 mcg/spray,

(cont.)

120 sprays/bottle (Omnaris). Nasal aerosol, 37 mcg/actuation, 60 actuations/canister (Zetonna).] ▶L ♀C ▶? $$$

FLUNISOLIDE—NASAL (*Nasalide, ✦Rhinalar*) Start 2 sprays per nostril two times per day. Max 8 sprays/nostril/day. [Generic only: Nasal soln 0.025%] ▶L ♀C ▶? $$$

FLUTICASONE—NASAL (*Flonase, Veramyst*) 2 sprays per nostril daily. [Generic/Trade: Flonase: Nasal spray 0.05%, 120 sprays/bottle. Trade only: (Veramyst): Nasal spray susp: 27.5 mcg/spray, 120 sprays/bottle.] ▶L ♀C ▶? $

MOMETASONE—NASAL (*Nasonex*) Adult: 2 sprays/nostril daily. Peds 2 to 11 yo: 1 spray/nostril daily. [Trade only: Nasal spray, 120 sprays/bottle.] ▶L ♀C ▶? $$$$

TRIAMCINOLONE—NASAL (*Nasacort AQ, Nasacort HFA, Tri-Nasal, AllerNaze*) Nasacort HFA, Tri-Nasal, AllerNaze: 2 sprays per nostril daily to two times per day. Max 4 sprays/nostril/day. Nasacort AQ: 1 to 2 sprays per nostril daily. [Trade only: Nasal inhaler 55 mcg/spray, 100 sprays/bottle (Nasacort HFA). Nasal spray, 55 mcg/spray, 120 sprays/bottle (Nasacort AQ). Nasal spray 50 mcg/spray, 120 sprays/bottle (Tri-Nasal, AllerNaze).] ▶L ♀C ▶— $$$$

Nasal Preparations—Other

AZELASTINE—NASAL (*Astelin, Astepro*) 1 to 2 sprays per nostril two times per day. [Generic/Trade: Nasal spray, 200 sprays/bottle. Trade only: Astepro 0.15% nasal spray 200 sprays/bottle.] ▶L ♀C ▶? $$$$

CETACAINE (benzocaine + tetracaine + butamben) Topical anesthesia of mucous membranes: Spray: Apply for no more than 1 sec. Liquid or gel: Apply with cotton applicator directly to site. [Generic/Trade: (14%/2%/2%) Spray 56 mL. Topical liquid 56 mL. Topical gel 5, 29 g.] ▶LK ♀C ▶? $$

CROMOLYN—NASAL (*NasalCrom*) 1 spray per nostril three to four times per day. [OTC Generic/Trade: Nasal inhaler 200 sprays/bottle 13, 26 mL.] ▶L ♀C ▶? $

DYMISTA (azelastine—nasal + fluticasone—nasal) 1 spray per nostril 2 times per day. [Trade only: Nasal spray: 137 mcg astelazine/50 mcg fluticasone/spray, 120 sprays/bottle.] ▶L— ♀C ▶? $$$

IPRATROPIUM—NASAL (*Atrovent Nasal Spray*) 2 sprays per nostril two to four times per day. [Generic/Trade: Nasal spray 0.03%, 345 sprays/bottle, 0.06%, 165 sprays/bottle.] ▶L ♀B ▶? $$

LEVOCABASTINE—NASAL (*✦Livostin*) Canada only. 2 sprays per nostril two times per day, increase prn to three to four times per day. [Trade only: Nasal spray 0.5 mg/mL, plastic bottles of 15 mL. 50 mcg/spray.] ▶L (but minimal absorption) ♀C ▶— $$

OLOPATADINE—NASAL (*Patanase*) 2 sprays per nostril two times per day. [Generic/Trade: Nasal spray, 240 sprays/bottle.] ▶L ♀C ▶? $$$

OXYMETAZOLINE (*Afrin, Dristan 12 Hr Nasal, Nostrilla, Vicks Sinex 12 Hr*) 2 to 3 gtts/sprays per nostril two times per day prn nasal congestion for no more than 3 days. [OTC Generic/Trade: Nasal spray 0.05% 15, 30 mL; Nose gtts 0.025%, 0.05% 20 mL with dropper.] ▶L ♀C ▶? $

PHENYLEPHRINE—NASAL (*Neo-Synephrine, Vicks Sinex*) 2 to 3 sprays or gtts per nostril q 4 h prn for 3 days. [OTC Generic/Trade: Nasal gtts/spray 0.25, 0.5, 1% (15 mL).] ▶L ♀C ▶? $

SALINE NASAL SPRAY (*SeaMist, Entsol, Pretz, NaSal, Ocean, ★hydraSense*) Nasal dryness: 1 to 3 sprays or gtts per nostril prn. [Generic/Trade: Nasal spray 0.4, 0.5, 0.65, 0.75%. Nasal gtts 0.4, 0.65%. Trade only: Preservative-free nasal spray 3% (Entsol).] ▶Not metabolized ♀A ▶+ $

GASTROENTEROLOGY

HELICOBACTER PYLORI THERAPY

- • Triple therapy PO for 10 to 14 days: clarithromycin 500 mg two times per day plus amoxicillin 1 g two times per day (or metronidazole 500 mg two times per day) plus PPI*

- • Quadruple therapy PO for 14 days: bismuth subsalicylate 525 mg (or 30 mL) three to four times per day plus metronidazole 500 mg three to four times per day plus tetracycline 500 mg three to four times per day plus a PPI* or an H2 blocker†

- • PPI or H2 blocker may need to be continued past 14 days to heal the ulcer.

*PPIs include esomeprazole 40 mg daily, lansoprazole 30 mg two times per day, omeprazole 20 mg two times per day, pantoprazole 40 mg two times per day, rabeprazole 20 mg two times per day.

†H2 blockers include cimetidine 400 mg two times per day, famotidine 20 mg two times per day, nizatidine 150 mg two times per day, ranitidine 150 mg two times per day. Adapted from Medical Letter Treatment Guidelines 2008:55.

Antidiarrheals

BISMUTH SUBSALICYLATE (*Pepto-Bismol, Kaopectate*) 2 tabs or caplets or 30 mL (262 mg/15 mL) PO q 30 min to 1 h up to 8 doses per day for up to 2 days. Peds: 5 mL (262 mg/15 mL) or $^1/_3$ tab, chew tab, or cap PO for age 3 to 6 yo, 10 mL (262 mg/15 mL) or $^2/_3$ tab, chew tab, or cap PO for age 6 to 9 yo. Risk of Reye's syndrome in children. OTC Generic/Trade: Chewable tabs 262 mg. Susp 262, 525, 750 mg/15 mL. OTC Trade only: Caplets 262 mg (Pepto-Bismol). Susp 87 mg/5 mL (Kaopectate Children's Liquid).] ▶K ♀D ▶? $

IMODIUM MULTI-SYMPTOM RELIEF (**loperamide + simethicone**) 2 tabs or caplets PO initially, then 1 tab or caplet PO after each unformed stool to a max of 4 tabs/caplets per day. Peds: 1 tab or caplet PO initially, then ½ caplet PO after each unformed stool (up to 2 tabs or caplets PO per day for age 6 to 8 yo or wt 48 to 59 lbs or up to 3 tabs or caplets PO per day for age 9 to 11 yo or wt 60 to 95 lbs). [OTC Generic/Trade: Caplets, Chewable tabs 2 mg loperamide/125 mg simethicone.] ▶L ♀C ▶– $

LOMOTIL (**diphenoxylate + atropine**) 2 tabs or 10 mL PO four times per day. [Generic/Trade: Oral soln or tab 2.5 mg/0.025 mg diphenoxylate/atropine per 5 mL or tab.] ▶L ♀C ▶– $

LOPERAMIDE (*Imodium, Imodium AD, ✦Loperacap, Diarr-Eze*) 4 mg PO initially, then 2 mg PO after each unformed stool to max 16 mg per day. Peds: 1 mg PO three times per day for wt 13 to 20 kg, 2 mg PO two times per day for age 6 to 8 yo or wt 21 to 30 kg, 2 mg PO three times per day for wt greater than 30 kg. [OTC Generic/Trade: Tabs 2 mg. Oral soln 1 mg/5 mL. Oral soln 1 mg/7.5 mL.] ▶L ♀C ▶+ $

MOTOFEN (**difenoxin + atropine**) 2 tabs PO initially, then 1 tab after each loose stool q 3 to 4 h prn (up to 8 tabs per day). [Trade only: Tabs difenoxin 1 mg + atropine 0.025 mg.] ▶L ♀C ▶– ©IV $$

GASTROENTEROLOGY

OPIUM (opium tincture, paregoric) Paregoric: 5 to 10 mL PO daily (up to four times). Opium tincture: 0.6 mL (range 0.3 to 1 mL) PO q 2 to 6 h, prn, to a max of 6 mL per day. Opium tincture contains 25 times more morphine than paregoric. [Trade only: Opium tincture 10% (deodorized opium tincture, 10 mg morphine equivalent/mL). Generic only: Paregoric (camphorated opium tincture, 2 mg morphine equivalent/5 mL).] ▶L ♀B (D with long-term use) ▶? ⊚II (opium tincture), III (paregoric) $$

Antiemetics—5-HT3 Receptor Antagonists

AKYNZEO (palonosetron + netupitant) Nausea with chemo: 1 capsule PO 1 h prior to chemo. [Trade only: Capsule (0.5 mg palonosetron + 300 mg netupitant).] ▶L ♀C ▶? $$$$$

DOLASETRON (Anzemet) Nausea with chemo: 100 mg PO single dose. [Trade only: Tabs 50, 100 mg. Injectable no longer available in Canada.] ▶LK ♀B ▶? $$$

GRANISETRON (Sancuso) Nausea with chemo: Transdermal (Sancuso): 1 patch to upper outer arm at least 24 h (but up to 48 h) before chemotherapy. Remove 24 h after completion of chemotherapy. Can be worn up to 7 days depending on the duration of chemo. [Trade only: Transdermal patch (Sancuso) 34.3 mg of granisetron delivering 3.1 mg/24 h.] ▶L ♀B ▶? $$$$

ONDANSETRON (Zofran, Zuplenz) Nausea with chemo: IV: 0.15 mg/kg/dose (max 16 mg) 30 min prior to chemo and repeated at 4 h and 8 h after 1st dose for age 6 mo or older. PO: 4 mg PO 30 min prior to chemo and repeat at 4 h and 8 h for age 4 to 11 yo, 8 mg PO and repeated 8 h later for age 12 yo or older. Prevention of post-op N/V: 4 mg IV over 2 to 5 min or 4 mg IM or 16 mg PO 1 h before anesthesia. Give 0.1 mg/kg IV over 2 min to 5 min as a single dose for age 1 mo to 12 yo if wt 40 kg or less; 4 mg IV over 2 min to 5 min as a single dose if wt greater than 40 kg. Prevention of N/V associated with radiotherapy: 8 mg PO three times per day. [Generic/Trade: Tabs 4, 8, 24 mg. Orally disintegrating tabs 4, 8 mg. Oral soln 4 mg/5 mL. Trade only: Oral film (Zuplenz) 4, 8 mg.] ▶L ♀B ▶? $$$$$

PALONOSETRON (Aloxi) Nausea with chemo: 0.25 mg IV over 30 sec, 30 min prior to chemo. Children 1 mo to 17 yo: 20 mcg/kg (max 1.5 mg) IV over 15 min, 30 min prior to chemo. Prevention of postop N/V: 0.075 mg IV over 10 sec just prior to anesthesia. [Trade only: injectable.] ▶L ♀B ▶? $$$$$

Antiemetics—Other

APREPITANT (Emend, fosaprepitant) Prevention of nausea with moderately to highly emetogenic chemo, in combination with a corticosteroid and a 5-HT3 antagonist: 125 mg PO on day 1 (1 h prior to chemo), then 80 mg PO q am on days 2 and 3. Alternative for 1st dose only is 115 mg IV (fosaprepitant) over 15 min given 30 min prior to chemo. Alternatively, single dose of 150 mg IV (fosaprepitant) over 20 to 30 min, with a corticosteroid and a 5-HT3 antagonist. Prevention of postop N/V: 40 mg PO within 3 h prior to anesthesia. [Trade only (aprepitant): Caps 40, 80, 125 mg. IV prodrug form is fosaprepitant.] ▶L ♀B ▶? $$$$$

DICLEGIS (doxylamine + pyridoxine, ✦*Diclectin*) N/V due to pregnancy: 2 tabs PO at bedtime. If not controlled, can increase to max 4 tabs daily (1 tab PO q am, 1 tab PO mid-afternoon, 2 tabs PO at bedtime). [Trade: Tabs doxylamine 10 mg and pyridoxine 10 mg.] ▶LK ♀A ▶– $$$$$

DIMENHYDRINATE (*Dramamine*, ✦*Gravol*) 50 to 100 mg PO/IM/IV q 4 to 6 h prn (max 400 mg/24 h PO, 600 mg/day IV/IM). Canada only: 50 to 100 mg/dose PR q 4 to 6 h prn. [OTC Generic/Trade: Tabs 50 mg. Trade only: Chewable tabs 25, 50 mg. Generic only: Oral soln 12.5 mg/5 mL. Canada only: Supp 25, 50, 100 mg.] ▶LK ♀B ▶– $

DOMPERIDONE Canada only. Postprandial dyspepsia: 10 to 20 mg PO three to four times per day, 30 min before a meal. N/V: 20 mg PO three to four times per day. [Canada only. Trade/Generic: Tabs 10, 20 mg.] ▶L ♀? ▶ $$

DOXYLAMINE (*Unisom Nighttime Sleep Aid, others*) N/V associated with pregnancy: 12.5 mg PO two to four times per day; often used in combination with pyridoxine. Do not use in children younger than 12 yo. [OTC, Generic/Trade: Tabs 25 mg.] ▶LK ♀A ▶? ♥

DRONABINOL (*Marinol*) Nausea with chemo: 5 mg/m² PO 1 to 3 h before chemo then 5 mg/m²/dose q 2 to 4 h after chemo for 4 to 6 doses/day. Anorexia associated with AIDS: Initially 2.5 mg PO two times per day before lunch and dinner. If indicated and tolerated, increase to 20 mg/day. [Generic/Trade: Caps 2.5, 5, 10 mg.] ▶L ♀C ▶– ©III $$$$$

DROPERIDOL (*Inapsine*) 0.625 to 2.5 mg IV or 2.5 mg IM. May cause fatal QT prolongation, even in patients with no risk factors. Monitor ECG before. ▶L ♀C ▶? $

METOCLOPRAMIDE (*Reglan, Metozolv ODT*, ✦*Maxeran*) GERD/diabetic gastroparesis: 10 mg IV/IM q 2 to 3 h prn. 10 to 15 mg PO four times per day, 30 min before meals and at bedtime. Caution with long-term (more than 3 months) use. Prevention of postop nausea: 10 to 20 mg IM/IV near end of surgical procedure, may repeat q 3 to 4 h prn. [Generic/Trade: Tabs 5, 10 mg. Trade: Orally disintegrating tabs 5, 10 mg (Metozolv). Generic only: Oral soln 5 mg/5 mL.] ▶K ♀B ▶? $

NABILONE (*Cesamet*) 1 to 2 mg PO two times per day, 1 to 3 h before chemotherapy. [Trade only: Caps 1 mg.] ▶L ♀C ▶– ©II $$$$$

PHOSPHORATED CARBOHYDRATES (*Emetrol*) 15 to 30 mL PO q 15 min prn, max 5 doses. Peds: 5 to 10 mL per dose. [OTC Generic/Trade: Soln containing dextrose, fructose, and phosphoric acid.] ▶L ♀A ▶+ $

PROCHLORPERAZINE (✦*Stemetil*) 5 to 10 mg IV over at least 2 min. 5 to 10 mg PO/IM three to four times per day. 25 mg PR q 12 h. Sustained-release: 15 mg PO q am or 10 mg PO q 12 h. Peds: 0.1 mg/kg/dose PO/PR three to four times per day or 0.1 to 0.15 mg/kg/dose IM three to four times per day. Brand name Compazine no longer available. [Generic only: Tabs 5, 10, 25 mg. Supp 25 mg.] ▶LK ♀C ▶? $

PROMETHAZINE (*Phenergan*) Adults: 12.5 to 25 mg PO/IM/PR q 4 to 6 h. Peds: 0.25 to 1 mg/kg PO/IM/PR q 4 to 6 h. Contraindicated if age younger than 2 yo; caution in older children. IV use common but not approved. Brand name Phenergan no longer available. [Generic only: Tabs/Supp 12.5, 25, 50 mg. Syrup 6.25 mg/5 mL.] ▶LK ♀C ▶– $

SCOPOLAMINE (*Transderm-Scop, Scopace, ✦Transderm-V*) Motion sickness: Apply 1 disc (1.5 mg) behind ear 4 h prior to event; replace q 3 days. Tab: 0.4 to 0.8 mg PO 1 h before travel and q 8 h prn. [Trade only: Topical disc 1.5 mg/72 h, box of 4. Oral tab 0.4 mg.] ▶L ♀C ▶+ $$

TRIMETHOBENZAMIDE (*Tigan*) 300 mg PO q 6 to 8 h, 200 mg IM q 6 to 8 h. [Generic/Trade: Cap 300 mg.] ▶LK ♀C ▶? $

Antiulcer—Antacids

ALKA-SELTZER (**acetylsalicylic acid + citrate + bicarbonate**) 2 regular-strength tabs in 4 oz water q 4 h PO prn (up to 8 tabs daily for age younger than 60 yo, up to 4 tabs daily for age 60 yo or older) or 2 extra-strength tabs in 4 oz water q 6 h PO prn (up to 7 tabs daily for age younger than 60 yo, up to 3 tabs daily for age 60 yo or older). [OTC Trade only: Regular-strength, original: aspirin 325 mg + citric acid 1000 mg + sodium bicarbonate 1916 mg. Regular-strength lemon-lime and cherry: 325 mg + 1000 mg + 1700 mg. Extra-strength: 500 mg + 1000 mg + 1985 mg. Not all forms of Alka-Seltzer contain aspirin (eg, Alka-Seltzer Heartburn Relief).] ▶LK ♀? (− 3rd trimester) ▶? $

ALUMINUM HYDROXIDE (*Alternagel, Amphojel, Alu-Tab, Alu-Cap, ✦Basaljel, Mucaine*) 5 to 10 mL or 300 to 600 mg PO up to 6 times per day. Constipating. [OTC Generic/Trade: Susp 320, 600 mg/ 5 mL.] ▶K ♀C ▶? $

GAVISCON (**aluminum hydroxide + magnesium carbonate**) 2 to 4 tabs or 15 to 30 mL (regular-strength) or 10 mL (extra-strength) PO four times per day prn. [OTC Trade only: Tabs: Regular-strength (Al hydroxide 80 mg + Mg carbonate 20 mg), Extra-strength (Al hydroxide 160 mg + Mg carbonate 105 mg). Liquid: Regular-strength (Al hydroxide 95 mg + Mg carbonate 358 mg per 15 mL), Extra-strength (Al hydroxide 254 mg + Mg carbonate 237.5 mg per 5 mL).] ▶K ♀? ▶? $

MAALOX (**aluminum hydroxide + magnesium hydroxide**) 10 mL to 20 mL or 1 to 2 tabs PO prn. [OTC Generic/Trade: Regular-strength chewable tabs (Al hydroxide + Mg hydroxide 200/200 mg). Susp (225/200 mg per 5 mL). Other strengths available.] ▶K ♀C ▶? $

MYLANTA (**aluminum hydroxide + magnesium hydroxide + simethicone**) 10 to 20 mL PO between meals and at bedtime prn. [OTC Generic/Trade: Liquid (various concentrations, eg, regular-strength, maximum-strength, supreme, etc.).] ▶K ♀C ▶? $

ROLAIDS (**calcium carbonate + magnesium hydroxide**) 2 to 4 tabs PO q 1 h prn, max 12 tabs/day (regular-strength) or 10 tabs/day (extra-strength). [OTC Trade only: Tabs regular-strength (Ca carbonate 550 mg, Mg hydroxide 110 mg), extra-strength (Ca carbonate 675 mg, Mg hydroxide 135 mg).] ▶K ♀? ▶? $

Antiulcer—H2 Antagonists

CIMETIDINE (*Tagamet, Tagamet HB*) 300 mg IV/IM/PO q 6 to 8 h, 400 mg PO two times per day, or 400 to 800 mg PO at bedtime. Erosive esophagitis: 800 mg PO two times per day or 400 mg PO four times per day. Continuous IV infusion 37.5 to 50 mg/h (900 to 1200 mg/day). [Tabs 200, 300, 400, 800 mg. Rx Generic only: Oral soln 300 mg/5 mL. OTC Generic/Trade: Tabs 200 mg.] ▶LK ♀B ▶+ $

FAMOTIDINE (*Pepcid, Pepcid AC, Maximum Strength Pepcid AC*) 20 mg IV q 12 h, 20 to 40 mg PO at bedtime, or 20 mg PO two times per day. [Generic/Trade: Tabs 10 mg (OTC, Pepcid AC Acid Controller), 20 mg (Rx and OTC, Maximum Strength Pepcid AC), 40 mg. Rx Generic/Trade: Susp 40 mg/5 mL.] ▶LK ♀B ▶? $

NIZATIDINE (*Axid, Axid AR*) 150 to 300 mg PO at bedtime, or 150 mg PO two times per day. [OTC (Axid AR): Tabs 75 mg. Rx Generic: Caps 150 mg. Oral soln 15 mg/mL (120, 480 mL). Caps 300 mg.] ▶K ♀B ▶? $$$$

PEPCID COMPLETE (**famotidine + calcium carbonate + magnesium hydroxide**) 1 tab PO prn. Max 2 tabs/day. [OTC trade/generic: Chewable tab, famotidine 10 mg with Ca carbonate 800 mg and Mg hydroxide 165 mg.] ▶LK ♀B ▶? $

RANITIDINE (*Zantac, Zantac EFFERdose, Zantac 75, Zantac 150, Peptic Relief*) 150 mg PO two times per day or 300 mg PO at bedtime. 50 mg IV/IM q 8 h, or continuous infusion 6.25 mg/h (150 mg/day). [Generic/Trade: Tabs 75 mg (OTC: Zantac 75), 150 mg (OTC and Rx: Zantac 150), 300 mg. Syrup 75 mg/5 mL. Rx Trade only: Effervescent tabs 25 mg. Rx Generic only: Caps 150, 300 mg.] ▶K ♀B ▶? $$$

Antiulcer—Helicobacter pylori Treatment

PREVPAC (**lansoprazole + amoxicillin + clarithromycin**, ✦*HP-Pac*) 1 dose PO two times per day for 10 to 14 days. [Generic/Trade: Each dose consists of lansoprazole 30 mg cap + amoxicillin 1 g (2 × 500 mg cap), + clarithromycin 500 mg tab.] ▶LK ♀C ▶? $$$$$

PYLERA (**bismuth subcitrate potassium + metronidazole + tetracycline**) 3 caps PO four times per day (after meals and at bedtime) for 10 days. Use with omeprazole 20 mg PO two times per day. [Trade only: Each cap contains bismuth subcitrate potassium 140 mg + metronidazole 125 mg + tetracycline 125 mg.] ▶LK ♀D ▶– $$$$$

Antiulcer—Proton Pump Inhibitors

DEXLANSOPRAZOLE (*Dexilant*) Take without regard to meals. Healing of erosive esophagitis: 60 mg PO once daily for up to 8 weeks. Maintenance of erosive esophagitis: 30 mg PO once daily for up to 6 months. Symptomatic nonerosive GERD: 30 mg PO once daily for 4 weeks. [Rx: Cap 30 mg, 60 mg.] ▶L ♀B ▶–

ESOMEPRAZOLE (*Nexium*) Erosive esophagitis: 20 to 40 mg PO daily for 4 to 8 weeks. Maintenance of erosive esophagitis: 20 mg PO daily. Zollinger-Ellison: 40 mg PO two times per day. GERD: 20 mg PO daily for 4 weeks. Prevention of NSAID-associated gastric ulcer: 20 to 40 mg PO daily for up to 6 months. *H. pylori* eradication: 40 mg PO daily with amoxicillin 1000 mg PO two times per day and clarithromycin 500 mg PO two times per day for 10 days. [Rx Generic/Trade: Caps, delayed-release 20, 40 mg. Trade only: Delayed-release granules for oral susp 2.5, 5, 10, 40 mg per packet. OTC/Trade: Caps, delayed-release 20 mg.] ▶L ♀B ▶? $$$$$

LANSOPRAZOLE (*Prevacid*) Heartburn: 15 mg PO daily. Duodenal ulcer: 15 mg daily for 4 weeks. Maintenance therapy after healing of duodenal ulcer: 15 mg

(cont.)

PO daily for up to 12 months. NSAID-induced gastric ulcer: 30 mg PO daily for 8 weeks (treatment), 15 mg PO daily for up to 12 weeks (prevention). GERD: 15 mg PO daily for up to 8 weeks. Gastric ulcer: 30 mg PO daily for up to 8 weeks. Erosive esophagitis: 30 mg PO daily for up to 8 weeks or 30 mg IV daily for 7 days or until taking PO. [OTC Generic/Trade: Caps 15 mg. Rx Generic/Trade: 15, 30 mg. Rx Trade only: Orally disintegrating tab 15, 30 mg.] ▶L ♀B ▶? $$$$

OMEPRAZOLE (*Prilosec*, *+Losec*) GERD, duodenal ulcer, erosive esophagitis: 20 mg PO daily. Heartburn (OTC): 20 mg PO daily for 14 days. Gastric ulcer: 40 mg PO daily. Hypersecretory conditions: 60 mg PO daily. [Rx Generic/Trade: Caps 10, 20, 40 mg. Trade only: Granules for oral susp 2.5 mg, 10 mg. OTC Trade only: Cap 20 mg.] ▶L ♀C ▶? OTC $, Rx $$$$

PANTOPRAZOLE (*Protonix*, *+Pantoloc, Tecta*) Treatment of erosive esophagitis associated with GERD: 40 mg PO daily for 8 to 16 weeks. Maintenance of erosive esophagitis: 40 mg PO once daily. Zollinger-Ellison syndrome and other hypersecretory conditions: 40 mg PO twice daily or 80 mg IV q 8 to 12 h for 7 days until taking PO. [Generic/Trade: Tabs 20, 40 mg. Trade only: Granules for susp 40 mg/packet.] ▶L ♀B ▶? $

RABEPRAZOLE (*AcipHex*, *+Pariet*) GERD, duodenal ulcer, erosive esophagitis: 20 mg PO daily. [Generic/Trade: Tabs 20 mg. Trade only: Sprinkle caps (open and sprinkle on soft food or liquid) 5 mg and 10 mg.] ▶L ♀C ▶? $$$$

ZEGERID (omeprazole + bicarbonate) Duodenal ulcer, GERD, erosive esophagitis: 20 mg PO daily for 4 to 8 weeks. Maintenance of erosive esophagitis: 20 mg PO daily. Gastric ulcer: 40 mg PO once daily for 4 to 8 weeks. Reduction of risk of upper GI bleed in critically ill (susp only): 40 mg PO, then 40 mg 6 to 8 h later, then 40 mg once daily thereafter for up to 14 days. [OTC Trade only: Omeprazole/sodium bicarbonate caps 20 mg/1.1 g. Rx Generic/Trade: Caps 20 mg/1.1 g and 40 mg/1.1 g. Trade only: Powder packets for susp 20 mg/1.1 g and 40 mg/1.68 g.] ▶L ♀C ▶? $$$$$

Antiulcer—Other

DICYCLOMINE (*Bentyl*, *+Bentylol*) 10 to 20 mg PO/IM four times per day up to 40 mg PO four times per day. [Generic/Trade: Tabs 20 mg. Caps 10 mg.] ▶LK ♀B ▶– $

DONNATAL (phenobarbital + hyoscyamine + atropine + scopolamine) 1 to 2 tabs/caps or 5 to 10 mL PO three to four times per day. 1 extended-release tab PO q 8 to 12 h. [Generic/Trade: Phenobarbital 16.2 mg + hyoscyamine 0.1 mg + atropine 0.02 mg + scopolamine 6.5 mcg in each tab or 5 mL. Trade only: Extended-release tab, 48.6 + 0.3111 + 0.0582 + 0.0195 mg.] ▶LK ♀C ▶– $$$

GI COCKTAIL (green goddess) Acute GI upset: Mixture of Maalox/Mylanta 30 mL + viscous lidocaine (2%) 10 mL + Donnatal 10 mL administered PO in a single dose. ▶LK ♀See individual ▶See individual $

HYOSCINE (*+Buscopan*) Canada: GI or bladder spasm: 10 to 20 mg PO/IV up to 60 mg daily (PO) or 100 mg daily (IV). [Canada Trade only: Tabs 10 mg.] ▶LK ♀C ▶? $$

HYOSCYAMINE (*Anaspaz, A-spaz, Cystospaz, ED Spaz, Hyosol, Hyospaz, Levbid, Levsin, Medispaz, NuLev, Spacol, Spasdel, Symax*) Bladder spasm, control

(cont.)

gastric secretion, GI hypermotility, irritable bowel syndrome: 0.125 to 0.25 mg PO/SL q 4 h or prn. Extended-release: 0.375 to 0.75 mg PO q 12 h. Max 1.5 mg/day. [Generic/Trade: Tabs 0.125. Sublingual tabs 0.125 mg. Chewable tabs 0.125 mg. Extended-release tabs 0.375 mg. Elixir 0.125 mg/5 mL. Gtts 0.125 mg/1 mL.] ▶LK ♀C ▶– $

MISOPROSTOL (*PGE1, Cytotec*) Prevention of NSAID-induced gastric ulcers: 100 mcg PO two times per day, then titrate as tolerated up to 200 mcg PO four times per day. Cervical ripening: 25 mcg intravaginally q 3 to 6 h (or 50 mcg q 6 h). First trimester pregnancy failure: 800 mcg intravaginally, repeat on day 3 if expulsion incomplete. [Generic/Trade: Oral tabs 100, 200 mcg.] ▶LK ♀X ▶– $$$$

PROPANTHELINE (*Pro-Banthine*) 7.5 to 15 mg PO 30 min after meals and 30 mg at bedtime. [Generic only: Tabs 15 mg.] ▶LK ♀C ▶– $$$

SIMETHICONE (*Mylicon, Gas-X, Phazyme, ✦Ovol*) 40 to 360 mg PO four times per day prn, max 500 mg/day. Infants: 20 mg PO four times per day prn. [OTC Generic/Trade: Chewable tabs 80, 125 mg. Gtts 40 mg/0.6 mL. Trade only: Softgels 166 mg (Gas-X) 180 mg (Phazyme). Strips, oral (Gas-X) 62.5 mg (adults), 40 mg (children).] ▶not absorbed ♀C but + ▶? $

SUCRALFATE (*Carafate, ✦Sulcrate*) 1 g PO 1 h before meals (2 h before other medications) and at bedtime. [Generic/Trade: Tabs 1 g. Susp 1 g/10 mL.] ▶not absorbed ♀B ▶? $$

Laxatives—Bulk-Forming

METHYLCELLULOSE (*Citrucel*) 1 heaping tablespoon in 8 oz water or 2 caplets PO daily (up to three times per day). [OTC Trade only: Regular and sugar-free packets and multiple-use canisters, Clear-mix soln, Caplets 500 mg.] ▶not absorbed ♀+ ▶? $

POLYCARBOPHIL (*FiberCon, Konsyl Fiber, Equalactin*) Laxative: 2 tabs (1250 mg) PO four times per day prn. Diarrhea: 2 tabs (1250 mg) PO q 30 min. Max daily dose 6 g. [OTC Generic/Trade: Tabs/Caps 625 mg. OTC Trade only: Chewable tabs 625 mg (Equalactin).] ▶not absorbed ♀+ ▶? $

PSYLLIUM (*Metamucil, Fiberall, Konsyl, Hydrocil*) 1 teaspoon in liquid, 1 packet in liquid, or 1 to 2 wafers with liquid PO daily (up to three times per day). [OTC Generic/Trade: Regular and sugar-free powder, Granules, Caps, Wafers, including various flavors and various amounts of psyllium.] ▶not absorbed ♀+ ▶? $

Laxatives—Osmotic

GLYCERIN (*Fleet*) 1 adult or infant supp or 5 to 15 mL as an enema PR prn. [OTC Generic/Trade: Supp, infant and adult. Soln (Fleet Babylax) 4 mL/applicator.] ▶not absorbed ♀C ▶? $

LACTULOSE (*Enulose, Kristalose*) Constipation: 15 mL to 30 mL (syrup) or 10 g to 20 g (powder for oral soln) PO daily. Hepatic encephalopathy: 30 mL to 45 mL (syrup) PO three to four times per day, or 300 mL retention enema. [Generic/Trade: Syrup 10 g/15 mL. Trade only (Kristalose): 10, 20 g packets for oral soln.] ▶not absorbed ♀B ▶? $$

MAGNESIUM CITRATE 150 to 300 mL PO once or in divided doses. 2 to 4 mL/kg/day once or in divided doses for age younger than 6 yo. [OTC Generic only: Soln 300 mL/bottle. Low-sodium and sugar-free available.] ▶K ♀C ▶? $

MAGNESIUM HYDROXIDE (*Milk of Magnesia*) Laxative: 30 to 60 mL regular-strength (400 mg per 5 mL) liquid PO. Antacid: 5 to 15 mL regular-strength liquid or 622 to 1244 mg PO four times per day prn. [OTC Generic/Trade: Susp 400 mg/5 mL. Trade only: Chewable tabs 311, 400 mg. Generic only: Susp 800 mg/5 mL, (concentrated) 1200 mg/5 mL, sugar-free 400 mg/5 mL.] ▶K ♀+ ▶? $

POLYETHYLENE GLYCOL (*MiraLax, GlycoLax, ♦Lax-A-Day, RestoroLAX*) 17 g (1 heaping tablespoon) in 4 to 8 oz water, juice, soda, coffee, or tea PO daily. [OTC Generic/Trade: Powder for oral soln 17 g/scoop, 17 g packets. Rx Generic/Trade: Powder for oral soln 17 g/scoop.] ▶not absorbed ♀C ▶? $

POLYETHYLENE GLYCOL WITH ELECTROLYTES (*GoLYTELY, Colyte, Suclear, Suprep, TriLyte, NuLYTELY, MoviPrep, HalfLytely, ♦Klean-Prep, Electropeg, Peg-Lyte*) Bowel prep: 240 mL q 10 min PO or 20 to 30 mL per NG until 4 L are consumed. MoviPrep, Suclear, Suprep: Follow specific instructions. [Generic/Trade: Powder for oral soln in disposable jug 4 L or 2 L (MoviPrep). Trade only: GoLYTELY Packet for oral soln to make 3.785 L. Suclear: Dose 1 (16 oz) and Dose 2 (2 L bottle) for reconstitution. Suprep: Two 6 oz bottles.] ▶not absorbed ♀C ▶? $

PREPOPIK (**sodium picosulfate**) Preferred method: 1 packet (diluted in 5 oz water) evening before the colonoscopy and 2nd packet (diluted in 5 oz water) morning prior to colonoscopy. Alternatively, 1st dose during afternoon or early evening before the colonoscopy and 2nd dose 6 h later in evening before colonoscopy. Additional clear liquids should be consumed. [Trade: 2 packets of 16 g powder for reconstitution.] ▶minimal absorption ♀B ▶? $

SODIUM PHOSPHATE (*Fleet enema, Fleet EZ-Prep, Accu-Prep, OsmoPrep, Visicol, ♦Enemol, Phoslax*) Constipation: 1 adult or pediatric enema PR or 20 to 30 mL of oral soln PO prn (max 45 mL/24 h). Prep prior to colonoscopy: Visicol: Evening before colonoscopy: 3 tabs with 8 oz clear liquid q 15 min until 20 tabs are consumed. Day of colonoscopy: Starting 3 to 5 h before procedure, 3 tabs with 8 oz clear liquid q 15 min until 20 tabs are consumed. OsmoPrep: 32 tabs PO with total of 2 quarts clear liquids as follows: evening before procedure: 4 tabs PO with 8 oz of clear liquids q 15 min for a total of 20 tabs; day of procedure: 3 to 5 h before procedure, 4 tabs with 8 oz of clear liquids q 15 min for a total of 12 tabs. [OTC Generic/Trade: Adult enema, oral soln. OTC Trade only: Pediatric enema, bowel prep. Rx Trade only: Visicol, OsmoPrep tab ($$$$) 1.5 g.] ▶not absorbed ♀C ▶? $ ▲

SORBITOL 30 to 150 mL (of 70% soln) PO or 120 mL (of 25 to 30% soln) PR as a single dose. Cathartic: 4.3 mL/kg PO. [Generic only: Soln 70%.] ▶not absorbed ♀C ▶? $

SUPREP (**sodium sulfate + potassium sulfate + magnesium sulfate**) Evening before colonoscopy: Dilute 1 bottle to 16 oz with water and drink, then drink 32 oz water over next hour. Next morning, repeat both steps. Compete 1 h before colonoscopy. [Trade: Two 6 oz bottles for dilution.] ▶not absorbed ♀C ▶? $

Laxatives—Stimulant

BISACODYL (*Correctol, Dulcolax, Feen-a-Mint, Fleet*) 5 to 15 mg PO prn, 10 mg PR prn, 5 to 10 mg PR prn if 2 to 11 yo. [OTC Generic/Trade: Tabs 5 mg, suppository 10 mg. OTC Trade only: Enema, 10 mg/30 mL.] ▶L ♀C ▶? $

CASCARA 5 mL of aromatic fluid extract PO at bedtime prn. [Rx Generic only: Liquid aromatic fluid extract.] ▶L ♀C ▶+ $

CASTOR OIL Children: 5 to 15 mL/dose of castor oil PO or 7.5 to 30 mL emulsified castor oil PO once a day. Adult: 15 to 60 mL castor oil or 30 to 60 mL emulsified castor oil PO once a day. [OTC Generic only: Oil 60, 120, 180, 480 mL.] ▶not absorbed ♀– ▶? $

SENNA (*Senokot, SenokotXTRA, Ex-Lax, Fletcher's Castoria*) 2 tabs or 1 teaspoon granules or 10 to 15 mL syrup PO. Max 8 tabs, 4 teaspoon granules, 30 mL syrup/day. Take granules with full glass of water. [OTC Generic/Trade (All dosing is based on sennosides content; 1 mg sennosides is equivalent to 21.7 mg standardized senna concentrate): Syrup 8.8 mg/5 mL. Liquid 33.3 mg concentrate/mL (Fletcher's Castoria). Tabs 8.6, 15, 17, 25 mg. Chewable tabs 10, 15 mg.] ▶L ♀C ▶+ $

Laxatives—Stool Softener

DOCUSATE (*Colace, Docu-Soft, DOK, Dulcolax, Docu-Liquid, Enemeez, Fleet Sof-Lax, Octycine, Silace*) Constipation: Docusate calcium: 240 mg PO daily. Docusate sodium: 50 to 500 mg/day PO divided in 1 to 4 doses. Peds: 10 to 40 mg/day for age younger than 3 yo, give 20 to 60 mg/day for age 3 to 6 yo, give 40 to 150 mg/day for age 6 to 12 yo. In all cases, doses are divided up to four times per day. Cerumen impaction: 1 mL in affected ear. [Docusate calcium OTC Generic/Trade: Caps 240 mg. Docusate sodium OTC Generic/Trade: Caps 50, 100, 250 mg. Liquid 50 mg/5 mL. Syrup 20 mg/5 mL. Docusate sodium OTC Trade only (Enemeez): Enema, rectal 283 mg/5 mL.] ▶L ♀C ▶? $

Laxatives—Other or Combinations

LUBIPROSTONE (*Amitiza*) Chronic idiopathic constipation: 24 mcg PO two times per day with food and water. Irritable bowel syndrome with constipation in women age 18 yo or older: 8 mcg PO two times per day. Opioid-induced constipation in adults with chronic, non-cancer pain: 24 mcg PO two times per day with food and water. [Trade only: Cap 8, 24 mcg.] ▶gut ♀C ▶? $$$$$

MINERAL OIL (*Kondremul, Fleet Mineral Oil Enema, Liqui-Doss, ✦Lansoyl*) 15 to 45 mL PO. Peds: 5 to 15 mL/dose PO. Mineral oil enema: 60 to 150 mL PR. Peds: 30 to 60 mL PR. [OTC Generic/Trade: Oil (30, 480 mL), Enema (Fleet). OTC Trade only: Oral liquid (Liqui-Doss) 13.5 mg/15 mL. Oral microemulsion (Kondremul) 2.5 mg/5 mL.] ▶not absorbed ♀C ▶? $

PERI-COLACE (docusate + sennosides) 2 to 4 tabs PO once daily or in divided doses prn. [OTC Generic/Trade: Tabs 50 mg docusate + 8.6 mg sennosides.] ▶L ♀C ▶? $

SENOKOT-S (senna + docusate) 2 tabs PO daily. [OTC Generic/Trade: Tabs 8.6 mg senna concentrate + 50 mg docusate.] ▶L ♀C ▶+ $

Ulcerative Colitis

BALSALAZIDE (*Colazal, Giazo*) Active mild to moderate ulcerative colitis: 2.25 g PO three times per day (Colazal) for 8 to 12 weeks or three 1.1 g (3.3 g) tabs PO twice per day (Giazo is for males only, not approved for use in females) for 8 weeks. [Generic/Trade (Colazal): Caps 750 mg. Trade only (Giazo): Tabs 1.1 g.] ▶minimal absorption ♀B ▶? $$$$$

MESALAMINE (**5-aminosalicylic acid**, *Apriso, 5-Aspirin, Lialda, Pentasa, Canasa, Rowasa, Delzicol, Asacol HD ✦Mesasal, Salofalk*) Apriso: 1.5 g (4 caps) PO q am. Delzicol: 800 mg PO three times a day (treatment) or 800 mg PO twice a day (maintenance). Pentasa: 1000 mg PO four times per day or two 800 mg tablets three times daily (4.8 g/day) with or without food for 6 weeks. Lialda: 2.4 to 4.8 g PO daily with a meal. Canasa: 500 mg PR two to three times per day or 1000 mg PR at bedtime. Susp: 4 g enema PR at bedtime (retain 8 h) for 3 to 6 weeks. Asacol HD: 1.6 g PO three times a day for 6 weeks. [Trade only: Delayed-release caps (Delzicol) 400 mg. Controlled-release caps 250, 500 mg (Pentasa). Delayed-release tabs 800 mg (Asacol HD), 1200 mg (Lialda). Rectal supp 1000 mg (Canasa). Generic/Trade: Rectal supp 0.375 g (Apriso). Generic/Trade: Rectal susp 4 g/60 mL (Rowasa).] ▶gut ♀C ▶? $$$$$

OLSALAZINE (*Dipentum*) Ulcerative colitis: 500 mg PO two times per day with food. [Trade only: Caps 250 mg.] ▶L ♀C ▶? $$$$$

SULFASALAZINE—GASTROENTEROLOGY (*Azulfidine, Azulfidine EN-tabs, ✦Salazopyrin En-tabs*) Ulcerative colitis: 500 to 1000 mg PO four times per day. Peds, age 6 yo and older: 30 to 60 mg/kg/day PO divided q 4 to 6 h. May turn body fluids, contact lenses, or skin orange-yellow. [Generic/Trade: Tabs 500 mg, scored. Enteric-coated, delayed-release (EN-tabs) 500 mg.] ▶L ♀B ▶? $$

Other GI Agents

ALOSETRON (*Lotronex*) Prescribers must be certified to prescribe. Diarrhea-predominant irritable bowel syndrome in women who have failed conventional therapy: 0.5 mg PO two times per day for 4 weeks; discontinue in patients who become constipated. If well tolerated and symptoms not controlled after 4 weeks, may increase to 1 mg PO two times per day. Discontinue if symptoms not controlled in 4 weeks on 1 mg PO two times per day. [Trade only: Tabs 0.5, 1 mg.] ▶L ♀B ▶? $$$$$ ■

ALPHA-GALACTOSIDASE (*Beano*) 5 gtts or 1 tab per ½ cup gassy food, 2 to 3 tabs PO (chew, swallow, crumble) or 1 melt-away tab or 10 gtts per typical meal. [OTC Trade only: Oral gtts, tabs, melt-away tabs.] ▶minimal absorption ♀? ▶? $

ALVIMOPAN (*Entereg*) Short-term (up to 15 doses) in hospitalized patients undergoing partial large or small bowel resection surgery with primary anastomosis: 12 mg PO 30 min to 5 h prior to surgery, then 12 mg PO two times per day starting the day after surgery for up to 7 days. [Trade only: Caps 12 mg.] ▶intestinal flora ♀B ▶? ? ■

BUDESONIDE (*Entocort EC, Uceris*) Mild to moderate Crohn's, induction of remission: 9 mg PO daily for up to 8 weeks. May repeat 8-week course for

(cont.)

recurring episodes. Maintenance: 6 mg PO daily for 3 months (Entocort only). Mild to moderate ulcerative colitis, induction of remission: 9 mg PO q am for up to 8 weeks. [Generic/Trade: Caps 3 mg. Trade only: Extended-release tabs (Uceris) 9 mg. (Uceris for ulcerative colitis, only).] ▶L ♀C ▶? $$$$$

CHLORDIAZEPOXIDE—CLIDINIUM 1 cap PO three to four times per day. [Generic: Caps, chlordiazepoxide 5 mg + clidinium 2.5 mg.] ▶K ♀D ▶– $$$

CONTRAVE (naltrexone + bupropion) 1 tab PO daily for 1 week, then 1 tab PO twice daily for 1 week 2, then 2 tabs PO q am and 1 tab PO q pm for 1 week, then 2 tabs PO twice daily. [Trade only: Tabs (naltrexone 8 mg + bupropion 90 mg).] ▶LK ♀X ▶? $$$$$ ■

CROFELEMER (*Fulyzaq*) Noninfectious AIDS diarrhea: 125 mg PO twice daily. [Trade: Delayed-release tab 125 mg.] ▶minimal absorption ♀C ▶? $$$$$

GLYCOPYRROLATE (*Robinul, Robinul Forte, Cuvposa*) Peptic ulcer disease: 1 to 2 mg PO two to three times per day. Chronic drooling in children (Cuvposa): 0.02 mg/kg PO three times per day. [Trade: Soln 1 mg/5 mL (480 mL, Cuvposa). Generic/Trade: Tabs 1, 2 mg.] ▶K ♀B ▶? $$$$

LACTASE (*Lactaid*) Swallow or chew 3 caplets (Original-strength), 2 tabs/caplets (Extra-strength), 1 caplet (Ultra) with 1st bite of dairy foods. Adjust dose based on response. [OTC Generic/Trade: Caplets, Chewable tabs.] ▶not absorbed ♀+ ▶+ $

LINACLOTIDE (*Linzess, ✦Constella*) IBS: 290 mcg PO daily. Chronic idiopathic constipation: 145 mcg PO once daily. Contraindicated in children 6 yo or younger. [Trade: Cap 145, 290 mcg.] ▶gut –♀C ▶? $$$$$ ■

LORCASERIN (*Belviq*) Obesity or overweight with comorbidities: 10 mg PO twice a day. [Trade: Tab 10 mg.] ▶L ♀X ▶– $$$

METHYLNALTREXONE (*Relistor*) Opioid-induced constipation: Less than 38 kg: 0.15 mg/kg SC every other day; 38 to 61 kg: 8 mg SC every other day; 62 to 114 kg: 12 mg SC every other day; 115 kg or greater: 0.15 mg/kg SC every other day. [Single-use vial 12 mg/0.6 mL soln for subcutaneous injection; single-use pre-filled syringe 0.8 mg/0.4 mL and 12 mg/0.6 mL soln for SC injection.] ▶unchanged ♀B ▶? $$$$$

NALOXEGOL (*Movantik*) Opioid-induced constipation: 25 mg PO once daily; if not tolerated, reduce dose to 12.5 mg. [Trade only: Tabs 12.5, 25 mg.] ▶L ♀C ▶– ⊙l $$$$$

NEOMYCIN—ORAL (*Neo-Fradin*) Hepatic encephalopathy: 4 to 12 g/day PO divided q 4 to 6 h. Peds: 50 to 100 mg/kg/day PO divided q 6 to 8 h. [Generic only: Tabs 500 mg. Trade only: Soln 125 mg/5 mL.] ▶minimal absorption ♀D ▶? $$$

OCTREOTIDE (*Sandostatin, Sandostatin LAR*) Variceal bleeding: Bolus 25 to 50 mcg IV followed by infusion 25 to 50 mcg/h. AIDS diarrhea: 25 to 250 mcg SC three times per day. [Generic/Trade: Injection vials 0.05, 0.1, 0.2, 0.5, 1 mg. Trade only: Long-acting injectable susp (Sandostatin LAR) 10, 20, 30 mg.] ▶LK ♀B ▶? $$$$$

ORLISTAT (*Alli, Xenical*) Weight loss: 60 to 120 mg PO three times per day with meals. [OTC Trade only (Alli): Caps 60 mg. Rx Trade only (Xenical): Caps 120 mg.] ▶gut ♀X ▶? $$$

PANCREATIN (*Creon, Ku-Zyme, ✦Entozyme*) 8000 to 24,000 units lipase (1 to 2 tabs/caps) PO with meals and snacks. [Tabs, Caps with varying amounts of lipase, amylase, and protease.] ▶gut ♀C ▶? $$$

PANCRELIPASE (*Creon, Pancreaze, Pancrecarb, Cotazym, Ku-Zyme HP, Ultresa, Viokace, Zenpep*) Varies by wt. Initial infant dose 2000 to 4000 lipase units PO per 120 mL formula or breastmilk. 12 mo or older to younger than 4 yo: 1000 lipase units/kg PO. 4 yo or older: 500 lipase units/kg per meal PO, max 2500 lipase units/kg per meal. [Tabs, Caps, Powder with varying amounts of lipase, amylase, and protease.] ▶gut ♀C ▶? $$$

QSYMIA (**phentermine + topiramate**) Obesity or overweight with comorbidities: 3.75 mg/23 mg PO once daily for 14 days, then increase to 7.5 mg/46 mg PO once daily. Max dose 15 mg/92 mg PO daily. [Trade: Tabs 3.75/23, 7.5/46, 11.25/69, 15/92 mg (phentermine/topiramate).] ▶KL ♀X ▶– ⊝IV $$$$

RECTIV (**nitroglycerin—rectal**) Painful chronic anal fissures: Apply 1 inch intra-anally q 12 for up to 3 weeks. [Oint 0.4% 30 g.] ▶L ♀C ▶? $$$$$

SECRETIN (*SecreFlo, ChiRhoStim*) Test dose 0.2 mcg IV. If tolerated, 0.2 to 0.4 mcg/kg IV over 1 min. ▶serum ♀C ▶? $$$$$

TEDUGLUTIDE (*Gattex*) Short bowel syndrome patients receiving IV TPN: 0.05 mg/kg (max 3.8 mg) SC daily. [Trade only: 5 mg/vial, powder for reconstitution.] ▶endrogeneous ♀B ▶? $$$$$

URSODIOL (*Actigall, URSO, URSO Forte*) Gallstone solution (Actigall): 8 to 10 mg/kg/day PO divided two to three times per day. Prevention of gallstones associated with rapid wt loss (Actigall): 300 mg PO two times per day. Primary biliary cirrhosis (URSO): 13 to 15 mg/kg/day PO divided in 2 to 4 doses. [Generic/Trade: Caps 300 mg, Tabs 250, 500 mg.] ▶bile ♀B ▶? $$$$

VEDOLIZUMAB (*Entyvio*) Ulcerative colitis and Crohn's disease: 300 mg IV over 30 min. Repeat in 2 and 6 weeks, then every 8 weeks. [Trade only: 300 mg single-use vials.] ▶proteolysis ♀B ▶? $$$$$ ■

HEMATOLOGY/ANTICOAGULANTS

Anticoagulants - Direct Thrombin Inhibitors

ARGATROBAN HIT: Start 2 mcg/kg/min IV infusion. Get PTT at baseline and 2 h after starting infusion. Adjust dose (max dose: 10 mcg/kg/min) until PTT is 1.5 to 3 times baseline (not more than 100 sec). ACCP recommends starting at max of 2 mcg/kg/min with lower doses of 0.5 to 1.2 mcg/kg/min in patients with heart failure, multi-organ failure, anasarca, or post-cardiac surgery. ▶L ♀B ▶– $$$$$

BIVALIRUDIN (*Angiomax*) Anticoagulation during PCI (patients with or at risk of HIT): 0.75 mg/kg IV bolus prior to intervention, then 1.75 mg/kg/h for duration of procedure (with provisional GPIIb/IIIa inhibition). For CrCl less than 30 mL/min, reduce infusion dose to 1 mg/kg/h after bolus. For patients on dialysis, reduce infusion to 0.25 mg/kg/h after bolus. Use with aspirin 300 to 325 mg PO daily. Additional bolus of 0.3 mg/kg if activated clotting time less than 225 sec. ▶proteolysis/K ♀B ▶? $$$$$

DABIGATRAN (*Pradaxa*) Stroke prevention in atrial fibrillation: CrCl greater than 30 mL/min: 150 mg PO two times per day; CrCL between 15 and 30 mL/min: 75 mg PO two times per day; CrCl less than 15 mL/min: contraindicated. Per ACCP CHEST guidelines, not recommended if CrCl is less than 30 mL/min. Treatment of DVT/PE: CrCl greater than 30 mL/min: 150 mg PO two times per day after 5 to 10 days of parenteral anticoagulation. Reduction in risk of DVT/PE: CrCl greater than 30 mL/min: 150 mg PO two times per day after previous treatment. [Trade only: caps 75, 150 mg.] ▶K ♀C ▶? $$$$$ ■

DESIRUDIN (*Iprivask*) DVT prophylaxis (hip replacement surgery): 15 mg SC q 12 h. (If CrCl is 31 to 60 mL/min, give 5 mg SC q 12 h; if CrCl less than 31 mL/min, give 1.7 mg SC q 12 h.) ▶K ♀C ▶? $$$$$ ■

Anticoagulants-Factor Xa Inhibitors

APIXABAN (*Eliquis*) Nonvalvular atrial fibrillation: 5 mg PO two times per day. If at least two of the following characteristics: age 80 yo or older, wt 60 kg or less, serum creatinine 1.5 mg/dL or greater, then decrease dose to 2.5 mg PO two times daily. DVT prophylaxis in hip or knee replacement: 2.5 mg PO two times per day. Treatment of DVT/PE: 10 mg PO two times daily for 7 days, then 5 mg PO two times daily. Reduction in risk of recurrence of DVT/PE: 2.5 mg PO two times daily after initial therapy for treatment. [Trade only: Tabs 2.5, 5 mg.] ▶LK ♀B ▶? $$$$$ ■

EDOXABAN (*Savaysa*) Nonvalvular atrial fibrillation: CrCl is greater than 50 up to and including 95 mL/min: 60 mg PO daily. CrCl 15 to 50 mL/min: 30 mg PO daily. Treatment of DVT/PE: 60 mg PO daily after 5 to 10 days of parenteral anticoagulation. CrCl 15 to 50 mL/min or body weight 60 kg or less or certain P-gp inhibitors: 30 mg PO daily after 5 to 10 days of parenteral anticoagulation. [Trade only: 15, 30, 60 mg tabs.] ▶K ♀C ▶? $$$$$ ■

FONDAPARINUX (*Arixtra*) DVT prophylaxis, hip/knee replacement or hip fracture surgery, abdominal surgery: 2.5 mg SC daily starting 6 to 8 h postop. DVT/PE

(cont.)

treatment based on wt: wt less than 50 kg: 5 mg SC daily; wt between 50 and 100 kg: 7.5 mg SC daily; wt greater than 100 kg: 10 mg SC daily for at least 5 days and therapeutic oral anticoagulation. [Generic/Trade: Prefilled syringes 2.5 mg/0.5 mL, 5 mg/0.4 mL, 7.5 mg/0.6 mL, 10 mg/0.8 mL.] ▶K ♀B ▶? $$$$$ ■

RIVAROXABAN (*Xarelto*) DVT prophylaxis in knee or hip replacement: 10 mg PO daily, if CrCl less than 30 mL/min avoid use. Nonvalvular atrial fibrillation: 20 mg PO daily if CrCl greater than 50 mL/min; reduce dose to 15 mg PO daily if CrCl 15 to 50 mL/min, avoid use if CrCl less than 15 mL/min. DVT/PE treatment and to reduce risk of DVT/PE recurrence: 15 mg PO two times daily with food for 21 days, then 20 mg PO daily with food. If CrCl 30 to 49 mL/min: 15 mg PO twice daily with food for 3 weeks, then 15 mg PO daily with food. [Trade only: Tabs 10, 15, 20 mg.] ▶K – ♀C ▶? $$$$$ ■

Anticoagulants—Low Molecular Weight Heparins (LWMH)

DALTEPARIN (*Fragmin*) DVT prophylaxis, acute medical illness with restricted mobility: 5000 units SC daily. DVT prophylaxis, abdominal surgery: 2500 units SC 1 to 2 h preop and daily postop. DVT prophylaxis, abdominal surgery in patients with malignancy: 5000 units SC evening before surgery and daily postop, or 2500 units 1 to 2 h preop and 12 h later, then 5000 units daily. DVT prophylaxis, hip replacement: Preop start (day of surgery): 2500 units SC given 2 h preop, 4 to 8 h postop, then 5000 units daily starting at least 6 h after 2nd dose, or 5000 units 10 to 14 h preop, 4 to 8 h postop, then daily (approximately 24 h between doses). Preop start (evening before surgery): 5000 units SC given evening before surgery then 5000 units daily starting at least 4 to 8 h postop (approximately 24 h between doses). Postop start: 2500 units 4 to 8 h postop, then 5000 units daily starting at least 6 h after 1st dose. Treatment of DVT/PE in cancer: 200 units/kg SC daily for 1 month, then 150 units/kg SC daily for 5 months; max 18,000 units/day. Unstable angina or non-Q-wave MI: 120 units/kg up to 10,000 units SC q 12 h with aspirin (75 to 165 mg/day PO) until clinically stable. [Trade only: Single-dose syringes 2500, 5000 units/0.2 mL, 7500 units/0.3 mL, 10,000 units/1 mL, 12,500 units/0.5 mL, 15,000 units/0.6 mL, 18,000 units/0.72 mL; multidose vial 10,000 units/mL, 9.5 and 25,000 units/mL, 3.8 mL.] ▶KL ♀B ▶+ $$$$$ ■

ENOXAPARIN (*Lovenox*) See table. [Generic/Trade: Syringes 30, 40 mg; graduated syringes 60, 80, 100, 120, 150 mg. Concentration is 100 mg/mL except for 120, 150 mg, which are 150 mg/mL. All strengths also available preservative free. Trade only: Multidose vial 300 mg.] ▶KL ♀B ▶+ $$$$$ ■

ENOXAPARIN ADULT DOSING

Indication	Dose	Dosing in Renal Impairment (CrCl less than 30 mL/min)*
DVT prophylaxis		
Abdominal surgery	40 mg SC once daily	30 mg SC once daily
Knee replacement	30 mg SC q 12 h	30 mg SC once daily
Hip replacement	30 mg SC q 12 h or 40 mg SC once daily	30 mg SC once daily
Medical patients	40 mg SC once daily	30 mg SC once daily
Acute DVT		
Inpatient treatment with or without PE	1 mg/kg SC q 12 h or 1.5 mg/kg SC once daily	1 mg/kg SC once daily
Outpatient treatment without PE	1 mg/kg SC q 12 h	1 mg/kg SC once daily
Acute coronary syndrome		
Unstable angina and non-Q-wave MI with aspirin	1 mg/kg SC q 12 h with aspirin	1 mg/kg SC once daily
Acute STEMI in patients younger than 75 yo with aspirin[†]	30 mg IV bolus with 1 mg/kg SC dose, then 1 mg/kg SC q 12 h (max 100 mg/dose for the 1st two doses)	30 mg IV bolus with 1 mg/kg SC dose, then 1 mg/kg SC once daily
Acute STEMI in patients 75 yo or older with aspirin[†]	No IV bolus, 0.75 mg/kg SC q 12 h (max 75 mg/dose for the 1st two doses)	No IV bolus, 1 mg/kg SC once daily

DVT = Deep vein thrombosis, PE = pulmonary embolism.

*Not FDA-approved in dialysis.

[†]If used with thrombolytics, SC dose should be started between 15 min before and 30 min after thrombolytic dose.

HEPARIN DOSING FOR ACUTE CORONARY SYNDROME (ACS)

ST elevation myocardial infarction (STEMI)	Adjunct to thrombolytics: For use with alteplase, reteplase, or tenecteplase: Bolus 60 units/kg IV load (max 4000 units), then initial infusion 12 units/kg/h (max 1000 units/h) adjusted to achieve target PTT 1.5 to 2 times control.
Unstable angina/non-ST elevation myocardial infarction (UA/NSTEMI)	Initial treatment: Bolus 60 to 70 units/kg IV load (max 4000 units), then initiate infusion at 12 to 15 units/kg/h (max 1000 units/h) and adjusted to achieve target PTT 1.5 to 2.5 times control.

(cont.)

HEPARIN DOSING FOR ACUTE CORONARY SYNDROME (ACS) (*continued*)

Percutaneous coronary intervention (PCI)	With prior anticoagulant therapy but *without* concurrent GPIIb/IIIa inhibitor planned: Additional heparin as needed (2000 to 5000 units) to achieve target ACT 250–300 seconds for HemoTec or 300–350 seconds for Hemochron.
	With prior anticoagulant therapy but *with* planned concurrent GPIIb/IIIa inhibitor: Additional heparin as needed (2000 to 5000 units) to achieve target ACT 200–250 seconds.
	Without prior anticoagulant therapy but *without* concurrent GPIIb/IIIa inhibitor planned: Bolus 70–100 units/kg with target ACT 250–300 seconds for HemoTec or 300–350 seconds for Hemochron.
	Without prior anticoagulant therapy but *with* planned concurrent GPIIb/IIIa inhibitor: Bolus 50–70 units/kg with target ACT 200–250 seconds.

J Am Coll Cardiol 2011;57:1946. *Circulation* 2011;124:e608. *Circulation* 2004;110:e82–292. *J Am Coll Cardiol* 2009;54:2235.

WEIGHT-BASED HEPARIN DOSING FOR DVT/PE*

Initial dose	80 units/kg IV bolus, then 18 units/kg/h; check PTT in 6 h
PTT less than 35 sec (less than 1.2 × control)	80 units/kg IV bolus, then increase infusion rate by 4 units/kg/h
PTT 35–45 sec (1.2–1.5 × control)	40 units/kg IV bolus, then increase infusion by 2 units/kg/h
PTT 46–70 sec (1.5–2.3 × control)	No change
PTT 71–90 sec (2.3–3 × control)	Decrease infusion rate by 2 units/kg/h
PTT greater than 90 sec (greater than 3 × control)	Hold infusion for 1 h, then decrease infusion rate by 3 units/kg/h

Adapted from *Ann Intern Med* 1993;119;874. *Chest* 2012;141:e28S, e154S. *Circulation* 2001;103:2994.

*PTT = Activated partial thromboplastin time. Reagent-specific target PTT may differ; use institutional nomogram when available. Consider establishing a max bolus dose/max initial infusion rate or use an adjusted body in obesity. Monitor PTT 6 h after heparin initiation and 6 h after each dosage adjustment. When PTT is stable within therapeutic range, monitor every morning. Therapeutic PTT range corresponds to anti-factor Xa activity of 0.3–0.7 units/mL. Check platelets between days 3 and 5. Can begin warfarin on 1 day of heparin; continue heparin for at least 4–5 days of combined therapy.

Anticoagulants—Other

HEPARIN Venous thrombosis/pulmonary embolus treatment: Load 80 units/kg IV, then initiate infusion at 18 units/kg/h. Adjust based on coagulation testing (PTT)—see Table. DVT prophylaxis: 5000 units SC q 8 to 12 h. Acute coronary syndromes with or without PCI: 60 units/kg IV, then 12 units/kg/h infusion, adjust according to aPTT or antiXa. See Table. Peds: Load 50 units/kg IV, then infuse 25 units/kg/h. [Generic only: 1000, 5000, 10,000, 20,000 units/mL in various vial and syringe sizes.] ▶Reticuloendothelial system ♀C but + ▶+ $$ ■

WARFARIN (*Coumadin, Jantoven*) Individualize dosing. Start 2 to 5 mg PO daily for 1 to 2 days, then adjust dose to maintain therapeutic INR. For healthy outpatients, 2012 ACCP CHEST guidelines recommend starting at 10 mg PO daily for 2 days, then adjust dose to maintain therapeutic INR. See product information if CYP2C9 or VKOR1C genotypes are known. [Generic/Trade: Tabs 1, 2, 2.5, 3, 4, 5, 6, 7.5, 10 mg.] ▶L ♀X, (D for mechanical heart valve replacement) ▶+ $$ ■

WARFARIN—SELECTED DRUG INTERACTIONS

Assume possible interactions with any new medication. When starting/stopping a chronic medication, the INR should be checked at least weekly for 2 to 3 weeks and dose adjusted accordingly. When starting an interacting anti-infective agent, the National Quality Forum recommends checking the INR within 3 to 7 days. Similarly, monitor if significant change in diet (including supplements) or illness resulting in decreased oral intake. For further information regarding mechanism or management, refer to the *Tarascon Pocket Pharmacopoeia* drug interactions database (mobile or Web edition).

INCREASED ANTICOAGULANT EFFECT OF WARFARIN / INCREASED RISK OF BLEEDING

Monitor INR when agents below started, stopped, or dosage changed. Consider alternative agent. Acetaminophen ≤2 g/day for ≥ 3 to 4 days, allopurinol, amiodarone*, amprenavir, anabolic steroids, ASA¶, cefixime, cefoperazone, cefotetan, celecoxib, chloramphenicol, cimetidine†, corticosteroids, danazol, danshen, disulfiram, dong quai, erlotinib, etravirine, fibrates, fish oil, fluconazole, fluoroquinolones, fluorouracil, fluvoxamine, fosphenytoin (acute), garlic supplements, gemcitabine, gemfibrozil, glucosamine-chondroitin, ginkgo, ifosfamide, imatinib, isoniazid, itraconazole, ketoconazole, leflunomide, lepirudin, levothyroxine#, macrolides‡, metronidazole, miconazole (intravaginal), neomycin (PO for >1 to 2 days), NSAIDs(P), olsalazine, omeprazole, paroxetine, penicillin (high-dose IV), pentoxifylline, phenytoin (acute), propafenone, propoxyphene, quinidine, quinine, statins§, sulfinpyrazone (with later inhibition), sulfonamides, tamoxifen, testosterones tetracyclines, tramadol, tigecycline, tipranavir, TCAs, valproate, voriconazole, vorinostat, vitamin A (high-dose), vitamin E, zafirlukast, zileuton

(cont.)

WARFARIN—SELECTED DRUG INTERACTIONS (*continued*)

DECREASED ANTICOAGULANT EFFECT OF WARFARIN / INCREASED RISK OF THROMBOSIS

Monitor INR when agents below started, stopped, or dosage changed. Consider alternative agent. Aprepitant, cefotetan, azathioprine, barbiturates, bosentan, carbamazepine, coenzyme Q-10, dicloxacillin, fosphenytoin (chronic), ginseng (American), griseofulvin, mercaptopurine, mesalamine, methimazole[#], mitotane, nafcillin, oral contraceptives**, phenytoin (chronic), primidone, propylthiouracil[#], raloxifene, ribavirin, rifabutin, rifampin, rifapentine, ritonavir, St. John's wort, vitamin C (high-dose).
Use alternative to agents below. Or give at different times of day and monitor INR when agent started, stopped, or dose/dosing schedule changed.
Cholestyramine, colestipol[††], sucralfate

Adapted from: Coumadin product information; *Am Fam Phys* 1999; 59:635; Chest 2004;126:204S; Hansen and Horn's Drug Interactions Analysis and Management; *Ann Intern Med* 2004; 141:23; Arch Intern Med 2005;165:1095. *Tarascon Pocket Pharmacopoeia* drug interactions database (Mobile or Web edition). National Quality Forum http://www.qualityforum.org.

*Interaction may be delayed; monitor INR for several weeks after starting and several months after stopping amiodarone. May need to decrease warfarin dose by 33 to 50%.
† Famotidine, nizatidine or ranitidine, are alternatives.
‡ Azithromycin appears to have lower risk of interaction than clarithromycin or erythromycin.
§ Pravastatin appears to have lower risk of interaction.
# Hyperthyroidism/thyroid replacement increases metabolism of clotting factors, increasing response to warfarin therapy and increased bleed risk (typically requires lowering warfarin dose). Reversal of hyperthyroidism (as with methimazole, propylthiouracil) will decrease metabolism of clotting factors and decrease response to warfarin (typically requires increasing warfarin dose).
¶ Does not necessarily increase INR, but increases bleeding risk. Check INR frequently and monitor for GI bleeding.
**Do not necessarily decreases INR, but may induce hypercoagulability.
†† Likely lower risk than cholestyramine

THERAPEUTIC GOALS FOR ANTICOAGULATION WITH WARFARIN

INR Range*	Indication
2.0–3.0	Atrial fibrillation, deep venous thrombosis, pulmonary embolism, bioprosthetic heart valve (mitral position), mechanical prosthetic heart valve (aortic position)
2.5–3.5	Mechanical prosthetic heart valve (mitral position)

Adapted from: *Chest* 2012; 141:e422S, e425S, e533S, e578S; see these guidelines for additional information and other indications.

*Aim for an INR in the middle of the INR range (eg, 2.5 for range of 2 to 3 and 3.0 for range of 2.5 to 3.5).

Colony-Stimulating Factors

DARBEPOETIN (*Aranesp, NESP*) Anemia of chronic renal failure: 0.45 mcg/kg IV/SC once a week, or 0.75 mcg/kg q 2 weeks in some nondialysis patients. Cancer chemo anemia: 2.25 mcg/kg SC weekly, or 500 mcg SC q 3 weeks. Adjust dose based on Hb. [Trade only: All forms are available with or without albumin. Single-dose vials: 25, 40, 60, 100, 200, 300, 500 mcg/1 mL, and 150 mcg/0.75 mL. Single-dose prefilled syringes or autoinjectors: 25 mcg/0.42 mL, 40 mcg/0.4 mL, 60 mcg/0.3 mL, 100 mcg/0.5 mL, 150 mcg/0.3 mL, 200 mcg/0.4 mL, 300 mcg/0.6 mL, 500 mcg/1 mL.] ▶cellular sialidases, L ♀C ▶? $$$$$ ■

EPOETIN ALFA (*Epogen, Procrit,* erythropoietin alpha, *Eprex*) Anemia: 1 dose IV/SC 3 times a week. Initial dose if renal failure is 50 to 100 units/kg, Zidovudine-induced anemia is 100 units/kg, or chemo-associated anemia is 150 units/kg. Alternate for chemo-associated anemia: 40,000 units SC once a week. Adjust dose based on Hb. [Trade only: Single-dose 1-mL vials 2000, 3000, 4000, 10,000, 40,000 units/mL. Multidose vials 10,000 units/mL 2 mL, 20,000 units/mL 1 mL.] ▶L ♀C ▶? $$$$$ ■

FILGRASTIM (filgrastim-sndz, tbo-filgrastim, *G-CSF, Neupogen, Granix, Zarxio*)** Neutropenia: 5 mcg/kg SC/IV daily. Bone marrow transplant: 10 mcg/kg/day SC/IV infusion. Concomitant myelosuppressive doses of radiation: 10 mcg/kg SC daily. [Trade: Single-dose vials (Neupogen): 300 mcg/1 mL, 480 mcg/1.6 mL. Biosimilars, Single-dose syringes: Granix, tbo-filgrastim: 300 mcg/0.5 mL, 480 mcg/0.8 mL; Zarxio, filgrastim-sndz: 300 mcg/0.5 mL, 480 mcg/0.8 mL.] ▶L ♀C ▶? $$$$$

OPRELVEKIN (*Neumega*) Chemotherapy-induced thrombocytopenia in adults: 50 mcg/kg SC daily. [Trade only: 5 mg single-dose vials with diluent.] ▶K ♀C ▶? $$$$$ ■

PEGFILGRASTIM (*Neulasta*) 6 mg SC once each chemo cycle. [Trade only: Single-dose syringes 6 mg/0.6 mL.] ▶plasma ♀C ▶? $$$$$

SARGRAMOSTIM (*GM-CSF, Leukine*) Specialized dosing for bone marrow transplant. ▶L ♀C ▶? $$$$$

Other Hematological Agents

AMINOCAPROIC ACID (*Amicar*) Hemostasis: 4 to 5 g PO/IV over 1 h, then 1 g/h prn. [Generic/Trade: Syrup 250 mg/mL, Tabs 500 mg. Trade only: Tabs 1000 mg.] ▶K ♀D ▶? $ IV $$$$$ Oral

ANAGRELIDE (*Agrylin*) Thrombocythemia due to myeloproliferative disorders: Start 0.5 mg PO four times per day or 1 mg PO two times per day, then after 1 week adjust to lowest effective dose. Max 10 mg/day. [Generic/Trade: Caps 0.5 mg. Generic only: Caps 1 mg.] ▶LK ♀C ▶? $$$$$

DEFERASIROX (*Exjade*) Chronic iron overload due to blood transfusions: 20 mg/kg PO daily; adjust dose q 3 to 6 months based on ferritin trends. Max 40 mg/kg/day. Chronic iron overload in non-transfusion-dependent thalassemia syndromes: 10 mg/kg PO daily; adjust dose based on ferritin and liver iron concentration. Max 20 mg/kg/day. [Trade only: Tabs for dissolving into oral susp 125, 250, 500 mg.] ▶L ♀B ▶? $$$$$ ■

HYDROXYUREA (*Hydrea, Droxia*) Sickle cell anemia (Droxia): Start 15 mg/kg PO daily while monitoring CBC q 2 weeks. If no marrow depression, then increase dose q 12 weeks by 5 mg/kg/day (max 35 mg/kg/day). Solid tumors (Hydrea): Intermittent therapy: 80 mg/kg PO for a single dose q 3 days. Continuous therapy: 20 to 30 mg/kg PO daily. Head and neck cancer with radiation (Hydrea): 80 mg/kg PO for a single dose q 3 days. Resistant chronic myelocytic leukemia: 20 to 30 mg/kg PO daily. Give concomitant folic acid. [Generic/Trade: Caps 500 mg. Trade only: (Droxia) Caps 200, 300, 400 mg.] ▶LK ♀D ▶− $ varies by therapy ■

PROTAMINE Reversal of heparin: Within 30 minutes of IV heparin: 1 mg antagonizes about 100 units heparin. If greater than 30 minutes since IV heparin: 0.5 mg antagonizes about 100 units heparin. Due to short half-life of heparin (60 to 90 min), use IV heparin doses only from last several hours to calculate dose of protamine. SC heparin may require prolonged administration of protamine. Reversal of low-molecular-weight heparin: If within 8 h of LMWH dose: Give 1 mg protamine per 100 anti-Xa units of dalteparin or 1 mg protamine per 1 mg enoxaparin. Smaller doses advised if greater than 8 h since LMWH administration. Give IV (max 50 mg) over 10 min. May cause allergy/anaphylaxis. ▶plasma ♀C ▶? $ ■

PROTHROMBIN COMPLEX CONCENTRATE (*Kcentra*) Vitamin K antagonist reversal with need for reversal due to acute major bleed or urgent surgery/invasive procedure: Individualized dosing based on pre-treatment INR and body weight. INR 2 to less than 4: 25 units of Factor IX/kg body weight (max: 2500 units); INR 4 to 6: 35 units of Factor IX/kg body weight (max: 3500 units); INR greater than 6: 50 units of Factor IX/kg body weight (max 5000 units). [Brand: 500, 1000 unit vial.] ▶N/A ♀C ▶? $$$$$ ■

HERBAL AND ALTERNATIVE THERAPIES

NOTE: *In the United States, herbal and alternative therapy products are regulated as dietary supplements, not drugs. Premarketing evaluation and FDA approval are not required unless specific therapeutic claims are made. Because these products are not required to demonstrate efficacy, it is unclearv whether many of them have health benefits. In addition, there may be considerable variability in content from lot to lot or between products.*

ALOE VERA (acemannan, burn plant) Topical: Efficacy unclear for seborrheic dermatitis, psoriasis, genital herpes, skin burns. Do not apply to surgical incisions; impaired healing reported. Oral: Efficacy unclear for mild to moderate active ulcerative colitis, type 2 diabetes. OTC laxatives containing aloe latex were removed from US market due to possible increased risk of colon cancer. [Not by prescription.] ▶LK♀ oral – topical + ? ▶ oral – topical + ? $

ALPHA LIPOIC ACID (lipoic acid, thioctic acid, ALA) Peripheral neuropathy (possibly effective): Usual dose is 600 mg PO daily. [Not by prescription] ▶intracellular ♀C ▶? $

ARTICHOKE LEAF EXTRACT (*Cynara scolymus*) May reduce total cholesterol, but clinical significance is unclear. Possibly effective for functional dyspepsia. [Not by prescription.] ▶? ♀? ▶? $

ASTRAGALUS (*Astragalus membranaceus*, huang qi, *Jin Fu Kang*, vetch) Used in combination with other herbs in traditional Chinese medicine for CAD, CHF, chronic liver disease, kidney disease, viral infections, and upper respiratory tract infection. Possibly effective for improving survival and performance status with platinum-based chemotherapy for non-small-cell lung cancer. However, astragalus-based herbal formula (Jin Fu Kang) did not affect survival or pharmacokinetics of docetaxel in phase II study of patients with non-small-cell lung cancer. [Not by prescription.] ▶? ♀? ▶? $

BUTTERBUR (*Petasites hybridus*, Petadolex) Migraine prophylaxis (effective): Petadolex 50 to 75 mg PO two times per day. Allergic rhinitis prophylaxis (possibly effective): Petadolex 50 mg PO two times per day. Efficacy unclear for asthma. [Not by prescription. Standardized pyrrolizidine-free extracts: Petadolex tabs 50, 75 mg.] ▶? ♀– ▶? $

CHAMOMILE (*Matricaria recutita*—German chamomile, *Anthemis nobilis*—Roman chamomile) Oral extract: Modest benefit in study for generalized anxiety disorder, but little to no benefit in study for primary chronic insomnia. Topical: Efficacy unclear for skin infections or inflammation. [Not by prescription.] ▶? ♀– ▶? $

CHASTEBERRY (*Vitex agnus castus* fruit extract, Femaprin) Premenstrual syndrome (possibly effective): 20 mg PO daily of extract ZE 440. [Not by prescription.] ▶? ♀– ▶– $

CHONDROITIN Does not appear effective for relief of OA pain overall. Chondroitin 400 mg PO three times per day + glucosamine may improve pain in subgroup of patients with moderate to severe knee OA. [Not by prescription.] ▶K ♀? ▶? $

COENZYME Q10 (*CoQ-10*, ubiquinone) Heart failure: 100 to 300 mg/day PO divided two to three times per day (conflicting clinical trials; AHA/ACC does not recommend). Statin-induced myalgia: 100 to 200 mg PO daily (efficacy unclear; conflicting clinical trials). Prevention of migraine (efficacy unclear): 100 mg PO three times per day. May be considered for migraine prevention per American Academy of Neurology and American Headache Society. Efficacy unclear for hypertension and improving athletic performance. Appears ineffective for diabetes. Did not improve cancer-related fatigue or quality of life in RCT of women with breast cancer. Does not slow functional decline in early Parkinson disease. [Not by prescription.] ▶Bile ♀– ▶– $$

CRANBERRY (*Cranactin*, *Vaccinium macrocarpon*) Prevention of UTI (possibly ineffective): 300 mL/day PO cranberry juice cocktail. Usual dose of cranberry juice extract caps/tabs is 300 to 400 mg PO two times per day. Insufficient data to assess efficacy for treatment of UTI. Potential increase in INR with warfarin. [Not by prescription.] ▶? ♀+ in food, – in supplements ▶+ in food, – in supplements $

CREATINE Promoted to enhance athletic performance. No benefit for endurance exercise; modest benefit for intense anaerobic tasks lasting less than 30 sec. Usual loading dose of 10 to 20 g/day PO for 4 to 7 days, then 2 to 5 g/day divided two times per day. Can slightly increase serum creatinine in young adults. [Not by prescription.] ▶LK ♀– ▶– $

DEHYDROEPIANDROSTERONE (*DHEA*, *Aslera*, *Fidelin*, *Prasterone*) To improve well-being in women with adrenal insufficiency: 50 mg PO daily (possibly effective; conflicting clinical trials). Does not improve cognition, quality of life, or sexual function in elderly. Not recommended as androgen replacement in late-onset male hypogonadism. [Not by prescription.] ▶Peripheral conversion to estrogens and androgens ♀– ▶– $

DEVIL'S CLAW (*Harpagophytum procumbens*, *Dolomethic*, *Harpadol*) OA, acute exacerbation of chronic low-back pain (possibly effective): 2400 mg extract/day (50 to 100 mg harpagoside/day) PO divided two to three times per day. [Not by prescription. Extracts standardized to harpagoside (iridoid glycoside) content.] ▶? ♀– ▶– $

ECHINACEA (*E. purpurea*, *E. angustifolia*, *E. pallida*, cone flower, *EchinaGuard*, *Echinacin Madaus*) Conflicting clinical trials for prevention or treatment of upper respiratory infections. Does not appear effective for treatment of common cold in adults. [Not by prescription.] ▶L ♀– ▶– $

ELDERBERRY (*Sambucus nigra*, *Rubini*, *Sambucol*) Efficacy unclear for influenza, sinusitis, and bronchitis. [Not by prescription.] ▶LK ♀– ▶– $

FENUGREEK (*Trigonella foenum-graecum*) Efficacy unclear for diabetes or hyperlipidemia. [Not by prescription.] ▶? ♀– ▶– $$

FEVERFEW (*Chrysanthemum parthenium*, *MigreLief*, *Tanacetum parthenium L.*) Prevention of migraine (probably effective): 50 to 100 mg extract PO daily. May take 1 to 2 months to be effective. [Not by prescription.] ▶? ♀– ▶– $

FLAVOCOXID (*Limbrel*) OA (efficacy unclear): 250 to 500 mg PO two times per day. Case reports of hepatotoxicity and hypersensitivity pneumonitis. [Caps 250, 500 mg. Marketed as medical food by prescription only (not all medical foods require a prescription).] ▶L ♀– ▶– $$$

GARLIC SUPPLEMENTS (*Allium sativum, Kwai, Kyolic*) Ineffective for hyperlipidemia. Small reductions in BP, but efficacy for HTN unclear. Does not appear effective for diabetes. Efficacy unclear for common cold. Significantly decreases saquinavir levels. May increase bleeding risk with warfarin with/without increase in INR. [Not by prescription.] ▶LK♀–▶– $

GINGER (*Zingiber officinale*) Acute chemotherapy-induced nausea (efficacy unclear as adjunct to standard antiemetics): 250 to 500 mg PO two times per day for 6 days, starting 3 days before chemo. American Society of Clinical Oncology and National Comprehensive Cancer Network guidelines do not support for chemo-induced N/V. Possibly ineffective for prevention of motion sickness. Does not appear effective for postop N/V. American Congress of Obstetricians and Gynecologists considers ginger 250 mg PO four times per day a nonpharmacologic option for N/V in pregnancy. Some experts advise pregnant women to limit dose to usual dietary amount (no more than 1 g/day). Some European countries advise pregnant women to avoid ginger supplements because it is cytotoxic in vitro. [Not by prescription.] ▶bile ♀? ▶? $

GINKGO BILOBA (*EGb 761, Ginkgold, Ginkoba*) Dementia (efficacy unclear): 40 mg PO three times per day of standardized extract containing 24% ginkgo flavone glycosides and 6% terpene lactones. The American Psychiatric Association and others find evidence too weak to recommend for Alzheimer's or other dementias. Does not prevent dementia in elderly or improve memory in people with normal cognitive function. Does not appear effective for prevention of acute high altitude sickness. Ineffective for intermittent claudication, tinnitus. Possible risk of stroke. [Not by prescription.] ▶K♀–▶– $

GINSENG—AMERICAN (*Panax quinquefolius L., Cold-FX, Cold-FX Extra*) Prevention of colds/flu (possible modest efficacy): 1 to 2 caps Cold-FX PO two times per day or 1 cap Cold-FX Extra PO two times per day during flu season. Ineffective for cold treatment. Cancer-related fatigue (possibly effective; conflicting data): 1000 mg PO two times per day in am and midafternoon. Postprandial hyperglycemia in type 2 diabetes (possibly effective): 3 g PO taken with or up to 2 h before meal. [Not by prescription.] ▶? ♀–▶– $

GINSENG—ASIAN (*Panax ginseng, Ginsana, G115, Korean red ginseng*) Promoted to improve vitality and well-being: 200 mg PO daily. Ginsana: 2 caps PO daily or 1 cap PO two times per day. Preliminary evidence of efficacy for erectile dysfunction. Efficacy unclear for improving physical or psychomotor performance, diabetes, herpes simplex infections, or cognitive or immune function. American Congress of Obstetricians and Gynecologists and North American Menopause Society recommend against use for postmenopausal hot flashes. [Not by prescription.] ▶? ♀–▶– $

GINSENG—SIBERIAN (*Eleutherococcus senticosus, Ci-wu-jia*) Does not appear effective for improving athletic endurance or chronic fatigue syndrome. May interfere with some digoxin assays. [Not by prescription.] ▶? ♀–▶– $

GLUCOSAMINE (*Cosamin DS, Dona*) OA: Glucosamine HCl 500 mg PO three times per day or glucosamine sulfate (Dona $$) 1500 mg PO once daily. Appears ineffective overall for OA pain, but glucosamine plus chondroitin may improve pain in moderate to severe knee OA. [Not by prescription.] ▶L♀–▶– $

GREEN TEA (*Camellia sinensis, Polyphenon E*) Efficacy unclear for cancer prevention, hypercholesterolemia. Efficacy for short-term weight loss is minimal. Large doses might decrease INR with warfarin due to vitamin K content. Can decrease nadolol exposure; avoid coadministration. May contain caffeine. [Not by prescription. Green tea extract available in caps standardized to polyphenol content.] ▶LK♀+ in moderate amount in food, – in supplements ▶+ in moderate amount in food, – in supplements $

HAWTHORN (*Crataegus laevigata, C. monogyna, C. oxyacantha, Crataegutt, HeartCare*) Mild heart failure (possibly effective): 80 mg PO two times per day to 160 mg PO three times per day of standardized extract (19% oligomeric procyanidins; HeartCare 80 mg tabs). [Not by prescription.] ▶? ♀– $

HONEY (*Medihoney*) Topical for burn/wound (including diabetic foot, stasis leg ulcers, pressure ulcers, 1st- and 2nd-degree partial thickness burns): Apply Medihoney for 12 to 24 h/day. Oral for nocturnal cough due to upper respiratory tract infection in children (effective): Give PO within 30 min before sleep. Dose is ½ tsp for 2 to 5 yo, 1 tsp for 6 to 11 yo, 2 tsp for 12 to 18 yo. Do not feed honey to children younger than 1 yo due to risk of infant botulism. [Mostly not by prescription. Medihoney is FDA approved.] ▶? ♀+ ▶+ $ for oral $$$ for Medihoney

HORSE CHESTNUT SEED EXTRACT (*Aesculus hippocastanum*, buckeye, *Venastat*) Chronic venous insufficiency (effective): 1 cap Venastat (16% aescin standardized extract) PO two times per day with water before meals. American College of Cardiology found evidence insufficient to recommend for peripheral arterial disease. [Not by prescription.] ▶? ♀– ▶– $

LICORICE (*Cankermelt, Glycyrrhiza glabra, Glycyrrhiza uralensis*) Chronic high doses can cause pseudoprimary aldosteronism (with HTN, edema, hypokalemia). Prevention of postop sore throat (possibly effective): Licorice 0.5 g in 30 mL water gargled 5 minutes before anesthesia. Aphthous ulcers (efficacy unclear): Apply CankerMelt oral patch to ulcer for 16 h/day until healed. [Not by prescription.] ▶bile ♀– ▶– $

MELATONIN (*N-acetyl-5-methoxytryptamine*) To reduce jet lag after flights over more than 5 time zones (effective): 0.5 to 5 mg PO at bedtime for 3 to 6 nights starting on day of arrival. [Not by prescription.] ▶L ♀– ▶– $

MILK THISTLE (*Silybum marianum, Legalon*, silymarin, *Thisilyn*) Hepatic cirrhosis (efficacy unclear): 100 to 200 mg PO three times per day of standardized extract with 70 to 80% silymarin. Does not appear effective for hepatitis C. [Not by prescription.] ▶LK♀– ▶– $

NONI (*Morinda citrifolia*) Promoted for many medical disorders; but insufficient data to assess efficacy. Potassium content comparable to orange juice; hyperkalemia reported in chronic renal failure. Case reports of hepatotoxicity. [Not by prescription.] ▶? ♀– ▶– $$$

PEPPERMINT OIL (*Mentha x piperita oil*) Irritable bowel syndrome (possibly effective): 0.2 to 0.4 mL enteric-coated caps PO three times per day. Peds, 8 yo or older: 0.1 to 0.2 mL enteric-coated caps PO three times per day. Take before meals. [Not by prescription.] ▶LK♀+ in food, ? in supplements ▶+ in food, ? in supplements $

PROBIOTICS (*Acidophilus, Align, Bacid, Bifantis, Bifidobacteria, BioGaia, Culturelle, Florastor, Gerber Soothe Colic drops, Intestinex, Lactobacillus, Power-Dophilus, Primadophilus, Saccharomyces boulardii, VSL#3*) Prevention of antibiotic-associated diarrhea (effective): *Saccharomyces boulardii* 500 mg PO two times per day (Florastor 2 caps PO two times per day) for adults; 250 mg PO two times per day (Floraster 1 cap/packet PO two times per day) for peds. For peds: *Lactobacillus* GG (Culturelle) 10 to 20 billion cells/day PO given 2 h before/after antibiotic. IDSA recommends against probiotics for prevention of *C. difficile*–associated diarrhea; safety and efficacy are unclear. Peds, acute gastroenteritis, adjunct to rehydration (effective): *Lactobacillus* GG at least 10 billion cells per day PO for 5 to 7 days or *Saccharomyces boulardii* 250 to 750 mg per day PO for 5 to 7 days. Infant colic (efficacy unclear; conflicting study results): 5 drops of *L. reuteri* DSM 17938 (Gerber Soothe Colic drops) PO once daily for 21 days. Ulcerative colitis (effective): VSL#3, 1 to 2 sachets/day PO for maintenance; 2 to 4 sachets/day PO for pouchitis; 4 to 8 sachets/day PO for mild to moderate active; peds dose based on age (see www.vsl3.com). Irritable bowel syndrome: VSL#3 either ½ to 1 packet PO daily or 2 to 4 caps PO daily to relieve gas/bloating. Align: 1 cap PO once daily to relieve abdominal pain/bloating. [Mostly not by prescription. Culturelle Kids contains *Lactobacillus* GG 5 billion cells per powder packet/chewable tab. Culturelle Digestive Health contains *Lactobacillus* GG 10 billion cells per cap/chewable tab (also contains inulin). Culturelle Health & Wellness contains *Lactobacillus* GG 15 billion cells/cap. Florastor and Florastor Kids contain *Saccharomyces boulardii* 250 mg per cap/powder packet (contains lactose). VSL#3 (nonprescription medical food) contains 225 billion cells/Junior packet, 450 billion cells/sachet, 900 billion cells/DS sachet (Rx only), 225 billion cells/2 caps (*Bifidobacterium breve, B. longum, B. infantis, Lactobacillus acidophilus, L. plantarum, L. casei, L. bulgaricus, Streptococcus thermophilus*). Align contains *Bifidobacterium* infantis 35624, 1 billion cells/cap. Gerber Soothe Colic drops contains Lactobacillus reuteri DSM 17938, 100 million cells per 5 drops. BioGaia ProTectis contains *Lactobacillus reuteri* DSM 17938, 100 million cells per chewable tab/straw.] ▶? ♀+ ▶+ $

PYGEUM AFRICANUM (African plum tree) BPH (may have modest efficacy): 50 to 100 mg PO two times per day or 100 mg PO daily of standardized extract containing 14% triterpenes. [Not by prescription.] ▶? ♀– ▶– $

RED CLOVER (red clover isoflavone extract, *Trifolium pratense*, trefoil, *Promensil, Trinovin*) Postmenopausal vasomotor symptoms (conflicting evidence; does not appear effective overall, but may have modest benefit for severe symptoms): Promensil 1 tab PO daily to two times per day with meals. [Not by prescription. Isoflavone content (genistein, daidzein, biochanin, formononetin) is 40 mg/tab in Promensil and Trinovin.] ▶Gut, L, K ♀– ▶– $$

RED YEAST RICE (*Monascus purpureus, Xuezhikang, Zhibituo, Hypocol*) Hyperlipidemia: Usual dose is 1200 mg PO two times per day. Efficacy depends on whether formulation contains lovastatin or other statins. In the US, red yeast rice should not contain more than trace amounts of statins, but some products contain up to 10 mg lovastatin per cap. Some clinicians consider red yeast rice an alternative for patients who develop myalgia with prescription statins. Can cause myopathy. Some formulations may contain citrinin, a potential nephrotoxin. [Not by prescription. Xuezhikang marketed in Asia, Norway (HypoCol).] ▶L♀– ▶? $$

S-ADENOSYLMETHIONINE (*SAM-e*) Mild to moderate depression (effective): 800 to 1600 mg/day PO in divided doses with meals. Efficacy unclear for OA. [Not by prescription.] ▶L♀? ▶? $$$

SOUR CHERRY (*Prunus cerasus*, tart cherry, *Montmorency cherry*) OA (efficacy unclear): 240 mL juice PO two times per day. Prevention of gout (efficacy unclear): 15 mL concentrate PO two times per day. Insomnia (possibly effective): 240 mL juice or 30 mL concentrate PO two times per day. Prevention of exercise-induced muscle damage/pain after strenuous exercise (efficacy unclear): 240 or 360 mL juice or 30 mL concentrate PO two times per day. Dilute concentrate before drinking. [Not by prescription.] ▶LK ♀ + for moderate amount in food, – in supplements ▶ + for moderate amount in food, – in supplements $$

SOY (*Genisoy, Healthy Woman, Novasoy, Phyto soya, Supro*) Postmenopausal vasomotor symptoms (modest benefit): Per North American Menopause Society, consider 50 mg/day or more of soy isoflavones for at least 12 weeks. Conflicting clinical trials for postmenopausal bone loss. [Not by prescription.] ▶Gut, L, K♀+ for food, ? for supplements▶+ for food, ? for supplements $

ST. JOHN'S WORT (*Hypericum perforatum*) Mild to moderate depression (effective): 300 mg PO three times per day of standardized extract (0.3% hypericin). Does not appear effective for ADHD. May decrease efficacy of other drugs (eg, ritonavir, oral contraceptives) by inducing liver metabolism. May cause serotonin syndrome with SSRIs, MAOIs. [Not by prescription.] ▶L♀– ▶– $

TEA TREE OIL (melaleuca oil, *Melaleuca alternifolia*) Not for oral use; CNS toxicity reported. Limited evidence for topical treatment of onychomycosis, tinea pedis, acne vulgaris, dandruff, pediculosis. [Not by prescription.] ▶? ♀– ▶– $

VALERIAN (*Valeriana officinalis, Alluna*) Insomnia (possibly modestly effective; conflicting clinical trials): 400 to 900 mg of standardized extract PO 30 min before bedtime. Alluna: 2 tabs PO 1 h before bedtime. [Not by prescription.] ▶? ♀– ▶– $

WILLOW BARK EXTRACT (*Salicis cortex*, salicin) OA, low-back pain (possibly effective): 60 to 240 mg/day salicin PO divided two to three times per day. [Not by prescription. Some products standardized to 15% salicin content.] ▶K♀–▶– $

IMMUNOLOGY

ADULT IMMUNIZATION SCHEDULE (for more information see CDC website at cdc.gov)

ADULT IMMUNIZATION SCHEDULE*
Tetanus, diphtheria (Td): For all ages, 1 dose booster q 10 years.
Pertussis: Consider single dose of pertussis in adults younger than 65 yo (as part of Tdap), at least 10 years since last tetanus dose. If patient has never received a pertussis booster, use Boostrix if 10 to 18 yo, Adacel if 11 to 64 yo. Administer 1 dose Tdap during each pregnancy.
Influenza: 1 yearly dose (trivalent or quadrivalent) if age 50 or older. If younger than 50 yo, then 1 yearly dose if healthcare worker, pregnant, chronic underlying illness, household contact of person with chronic underlying illness or household contact with children younger than 5 yo, or those who request vaccination. Intranasal vaccine indicated for healthy adults younger than 50 yo. High dose vaccine indicated for 65 yrs or older.
Pneumococcal (polysccharide, Pneumovax 23): 1 dose if age 65 yo or older. If younger than 65 yo, consider immunizing if chronic underlying illness, nursing home resident. Consider revaccination 5 years later if high risk or if age 65 yo or older and received primary dose before age 65 yo.
Pneumococcal (conjugate, Prevnar 13): 1 dose in high-risk adolescents and adults such as those who are immunocpmpromised, those with asplenia, sickle cell/hemoglobinopathies, renal failure, CSF leak, Cochlear implant, as an adjunct to the polysaccharide vaccine.
Hepatitis A: For all ages with clotting factor disorders, chronic liver disease, or exposure risk (travel to endemic areas, illegal drug use, men having sex with men), 2 doses (0, 6 to 12 months). Twinrix (hepatitis A + B) requires 3-dose series.
Hepatitis B: For all ages with medical (hemodialysis, clotting factor recipients, chronic liver disease), occupational (healthcare or public safety workers with blood exposure), behavioral (illegal drug use, multiple sex partners, those seeking evaluation or treatment of sexually transmitted disease, men having sex with men), or other (household/sex contacts of those with chronic HBV or HIV infections, clients/staff of developmentally disabled, more than 6 months of travel to high-risk areas, inmates of correctional facilities) indications, 3 doses (0, 1–2, 4–6 months). Hemodialysis patients require 4 doses and higher dose (40 mcg).
Measles, mumps, rubella (MMR): If born during or after 1957 and immunity in doubt, see www.cdc.gov.
Varicella: For all ages if immunity in doubt, age 13 yo or older, 2 doses separated by 4 to 8 weeks.

IMMUNOLOGY

CHILDHOOD IMMUNIZATION SCHEDULE*

				Months						Years		
Age	Birth	1	2	4	6	12	15	18	2	4–6	11–12
Hepatitis B	HB	HB				HB					
Rotavirus			Rota	Rota	Rota@						
DTP			DTaP	DTaP	DTaP		DTaP			DTaP	
H influenzae b			Hib	Hib	Hibˣ	HibˣΔ					
Pneumococcal**			PCV	PCV	PCV	PCV					
Polio			IPV	IPV		IPV				IPV#	
Influenza†					Influenza (yearly)†						
MMR						MMR				MMR	
Varicella						Varicella				Varicella	
Hepatitis A¶						Hep A × 2¶					
Papillomavirus§,¶											HPV × 3§
Meningococcal^											MCV^

*2015 schedule from the CDC, ACIP, AAP, & AAFP, see CDC website (www.cdc.gov).

**Administer 1 dose Prevnar 13 to all healthy children 24 to 59 mo having an incomplete schedule.

***When immunizing adolescents 10 yo or older, consider Tdap if patient has never received a pertussis booster. (Boostrix if 10 yo or older, Adacel if 11 to 64 yo).

@ If using Rotarix, give at 2 and 4 mo (no earlier than 6 weeks). Give at 2, 4, and 6 mo if using Rotateq. Max age for final dose is 8 mo.

Δ Last IPV on or after 4th birthday, and at least 6 months since last dose.

ˣ if using PedvaxHib or Comvax, dose at 6 mo not necessary, but booster at 12 to 15 mo indicated.

† For healthy patients age 2 yo or older can use intranasal form. If age younger than 9 yo and receiving for first time, administer 2 doses 4 or more weeks apart for injected form and 6 or more weeks apart for intranasal form. FluLaval, Fluarix, and single-dose Fluzone syringe not indicated in younger than 3 years. Fluvirin not indicated in younger than 4 years. Do not use Afluria in younger than 9 years. Do not use Flucelvax, Fluzone ID or Fluzone HD in children.

¶ Two doses 6 to 18 months apart. Twinrix (hep A + hep B) requires 3 doses.

§ Second and third doses 2 and 6 months after 1st dose. Also approved (Gardasil only) for males 9 to 26 yo to reduce risk of genital warts. Either the quadrivalent or 9-valent or 2-valent (females only) vaccine can be used. Vaccination may begin as early as 9 years of age.

^ Vaccinate all children at age 11 to 12 years with a single dose of Menactra or Menveo, with a booster dose at age 16. For high-risk younger children, refer to CDC recommendations. Consider Trumendat or Bexero in children 10 years or older who are at risk for meningococcal disease.

TETANUS WOUND CARE (www.cdc.gov)

	Unknown or less than 3 prior tetanus immunizations	*3 or more prior tetanus immunizations*
Non-tetanus-prone wound (eg, clean and minor)	Td (DT age younger than 7 yo)	Td if more than 10 years since last dose
Tetanus-prone wound (eg, dirt, contamination, punctures, crush components)	Td (DT age younger than 7 yo), tetanus immune globulin 250 units IM at site other than Td	Td if more than 5 years since last dose

If patient age 10 yo or older has never received a pertussis booster consider DTaP (Boostrix if 10 yo or older, Adacel if 11–64 yo).

Immunizations

NOTE: *For vaccine info see CDC website (www.cdc.gov).*

BCG VACCINE 0.2 to 0.3 mL percutaneously. ▶immune system ♀C ▶? $$$$ ■

COMVAX **(haemophilus B vaccine + hepatitis B vaccine)** Infants born of HBsAg (negative) mothers: 0.5 mL IM for 3 doses, given at 2, 4, and 12 to 15 months. ▶immune system ♀C ▶? $$$

DIPHTHERIA, TETANUS, AND ACELLULAR PERTUSSIS VACCINE (***DTaP, Tdap, Infanrix, Daptacel, Boostrix, Adacel, ✢Tripacel***) 0.5 mL IM. Do not use Boostrix or Adacel for primary childhood vaccination series. ACIP recommends TDAP in every pregnancy, preferably between 27 and 35 weeks' gestation. ▶immune system ♀C ▶– $$

DIPHTHERIA-TETANUS TOXOID (***Td, DT, ✢D2T5***) 0.5 mL IM. [Injection DT (Peds: 6 weeks to 6 yo). Td (adult and children at least 7 yo).] ▶immune system ♀C ▶? $

HAEMOPHILUS B VACCINE (***ActHIB, Hiberix, PedvaxHIB***) 0.5 mL IM. Dosing schedule varies depending on formulation used and age of child at 1st dose. ▶immune system ♀C ▶? $$

HEPATITIS A VACCINE (***Havrix, Vaqta, ✢Avaxim, Epaxal***) Adult formulation 1 mL IM, repeat in 6 to 12 months. Peds: 0.5 mL IM for age 1 yo or older, repeat 6 to 18 months later. [Single-dose vial (specify pediatric or adult).] ▶immune system ♀C ▶+ $$$

HEPATITIS B VACCINE (***Engerix-B, Recombivax HB***) Adults: 1 mL IM, repeat 1 and 6 months later. ACIP recommends hepatitis B vaccine for all previously unvaccinated diabetics age 19 through 59 years; vaccinate as soon as possible after diabetes diagnosis. Children: Dosing based on age and maternal HBsAg status. ▶immune system ♀C ▶+ $$$

HUMAN PAPILLOMAVIRUS RECOMBINANT VACCINE (***Cervarix, Gardasil***) 0.5 mL IM at time 0, 2, and 6 months. ▶immune system ♀B ▶? $$$$$

INFLUENZA VACCINE—INACTIVATED INJECTION (***Afluria, Fluarix, FluLaval, Fluzone, Fluvirin, Flucelvax, Flublok, ✢Fluviral, Vaxigrip***) 0.5 mL IM or ID (Fluzone ID). Fluarix, FluLaval not indicated in children younger than 3 yo. Fluvirin

(cont.)

not indicated in children younger than 4 yo. Afluria not indicated in children younger than 9 yo. Flublok for 18 to 49 yo. Flucelvax for 18 yo and older. Fluzone ID for 18 to 64 yo. Fluzone HD for 65 yo and older. ▸immune system ♀C ▶+ $

INFLUENZA VACCINE—LIVE INTRANASAL (*FluMist*) 1 dose (0.2 mL) intranasally. Use only if 2 to 49 yo. If available, live, intranasal vaccine should be preferentially used for healthy children age 2 through 8 yo who have no contraindications or precautions. ▸immune system ♀C ▶+ $

JAPANESE ENCEPHALITIS VACCINE (*Ixiaro*) 1 mL SC for 3 doses on day 0, 7, and 30. ▸immune system ♀C ▶? $$$$

MEASLES, MUMPS, AND RUBELLA VACCINE (*M-M-R II, ✦Priorix*) 0.5 mL (1 vial) SC. ▸immune system ♀C ▶+ $$$

MENINGOCOCCAL VACCINE (*Menveo, Menomune-A/C/Y/W-135, Menactra, Trumenba, Bexsero,✦Menjugate*) 0.5 mL SC or IM (depending on product) to high-risk individuals (asplenia, etc), repeat in 2 months. Menveo: Four-dose series starting at 2 mo at 2, 4, 6, and 12 months. Menactra: Vaccinate all children 11 to 12 yo, and 16 yo. One dose only if between 13 and 18 yo and previously unvaccinated. Trumenba: Three-dose series starting at 0, 2, and 6 months in children 10 yo or older. Bexsero: 2 doses at 0 and 1 month in children 10 yo or older. ▸immune system ♀C ▶? $$$$

PEDIARIX (diphtheria tetanus and acellular pertussis vaccine + hepatitis B vaccine + polio vaccine) 0.5 mL IM at 2, 4, 6 mo. ▸immune system ♀C ▶? $$$

PNEUMOCOCCAL 13-VALENT CONJUGATE VACCINE (*Prevnar 13*) 0.5 mL IM for 3 doses at 2 mo, 4 mo, and 6 mo, followed by a 4th dose at 12 to 15 mo. Indicated for some high-risk adolescents and adults (immunocompromised adults, asplenic state, sickle cell/hemoglobinopathy, renal failure, CSF leak, Cochlear implant) as an adjunct to the 23-valent pneumococcal vaccine. Delay 13-valent vaccine at least 1 year after 23-valent vaccine or delay 23-valent vaccine 8 weeks after 13-valent vaccine. ▸immune system ♀C ▶? $$$

PNEUMOCOCCAL 23-VALENT VACCINE (*Pneumovax, ✦Pneumo 23*) 0.5 mL IM or SC. ▸immune system ♀C ▶+ $$

POLIO VACCINE (*IPOL*) 0.5 mL IM or SC. ▸immune system ♀C ▶? $$

ProQuad (measles, mumps, and rubella vaccine + varicella vaccine) 0.5 mL (1 vial) SC for age 12 mo to 12 yo. ▸immune system ♀C ▶? $$$$

RABIES VACCINE (*RabAvert, Imovax Rabies, BioRab, Rabies Vaccine Adsorbed*) 1 mL IM in deltoid region on days 0, 3, 7, 14, 28. ▸immune system ♀C ▶? $$$$$

ROTAVIRUS VACCINE (*RotaTeq, Rotarix*) RotaTeq: 1st dose (2 mL PO) between 6 and 12 weeks of age, and then 2nd and 3rd doses at 4- to 10-week intervals thereafter (last dose no later than 32 weeks). Rotarix: 1st dose (1 mL) at 6 weeks of age, 2nd dose (1 mL) at least 4 weeks later, and last dose prior to 24 weeks of age. [Trade only: Oral susp 2 mL (RotaTeq), 1 mL (Rotarix).] ▸immune system ♀not applicable ▶? $$$$$

TETANUS TOXOID 0.5 mL IM or SC. ▸immune system ♀C ▶+ $$

TWINRIX (hepatitis A vaccine + hepatitis B vaccine Adsorbed): Adults: 1 mL IM in deltoid, repeat 1 and 6 months later. All 3 doses required for hepatitis A immunity. Accelerated dosing schedule: 0, 7, 21, and 30 days and booster dose at 12 months. ▸immune system ♀C ▶? $$$$

TYPHOID VACCINE—INACTIVATED INJECTION (*Typhim Vi*, *◆Typherix*) 0.5 mL IM single dose. May revaccinate q 2 to 5 years if high risk. ▶immune system ♀C ▶? $$

TYPHOID VACCINE—LIVE ORAL (*Vivotif Berna*) 1 cap every other day for 4 doses. May revaccinate every 2 to 5 years if high risk. [Trade only: Caps.] ▶immune system ♀C ▶? $$

VARICELLA VACCINE (*Varivax*, *◆Varilrix*) Children 1 to 12 yo: 0.5 mL SC. Repeat dose at ages 4 to 6 yo. Age 13 yo or older: 0.5 mL SC, repeat 4 to 8 weeks later. ▶immune system ♀C ▶+ $$

YELLOW FEVER VACCINE (*YF-Vax*) 0.5 mL SC. ▶immune system ♀C ▶+ $$$

ZOSTER VACCINE—LIVE (*Zostavax*) 0.65 mL SC single dose for age 50 yo or older. However, ACIP recommends immunizing those 60 yo and older. ▶immune system ♀C ▶? $$$$

Immunoglobulins

BOTULISM IMMUNE GLOBULIN (*BabyBIG*) Infant botulism: Give 1 mL/kg (50 mg/kg) IV for age younger than 1 yo. ▶L ♀? ▶? $$$$$

HEPATITIS B IMMUNE GLOBULIN (*H-BIG, HyperHep B, HepaGam B, NABI-HB*) 0.06 mL/kg IM within 24 h of needlestick, ocular, or mucosal exposure to Hepatitis B, repeat in 1 month. ▶L ♀C ▶? $$$$

IMMUNE GLOBULIN—INTRAMUSCULAR (*Baygam*, *◆Gamastan*) Hepatitis A prophylaxis: 0.02 to 0.06 mL/kg IM depending on length of travel to endemic area. Measles (within 6 days postexposure): 0.2 to 0.25 mL/kg IM. ▶L ♀C ▶? $$$

IMMUNE GLOBULIN—INTRAVENOUS (*Carimune, Flebogamma, Gammagard, Gammaplex, Gamunex, Octagam, Privigen*) IV dosage varies by indication and product. ▶L ♀C ▶? $$$$$ ■

IMMUNE GLOBULIN—SUBCUTANEOUS (*Vivaglobulin, Hizentra*) 100 to 200 mg/kg SC weekly. ▶L ♀C ▶? $$$$$ ■

LYMPHOCYTE IMMUNE GLOBULIN (*Atgam*) Specialized dosing. ▶L ♀C ▶? $$$$$

RABIES IMMUNE GLOBULIN HUMAN (*Imogam Rabies-HT, HyperRAB S/D*) 20 units/kg, as much as possible infiltrated around bite, the rest IM. ▶L ♀C ▶? $$$$$

RSV IMMUNE GLOBULIN (*RespiGam*) IV infusion for RSV. ▶plasma ♀C ▶? $$$$$

Immunosuppression

BASILIXIMAB (*Simulect*) Specialized dosing for organ transplantation. ▶plasma ♀B ▶? $$$$$

BELATACEPT (*Nulojix*) Specialized dosing for organ transplantation. ▶serum ♀C ▶— $$$$$

CYCLOSPORINE (*Sandimmune, Neoral, Gengraf*) Specialized dosing for organ transplantation, RA, and psoriasis. [Generic/Trade: Microemulsion Caps 25, 100 mg. Generic/Trade: Caps (Sandimmune) 25, 100 mg. Soln (Sandimmune) 100 mg/mL. Microemulsion soln (Neoral, Gengraf) 100 mg/mL.] ▶L ♀C ▶— $$$$$ ■

EVEROLIMUS (*Zortress*) Specialized dosing for organ transplantation. [Trade: Tabs 0.25, 0.5, 0.75 mg.] ▶L — ♀C ▶— $$$$$

MYCOPHENOLATE MOFETIL (*CellCept, Myfortic*) Specialized dosing for organ transplantation. [Generic/Trade: Caps 250 mg. Tabs 500 mg. Tabs, extended-release (Myfortic): 180, 360 mg. Trade only (CellCept): Susp 200 mg/mL (160 mL).] ▶? ♀D ▶– $$ ■

SIROLIMUS (*Rapamune*) Specialized dosing for organ transplantation. [Generic/Trade: Tabs 0.5, 1, 2 mg. Trade only: Soln 1 mg/mL (60 mL).] ▶L ♀C ▶– $$$$$

TACROLIMUS (*Astagraf XL, Hecoria, Prograf, FK 506, Envarsus XR, ★Advagraf*) Specialized dosing for organ transplantation. [Generic/Trade: Caps 0.5, 1, 5 mg. Trade only: Extended-release caps (Astagraf XL) 0.5, 1, 5 mg. (Envarsus XR) 0.75, 1, 4 mg.] ▶L ♀C ▶– $$$$$

Other

TUBERCULIN PPD (*Aplisol, Tubersol, Mantoux, PPD*) 5 tuberculin units (0.1 mL) intradermally, read 48 to 72 h later. ▶L ♀C ▶+ $

NEUROLOGY

Dermatomes

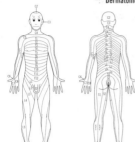

MOTOR FUNCTION BY NERVE ROOTS

Level	Motor Function
C3/C4/C5	Diaphragm
C5/C6	Deltoid/biceps
C7/C8	Triceps
C8/T1	Finger flexion/ intrinsics
T1–T12	Intercostal/ abd muscles
L2/L3	Hip flexion
L2/L3/L4	Hip adductor/quads
L4/L5	Ankle dorsiflexion
S1/S2	Ankle plantarflexion
S2/S3/S4	Rectal tone

LUMBOSACRAL NERVE ROOT COMPRESSIONS

Root	Motor	Sensory	Reflex
L4	quadriceps	medial foot	knee-jerk
L5	dorsiflexors	dorsum of foot	medial hamstring
S1	plantarflexors	lateral foot	ankle-jerk

GLASGOW COMA SCALE

Eye Opening	Verbal Activity	Motor Activity
4. Spontaneous	5. Oriented	6. Obeys commands
3. To command	4. Confused	5. Localizes pain
2. To pain	3. Inappropriate	4. Withdraws to pain
1. None	2. Incomprehensible	3. Flexion to pain
	1. None	2. Extension to pain
		1. None

Alzheimer's Disease—Cholinesterase Inhibitors

DONEPEZIL (*Aricept*) Start 5 mg PO at bedtime. May increase to 10 mg PO at bedtime in 4 to 6 weeks. Max 10 mg/day for mild to moderate disease. For moderate to severe disease (MMSE 10 or less): May increase after 3 months to 23 mg/day. [Generic/Trade: Tabs 5, 10, 23 mg.] ▶LK ♀C ▶? $

GALANTAMINE (*Razadyne, Razadyne ER, ✦Reminyl*) Extended-release: Start 8 mg PO every am with food; increase to 16 mg after 4 weeks. May increase to 24 mg after another 4 weeks. Immediate-release: Start 4 mg PO two times per day

(cont.)

NEUROLOGY

with food; increase to 8 mg two times per day after 4 weeks. May increase to 12 mg two times per day after another 4 weeks. [Generic/Trade: Tabs 4, 8, 12 mg. Extended-release caps 8, 16, 24 mg. Oral soln 4 mg/mL. Prior to April 2005 was called Reminyl in the US.] ▶LK ♀B ▷? $$$$

RIVASTIGMINE (*Exelon, Exelon Patch*) Alzheimer's disease: Start 1.5 mg PO two times per day with food. Increase to 3 mg two times per day after 2 weeks. Max 12 mg/day. Patch: Start 4.6 mg/24 h once daily; may increase after 1 month or more to recommended dose of 9.5 mg/24 h, max 13.3 mg/24 h. Rotate sites. Dementia in Parkinson's disease: Start 1.5 mg PO two times per day with food. Increase by 3 mg/day at intervals greater than 4 weeks to max 12 mg/day. Patch: Use dosing for Alzheimer's disease. [Generic/Trade: Caps 1.5, 3, 4.5, 6 mg. Trade only: Transdermal patch: 4.6 mg/24 h, 9.5 mg/24 h, 13.3 mg/24 h] ▶K ♀B ▷? $$$$$

Alzheimer's Disease—NMDA Receptor Antagonists

MEMANTINE (*Namenda, Namenda XR, ✦Ebixa*) Start 5 mg PO daily. Increase by 5 mg/day at weekly intervals to max 20 mg/day. Doses greater than 5 mg/day should be divided two times per day. Extended-release: start 7 mg once daily. Increase at weekly intervals to target dose of 28 mg/day. Reduce to 14 mg/day in renal impairment. [Trade only: Tabs 5, 10 mg. Oral soln 2 mg/mL. Extended-release caps 7, 14, 21, 28 mg.] ▶LK ♀B ▷? $$$$$

NAMZARIC (menatine extended-release + donepezil) For patients stabilized on memantine + donepezil: 28 mg/10 mg PO once daily in the evening. Reduce to 14/10 mg for severe renal insufficiency (ClCr 5 to 29 mL/min). [Trade only: Caps, extended-release memantine + donepezil 14/10, 28/10 mg.] ▶KL ♀C ▷?

Anticonvulsants

NOTE: *Avoid rapid discontinuation of anticonvulsants because this can precipitate seizures or other withdrawal symptoms. Recent data suggest an increased risk of suicidal ideation or behaviors with antiepileptic drugs. Monitor closely for signs of depression, anxiety, hostility, hypomania/mania, or suicidality. Symptoms may develop within 1 week of initiation, and risk continues for at least 24 weeks.*

CARBAMAZEPINE (*Tegretol, Tegretol XR, Carbatrol, Epitol, Equetro*) Epilepsy: Ages 13 yo and older: 200 mg PO twice daily, then increase by 200 mg/day at weekly intervals divided into three or four doses (immediate-release tabs) or two times per day (extended-release). Max 1,600 mg/day. Age 6 to 12 yo: Start 100 mg PO twice daily (immediate-release or extended-release) or ½ teaspoon (50 mg) susp four times daily. Increase by 100 mg/day at weekly intervals divided into three or four daily doses (immediate-release tabs or susp) or two times per day (extended-release). Max 1,000 mg/day. Age younger than 6 yo: Start 10 to 20 mg/kg/day PO divided into two to three doses per day (immediate-release tabs) or four times per day (susp). Increase weekly prn. Max 35 mg/kg/day. Bipolar disorder, acute manic/mixed episodes (Equetro): Start 200 mg PO two times per day; increase

(cont.)

by 200 mg/day to max 1600 mg/day. Trigeminal neuralgia: Start 100 mg PO two times per day (regular and XR tabs) or 50 mg PO four times per day (susp). May increase by 200 mg/day until pain relieved or max 1200 mg/day. Aplastic anemia, agranulocytosis, many drug interactions. [Generic/Trade: Tabs 200 mg, Chewable tabs 100 mg, Susp 100 mg/5 mL. Extended-release tabs (Tegretol XR) 100, 200, 400 mg. Extended-release caps (Carbatrol): 100, 200, 300 mg. Trade only: Extended-release caps (Equetro): 100, 200, 300 mg.] ▶LK ♀D ▶+ $$ ■

CLOBAZAM (*ONFI, ✦Frisium*) US, adults and children 2 yo and older, weight greater than 30 kg: Start 5 mg PO twice per day. Increase to 10 mg PO twice daily after 1 week, then to 20 mg PO twice daily after 2 weeks. Wt 30 kg or less: Start 5 mg PO daily. Increase to 5 mg PO twice per day after 1 week, then 10 mg PO twice per day after 2 weeks. Canada, adults: Start 5 to 15 mg PO daily. Increase prn to max 80 mg/day. Children younger than 2 yo: 0.5 to 1 mg/kg PO daily. Children age 2 to 16 yo: Start 5 mg PO daily. May increase prn to max 40 mg/day. [Trade only: Tabs 5, 10, 20 mg. Oral susp 2.5 mg/mL.] ▶L ♀C ▶– ⊙IV $$$$$

ESLICARBAZEPINE (*Aptiom*) Start 400 mg PO once daily. Increase after 1 week to 800 mg PO once daily. May increase weekly to max 1200 mg/day. [Trade only: Tabs 200, 400, 600, 800 mg.] ▶L ♀C ▶? Enters breastmilk

ETHOSUXIMIDE (*Zarontin*) Age 3 to 6 yo: Start 250 mg PO daily (or divided two times per day). Age older than 6 yo: Start 500 mg PO daily (or divided two times per day). Max 1.5 g/day. The optimal dose for most pediatric patients is 20 mg/kg/day. [Generic/Trade: Caps 250 mg. Syrup 250 mg/5 mL.] ▶LK ♀C ▶+ $$$$

EZOGABINE (*POTIGA*) Start 100 mg PO three times per day. Increase weekly by no more than 50 mg three times daily to usual maintenance dose of 200 to 400 mg PO three times daily or max of 250 mg three times daily if older than 65 yo. Reduce dose for moderate to severe renal or hepatic impairment. [Trade: Tabs 50, 200, 300, 400 mg.] ▶KL – ♀C ▶? ■

FOSPHENYTOIN (*Cerebyx*) Load: 15 to 20 mg "phenytoin equivalents" (PE) per kg IM/IV no faster than 150 mg PE/min. Maintenance: 4 to 6 mg PE/kg/day. ▶L ♀D ▶+ $$$$$

GABAPENTIN (*Neurontin, Horizant, Gralise*) Partial seizures, adjunctive therapy: Start 300 mg PO at bedtime. Increase gradually to 300 to 600 mg PO three times per day. Max 3600 mg/day divided three times per day. Postherpetic neuralgia, immediate-release tabs: Start 300 mg PO on day 1; increase to 300 mg two times per day on day 2, and to 300 mg three times per day on day 3. Max 1800 mg/day divided three times per day. Postherpetic neuralgia (Gralise): Start 300 mg PO once daily with evening meal. Increase to 600 mg on day 2, 900 mg on days 3 to 6, 1200 mg on days 7 to 10, 1500 mg on days 11 to 14, and 1800 mg on day 15. Max 1800 mg/day. Postherpetic neuralgia (Horizant): Start 600 mg PO q am for 3 days, then increase to 600 mg PO twice per day. Max 1200 mg/day. Partial seizures, initial monotherapy: Titrate as above. Usual effective dose is 900 to 1800 mg/day. Restless legs syndrome (Horizant): 600 mg PO once daily around 5 pm taken with food. [Generic only: Tabs 100, 300, 400 mg. Generic/Trade: Caps 100, 300, 400 mg. Tabs 100, 300, 400, 600, 800 mg. Soln 50 mg/mL. Trade only: Tabs, extended-release 300, 600 mg (gabapentin enacarbil, Horizant). Trade only (Gralise): Tabs 300, 600 mg.] ▶K ♀C ▶? $$$$

LACOSAMIDE (*Vimpat*) Adjunctive therapy: Start 50 mg PO/IV two times per day. Increase weekly by 50 mg two times per day to recommended dose of 100 to 200 mg two times per day. Max recommended 400 mg/day (max 300 mg/day in mild/moderate hepatic or severe renal impairment). Alternative initiation: Load with 200 mg PO/IV followed 12 h later by 100 mg PO two times per day for 1 week. May then increase weekly as required by 50 mg two times per day to max recommended dose of 400 mg/day. Monotherapy: Start 100 mg PO/IV two times per day. May increase weekly by 50 mg two times per day to recommended range of 150 to 200 mg two times per day. Alternative initiation: Load with 200 mg PO/IV followed 12 h later by 100 mg twice daily for 1 week. May then increase weekly as required by 50 mg two times per day to recommended range of 150 to 200 mg two times per day. Conversion to monotherapy: Initiate and titrate lacosamide to usual dose of 150 mg to 200 mg twice daily and maintain for at least 3 days before tapering off the concomitant drug. Loading and IV dosing should be monitored. Doses of 600 mg/day are not more effective than 400 mg/day. [Trade only: Tabs 50, 100, 150, 200 mg.] ▶KL ♀C ▶? ⊙V $$$$$

LAMOTRIGINE (*Lamictal, Lamictal CD, Lamictal ODT, Lamictal XR*) Partial seizures, Lennox-Gastaut syndrome, or generalized tonic-clonic seizures adjunctive therapy with a single enzyme-inducing anticonvulsant: Age 2 to 12 yo: Dosing is based on wt and concomitant meds (see package insert). Age older than 12 yo: 50 mg PO daily for 2 weeks, then 50 mg two times per day for 2 weeks, then gradually increase to 300 to 500 mg/day divided twice daily. Extended-release (generalized tonic-clonic and partial seizures): Start 50 mg PO daily for weeks 1 to 2, then increase to 100 mg PO daily for weeks 3 to 4. Then increase by 100 mg/day at weekly intervals to target dose of 400 to 600 mg/day. Partial seizures, Lennox-Gastaut syndrome, or generalized tonic-clonic seizures, adjunctive therapy (NOT with valproate or enzyme-inducing anticonvulsant (age older than 12 yo): Start 25 mg PO q day for weeks 1 to 2, then increase to 50 mg/day for weeks 3 to 4. Then increase by 50 mg/day q 1 to 2 weeks to target dose of 225 to 375 mg/day divided twice daily. Extended-release (generalized tonic-clonic and partial seizures): Start 25 mg PO daily for weeks 1 to 2, then increase to 50 mg/day for weeks 3 to 4. Then increase weekly by 50 mg/day to target dose of 300 to 400 mg/day. Partial seizures, Lennox-Gastaut syndrome, or generalized tonic-clonic seizures, adjunctive therapy with valproate (age older than 12 yo): Start 25 mg PO every other day for 2 weeks, then 25 mg PO daily for 2 weeks. Increase by 25 to 50 mg/day q 1 to 2 weeks to usual maintenance dose of 100 to 400 mg/day (when used with valproate + other inducers of glucuronidation) or 100 to 200 mg/day (when used with valproate alone) given once daily or divided twice per day. Extended-release (generalized tonic-clonic and partial seizures): Start 25 mg PO every other day for weeks 1 to 2, then increase to 25 mg/day for weeks 3 to 4. Then increase to 50 mg/day on week 5 and increase weekly by 50 mg/day to target dose of 200 to 250 mg/day. Conversion to monotherapy (age 16 yo or older): See package insert. Drug interaction with valproate (see package insert for adjusted dosing guidelines). Potentially life-threatening rashes reported in

(cont.)

0.3% of adults and 0.8% of children; discontinue at 1st sign of rash. [Generic/Trade: Tabs 25, 100, 150, 200 mg. Chewable dispersible tabs (Lamictal CD) 5, 25 mg. Extended-release tabs (Lamictal XR) 25, 50, 100, 200, 250, 300 mg. Trade only: Orally disintegrating tabs (Lamictal ODT) 25, 50, 100, 200 mg.] ▶LK ♀C (see notes)▶– $$$$ ■

LEVETIRACETAM (*Elepsia XR, Keppra, Keppra XR*) Partial seizures, juvenile myoclonic epilepsy (JME), or primary generalized tonic-clonic seizures (GTC), adjunctive: Start 500 mg PO/IV twice per day (Keppra) or 1000 mg PO once daily (Keppra XR and Elepsia XR, partial seizures only); increase by 1000 mg/day every 2 weeks prn to max 3000 mg/day (partial seizures) or to target dose of 3000 mg/day (JME or GTC). IV route not approved for GTC or if age younger than 16 yo. [Generic/Trade: Tabs 250, 500, 750, 1000 mg. Oral soln 100 mg/mL. Tabs, extended-release 500, 750, 1000 mg.] ▶K ♀C ▶? $$$

OXCARBAZEPINE (*Trileptal, Oxtellar XR*) Immediate-release: Start 300 mg PO two times per day. Titrate to 1200 mg/day (adjunctive) or 1200 to 2400 mg/day (monotherapy). Extended-release (adjunctive): Start 600 mg PO daily. Increase by 600 mg/day weekly if needed, max 2400 mg/day. Peds 2 to 16 yo: Immediate-release: Start 8 to 10 mg/kg/day divided two times per day. Extended-release (adjunctive for 6 to 17 yo): Start 8 mg/kg to 10 mg/kg PO once daily not to exceed 600 mg/day. May increase weekly by 8 mg/kg to 10 mg/kg once daily if needed to max based on wt of 900 mg/day (20 to 29 kg), 1200 mg/day (29.1 to 39 kg), or 1800 mg/day (greater than 39 kg). Life-threatening rashes and hypersensitivity reactions. [Generic/Trade: Tabs (scored) 150, 300, 600 mg. Oral susp 300 mg/5 mL. Trade only: Extended-release tabs (Oxtellar XR) 150, 300, 600 mg.] ▶LK ♀C ▶– $$$$$

PERAMPANEL (*Fycompa*) Partial-onset seizures: Without other enzyme-inducing drugs: Start 2 mg PO once daily at bedtime. Increase by 2 mg/day weekly to usual range of 8 to 12 mg/day. Max 12 mg/day. With enzyme-inducing drugs: Start 4 mg PO once daily at bedtime. May increase weekly by 2 mg/day to max 12 mg/day. Mild to moderate hepatic impairment: Start 2 mg PO once daily at bedtime. May increase by 2 mg/day q 2 weeks to max 6 mg/day for mild disease and 4 mg/day for moderate. Avoid in severe hepatic impairment. Generalized tonic-clonic seizures, adjunctive: Without other enzyme inducing drugs: Start 2 mg PO once daily at bedtime. Increase by 2 mg/day weekly to usual range of 8 to 12 mg/day. Max 12 mg/day. With enzyme-inducing drugs: Start 4 mg PO once daily at bedtime. May increase weekly by 2 mg/day to max 12 mg/day. Mild to moderate hepatic impairment: Start 2 mg PO once daily at bedtime. May increase by 2 mg/day q 2 weeks to max 6 mg/day for mild disease and 4 mg/day for moderate. Avoid in severe hepatic impairment. [Tabs 2, 4, 6, 8, 10, 12 mg.] ▶L ♀C ▶? ⊚III $$$$$ ■

PHENOBARBITAL (*Luminal*) Load: 20 mg/kg IV at rate no faster than 60 mg/min. Maintenance: 100 to 300 mg/day PO given once daily or divided two times per day. Peds 3 to 5 mg/kg/day PO divided two to three times per day. Many drug interactions. [Generic only: Tabs 15, 16.2, 30, 32.4, 60, 100 mg. Elixir 20 mg/5 mL.] ▶L ♀D– ⊚IV $

PHENYTOIN (*Dilantin, Phenytek*) Status epilepticus: Load 15 to 20 mg/kg IV no faster than 50 mg/min, then 100 mg IV/PO q 6 to 8 h. Epilepsy: Oral load: 400 mg PO initially, then 300 mg in 2 h and 4 h. Maintenance: 5 mg/kg (or 300 mg PO) given once daily (extended-release) or divided three times per day (susp and chew tabs) and titrated to a therapeutic level. Limit dose increases to 10% or less due to saturable metabolism. [Generic/Trade: Extended-release caps 100 mg (Dilantin). Susp 125 mg/5 mL. Extended-release caps 200, 300 mg (Phenytek). Chewable tabs 50 mg (Dilantin Infatabs). Trade only: Extended-release caps 30 mg (Dilantin).] ▶L ♀D ▶+ $$

PREGABALIN (*Lyrica*) Painful diabetic peripheral neuropathy: Start 50 mg PO three times per day; may increase within 1 week to max 100 mg PO three times per day. Postherpetic neuralgia: Start 150 mg/day PO divided two to three times per day. May increase within 1 week to 300 mg/day divided two to three times per day; max 600 mg/day. Partial seizures (adjunctive): Start 150 mg/day PO divided two to three times per day; increase prn to max 600 mg/day divided two to three times per day. Fibromyalgia: Start 75 mg PO two times per day; may increase to 150 mg two times per day within 1 week; max 225 mg two times per day. Neuropathic pain associated with spinal cord injury: Start 75 mg PO two times per day; may increase to 150 mg two times per day within 1 week and then to 300 mg two times per day after 2 to 3 weeks if tolerated. [Trade only: Caps 25, 50, 75, 100, 150, 200, 225, 300 mg. Oral soln 20 mg/mL (480 mL).] ▶K ♀C ▶? ⊙V $$$$$

PRIMIDONE (*Mysoline*) Epilepsy: Start 100 to 125 mg PO at bedtime. Increase over 10 days to 250 mg three to four times per day. Max 2 g/day. Metabolized to phenobarbital. Essential tremor (unapproved): Up to 750 mg/day. [Generic/Trade: Tabs 50, 250 mg.] ▶LK ♀D ▶− $$$$

RUFINAMIDE (*Banzel*) Start 400 to 800 mg/day PO divided two times per day. Increase by 400 to 800 mg/day every 2 days to max 3200 mg/day. [Trade only: Tabs 200, 400 mg. Susp 40 mg/mL.] ▶K ♀C ▶? $$$$$

TIAGABINE (*Gabitril*) Start 4 mg PO daily. Increase by 4 to 8 mg/day at weekly intervals prn to max 32 mg/day (age 12 to 18 yo) or max 56 mg/day (age older than 18 yo) divided two to four times per day. Avoid off-label use. [Trade only: Tabs 2, 4, 12, 16 mg.] ▶L ♀C ▶? $$$$$

TOPIRAMATE (*Qudexy XR, Topamax, Trokendi XR*) Partial seizures or primary generalized tonic-clonic seizures, monotherapy (standard tabs): Start 25 mg PO two times per day (week 1), 50 mg two times per day (week 2), 75 mg two times per day (week 3), 100 mg two times per day (week 4), 150 mg two times per day (week 5), then 200 mg two times per day as tolerated. Extended-release (Trokendi XR and Qudexy XR): Start 50 mg PO daily. Increase weekly by 50 mg/day for 4 weeks then by 100 mg/day for weeks 5 and 6 to recommended dose of 400 mg once daily. Partial seizures, primary generalized tonic-clonic seizures or Lennox-Gastaut syndrome, adjunctive therapy: Start 25 to 50 mg PO at bedtime. Increase weekly by 25 to 50 mg per day to usual effective dose of 200 mg PO two times per day. Doses greater than 400 mg per day found to be more effective. Extended-release (Trokendi XR and Qudexy XR): Start 25 to 50 mg PO once daily. Increase weekly by 25 to 50 mg/day to effective dose. Recommended dose 200

(cont.)

to 400 mg/day for partial seizures or Lennox-Gastaut syndrome or 400 mg/day for generalized tonic-clonic seizures. Migraine prophylaxis: Start 25 mg PO at bedtime (week 1), then 25 mg two times per day (week 2), then 25 mg every am and 50 mg every pm (week 3), then 50 mg two times per day (week 4 and thereafter). Bipolar disorder (unapproved): Start 25 to 50 mg per day PO. Titrate prn to max 400 mg per day divided two times per day. [Generic/Trade: Tabs 25, 50, 100, 200 mg. Sprinkle caps 15, 25 mg. Trade only: Extended-release caps (Trokendi XR and Qudexy XR) 25, 50, 100, 200 mg, (Qudexy XR) 150 mg.] ▶K ⊙D? $$$$$

VALPROIC ACID (*Depakene, Depakote, Depakote ER, Depacon, Stavzor, divalproex, sodium valproate, ✦Epival, Deproic*) Epilepsy: 10 to 15 mg/kg/day PO/IV divided two to four times per day (standard-release, delayed-release, or IV) or given once daily (Depakote ER). Titrate to max 60 mg/kg/day. Use rate no faster than 20 mg/min when given IV. Migraine prophylaxis: Start 250 mg PO two times per day (Depakote or Stavzor) or 500 mg PO daily (Depakote ER) for 1 week, then increase to max 1000 mg/day PO divided two times per day (Depakote or Stavzor) or given once daily (Depakote ER). Hepatotoxicity, drug interactions, reduce dose in elderly. Simple and complex absence seizures (age 10 yo and older): Start 15 mg/kg/day and increase as needed by 5 to 10 mg/kg/day to max dose 60 mg/kg/day. Doses above 250 mg/day should be divided in two to three doses. [Generic/Trade: Immediate-release caps 250 mg (Depakene), syrup (Depakene, valproic acid) 250 mg/5 mL. Delayed-release tabs (Depakote) 125, 250, 500 mg. Extended-release tabs (Depakote ER) 250, 500 mg. Delayed-release sprinkle caps (Depakote) 125 mg. Trade only (Stavzor): Delayed-release caps 125, 250, 500 mg.] ▶L ⊙D Category X when used for migraine prevention ▶+ $$$$ ■

ZONISAMIDE (*Zonegran*) Start 100 mg PO daily. Titrate every 2 weeks to 200 to 400 mg/day given once daily or divided two times per day. Max 600 mg/day. Drug interactions. Contraindicated in sulfa allergy. [Generic/Trade: Caps 25, 50, 100 mg.] ▶LK ⊙C ▶? $$$$

Migraine Therapy—Triptans (5-HT1 Receptor Agonists)

NOTE: *May cause vasospasm. Avoid in ischemic or vasospastic heart disease, cerebrovascular syndromes, peripheral arterial disease, uncontrolled HTN, and hemiplegic or basilar migraine. Do not use within 24 h of ergots or other triptans. Risk of serotonin syndrome if used with SSRIs or MAOIs. May be associated with medication overuse headaches if used 10 or more days per month.*

ALMOTRIPTAN (*Axert*) 6.25 to 12.5 mg PO. May repeat in 2 h prn. Max 25 mg/day. Avoid MAOIs. [Trade only: Tabs 6.25, 12.5 mg.] ▶LK ⊙C ▶? $$

ELETRIPTAN (*Relpax*) 20 to 40 mg PO. May repeat in 2 h prn. Max 40 mg/dose or 80 mg/day. Drug interactions. Avoid MAOIs. [Trade only: Tabs 20, 40 mg.] ▶LK ⊙C ▶? $$$

FROVATRIPTAN (*Frova*) 2.5 mg PO. May repeat in 2 h prn. Max 7.5 mg/24 h. [Trade only: Tabs 2.5 mg.] ▶LK ⊙C ▶? $

NARATRIPTAN (*Amerge*) 1 to 2.5 mg PO. May repeat in 4 h prn. Max 5 mg/ 24 h. [Generic/Trade: Tabs 1, 2.5 mg.] ▶KL ⊙C ▶? $$$

RIZATRIPTAN (*Maxalt, Maxalt MLT*) 5 to 10 mg PO. May repeat in 2 h prn. Max 30 mg/24 h. MLT form dissolves on tongue without liquids. Avoid MAOIs. [Generic/Trade: Tabs 5, 10 mg. Orally disintegrating tabs 5, 10 mg.] ▶LK ♀C ▶? $$$

SUMATRIPTAN (*Imitrex, Alsuma, Sumavel, Zecuity*) Migraine treatment: 4 to 6 mg SC. May repeat in 1 h prn. Max 12 mg/24 h. Tabs: 25 to 100 mg PO (50 mg most common). May repeat q 2 h prn with 25 to 100 mg doses. Max 200 mg/24 h. Intranasal spray: 5 to 20 mg q 2 h. Max 40 mg/24 h. Transdermal: 1 patch topically, max two patches/24 h with no less than 2 h before 2nd application. No evidence of increased benefit with 2nd patch. Cluster headache treatment: 6 mg SC. May repeat after 1 h or longer prn. Max 12 mg/24 h. Initial oral dose of 50 mg appears to be more effective than 25 mg. If HA returns after initial SC injection, then tabs may be used q 2 h prn, max 100 mg/24 h. Avoid MAOIs. [Generic/Trade: Tabs 25, 50, 100 mg. Injection (STATdose System) 4, 6 mg prefilled cartridges. Trade only: Nasal spray (Imitrex Nasal) 5, 20 mg (box of #6). Alsuma, Sumavel: Injection 6 mg prefilled cartridge. Zecuity Transdermal Patch: 6.5 mg/4 h. Generic only: Nasal spray 5, 20 mg (box of #6).] ▶LK ♀C ▶+ $

***TREXIMET* (sumatriptan + naproxen)** 1 tab PO at onset of headache. Efficacy of more than 1 tab not established. Max 2 tabs/24 h separated by at least 2 h. [Trade only: Tabs 85 mg sumatriptan + 500 mg naproxen sodium and 10 mg sumatriptan + 60 mg of naproxen sodium.] ▶LK ♀C ▶– $$

ZOLMITRIPTAN (*Zomig, Zomig ZMT*) 1.25 to 2.5 mg PO every 2 h. Max 10 mg/24 h. Orally disintegrating tabs (ZMT) 2.5 mg PO. May repeat in 2 h prn. Max 10 mg/24 h. Nasal spray: 5 mg (1 spray) in 1 nostril. May repeat in 2 h. Max 10 mg/24 h. [Generic/Trade: Tabs 2.5, 5 mg. Orally disintegrating tabs (ZMT) 2.5, 5 mg. Trade only: Nasal spray 5 mg/spray.] ▶L ♀C ▶? $$$$

Migraine Therapy—Other

***CAFERGOT* (ergotamine + caffeine)** 2 tabs PO at onset, then 1 tab every 30 min prn. Max 6 tabs/attack or 10/week. Drug interactions. Fibrotic complications. [Trade only: Tabs 1/100 mg ergotamine/caffeine.] ▶L ♀X ▶– $ ■

DIHYDROERGOTAMINE (*D.H.E. 45, Migranal*) Soln (D.H.E. 45) 1 mg IV/IM/SC. May repeat in 1 h prn. Max 2 mg (IV) or 3 mg (IM/SC) per day. Nasal spray (Migranal): 1 spray in each nostril. May repeat in 15 min prn. Max 6 sprays/24 h or 8 sprays/week. Drug interactions. Fibrotic complications. [Trade only: Nasal spray 0.5 mg/spray (Migranal). Self-injecting soln (D.H.E. 45): 1 mg/mL.] ▶L ♀X ▶– $$ ■

FLUNARIZINE Canada only. 10 mg PO at bedtime. [Generic/Trade: Caps 5 mg.] ▶L ♀C ▶– $$

Multiple Sclerosis

ALEMTUZUMAB (*Lemtrada*) First course: 12 mg/day by IV infusion over 4 h for 5 consecutive days. Second course (12 months after 1st course): 12 mg/day by IV infusion over 4 h for 3 consecutive days. Refer to package insert for infusion instructions and premedications required prior to infusions. [Trade: Injection 12 mg/1.2 mL] ▶proteolysis ♀C ▶? ■

DALFAMPRIDINE (*Ampyra*, ✦*Fampyra*) 10 mg PO two times per day. Contraindicated in seizure disorders or moderate to severe renal impairment. [Trade: Extended-release tabs 10 mg.] ▶K – ♀C ▶? $$$$$

DIMETHYL FUMARATE (*Tecfidera*) Start 120 mg PO twice per day. Increase to maintenance dose after 7 days to 240 mg twice per day. [Delayed-release capsules 120, 240 mg.] ▶esterases – ♀C ▶? $$$$$

FINGOLIMOD (*Gilenya*) 0.5 mg PO once daily. Contraindicated in cerebral or cardiovascular disease. [Trade only: Caps 0.5 mg.] ▶L – ♀C ▶?

GLATIRAMER (*Copaxone*, *Glatopa*) Glatiramer acetate 20 mg/mL: 20 mg SC daily. Copaxone 40 mg/mL: 40 mg SC three times weekly. [Trade and generic: Pre-filled syringes 20 mg per mL for injection. Trade only (Copaxone): 40 mg/mL. The 20 mg/mL and 40 mg/mL are not interchangeable.] ▶tissues local hydrolysis ♀B ▶? $$$$$

INTERFERON BETA-1A (*Avonex*, *Rebif*) Avonex 30 mcg (6 million units) IM q week. Rebif: For 22 mcg maintenance dose, start 4.4 SC mcg three times weekly for 2 weeks, then increase to 11 mcg three times weekly for 2 weeks, then increase to 22 mcg three times weekly. For 44 mcg maintenance dose, start 8.8 mcg SC three times weekly for 2 weeks, then increase to 22 mcg three times weekly for 2 weeks, then increase to 44 mcg three times weekly. Follow LFTs and CBC. [Trade only (Avonex): Injection 30 mcg single-dose vial with or without albumin. Prefilled syringe 30 mcg. Trade only (Rebif): Starter kit 20 mcg prefilled syringe. Prefilled syringe 22, 44 mcg.] ▶L ♀C ▶? $$$$$

INTERFERON BETA-1B (*Betaseron*) Start 0.0625 mg SC every other day; titrate over 6 weeks to 0.25 mg (8 million units) SC every other day. Suicidality, hepatotoxicity, blood dyscrasias. Follow LFTs. [Trade only: Injection 0.3 mg (9.6 million units) single-dose vial.] ▶L ♀C ▶? $$$$$

NATALIZUMAB (*Tysabri*) Refractory, relapsing multiple sclerosis (monotherapy) and Crohn's disease: 300 mg IV infusion over 1 h every 4 weeks. ▶ Serum ♀C ▶? $$$$$ ∎

Myasthenia Gravis

PYRIDOSTIGMINE (*Mestinon*, *Mestinon Timespan*, *Regonol*) 60 to 200 mg PO three times per day (standard-release) or 180 mg PO daily or divided two times per day (extended-release). [Generic/Trade: Tabs 60 mg. Extended-release tabs 180 mg. Trade only: Syrup 60 mg/ 5 mL.] ▶plasma, K ♀C ▶+ $$$$$

Parkinsonian Agents—Anticholinergics

BENZTROPINE MESYLATE (*Cogentin*) Parkinsonism: 0.5 to 2 mg IM/PO/IV given once daily or divided two times per day. Drug-induced extrapyramidal disorders: 1 to 4 mg PO/IM/IV given once daily or divided two times per day. [Generic only: Tabs 0.5, 1, 2 mg.] ▶LK ♀C ▶? $

BIPERIDEN (*Akineton*) 2 mg PO three to four times per day, max 16 mg/day. [Trade only: Tabs 2 mg.] ▶LK ♀C ▶? $$$$$

TRIHEXYPHENIDYL (*Artane*) Start 1 mg PO daily. Gradually increase to 6 to 10 mg/day divided three times per day. Max 15 mg/day. [Generic only: Tabs 2, 5 mg. Elixir 2 mg/5 mL.] ▶LK ♀C ▶? $

Parkinsonian Agents—COMT Inhibitors

ENTACAPONE (*Comtan*) Start 200 mg PO with each dose of carbidopa-levodopa. Max 8 tabs (1600 mg)/day. [Generic/Trade: Tabs 200 mg.] ▶L ♀C ▶? $$$$$

Parkinsonian Agents—Dopaminergic Agents and Combinations

APOMORPHINE (*Apokyn*) Start 0.2 mL SC prn. May increase in 0.1 mL increments every few days. Monitor for orthostatic hypotension after initial dose and with dose escalation. Max 0.6 mL/dose or 2 mL/day. Potent emetic, pretreat with trimethobenzamide 300 mg PO three times per day starting 3 days prior to use and continue for at least 6 weeks. Contains sulfites. [Trade only: Cartridges (for injector pen, 10 mg/mL) 3 mL. Ampules (10 mg/mL) 2 mL.] ▶L ♀C ▶? $$$$$

CARBIDOPA/LEVODOPA (*Rytary, DUOPA, Sinemet, Sinemet CR, Parcopa*) Start 1 tab (25/100 mg) PO three times per day. Increase every 1 to 4 days prn. Controlled-release: Start 1 tab (50/200 mg) PO two times per day; increase every 3 days prn. Extended-release caps (Rytary): Start 23.75/95 mg PO three times daily for 3 days. May then increase to 36.25/145 mg three times daily. Max daily dose 97.5/390 mg three times daily. Some patients may require shorter dosing intervals of up to 5 times per day with a max recommended dose of 612.5/2450 mg per day. Enteral susp (DUOPA): Dose is based on the amount of immediate-release carbidopa-levodopa the patient is taking and is administered via enteral feeding tube. Refer to the package insert for full dosing calculation information. [Generic/Trade: Tabs (carbidopa-levodopa) 10/100, 25/100, 25/250 mg. Tabs, sustained-release (Sinemet CR, carbidopa-levodopa ER) 25/100, 50/200 mg. Trade only: Orally disintegrating tabs (Parcopa) 10/100, 25/100, 25/250 mg. Enteral susp (DUOPA): 4.63 mg carbidopa/20 mg levodopa per mL. Caps, extended-release (Rytary): 23.75/95, 36.25/145, 48.75/195, 61.25/245 mg.] ▶L ♀C ▶— $$$$

PRAMIPEXOLE (*Mirapex, Mirapex ER*) Parkinson's disease: Start 0.125 mg PO three times per day. Increase weekly by 0.25 mg/dose (0.75 mg/day) to 0.5 to 1.5 mg PO three times per day. When discontinuing reduce dose by 0.75 mg/day until the daily dose is 0.75 mg/day, then reduce the dose by 0.375 mg/day. Extended-release: Start 0.375 mg PO daily. May increase after 5 to 7 days to 0.75 mg daily, then by 0.75 mg/day increments q 5 to 7 days to max 4.5 mg/day. When discontinuing, reduce dose by 0.75 mg/day until the daily dose is 0.75 mg/day, then reduce the dose by 0.375 mg/day. Restless legs syndrome: Start 0.125 mg PO 2 to 3 h before to bedtime. May increase every 4 to 7 days to max 0.5 mg/day given 2 to 3 h before bedtime. [Generic/Trade: Tabs 0.125, 0.25, 0.5, 0.75, 1, 1.5 mg. Trade only: Tabs, extended-release 0.375, 0.75, 1.5, 2.25, 3, 3.75, 4.5 mg.] ▶K ♀C ▶? $$$$$

ROPINIROLE (*Requip, Requip XL*) Parkinson's disease: Start 0.25 mg PO three times per day, then gradually increase over 4 weeks to 1 mg PO three times per day. Max 24 mg/day. Extended-release: Start 2 mg PO daily for 1 to 2 weeks, then gradually increase by 2 mg daily at weekly or longer intervals. Max 24 mg/day. Restless legs syndrome: Start 0.25 mg PO 1 to 3 h before bedtime for 2 days, then increase to 0.5 mg/day on days 3 to 7. Increase by 0.5 mg/day at weekly

(cont.)

intervals prn to max 4 mg/day given 1 to 3 h before bedtime. [Generic/Trade: Tabs, immediate-release 0.25, 0.5, 1, 2, 3, 4, 5 mg. Tabs, extended-release 2, 4, 6, 8, 12 mg.] ▶L ♀C ▷? $$$

ROTIGOTINE (*Neupro*) Early-stage Parkinson's disease: Start 2 mg/24 h patch daily; may increase by 2 mg/24 h at weekly intervals to max 6 mg/24 h. Advanced-stage Parkinson's disease: Start 4 mg/24 h patch daily; may increase by 2 mg/24 h at weekly intervals to max 8 mg/24 h. Restless legs syndrome: Start 1 mg/24 h patch daily; may be increased by 1 mg/24 h at weekly intervals to max 3 mg/24 h. [Trade: Transdermal patch 1, 2, 3, 4, 6, 8 mg/24 h.] ▶L – ♀C ▷?

***STALEVO* (carbidopa + levodopa + entacapone)** (Conversion from carbidopa-levodopa with or without entacapone): Start Stalevo tab that contains the same amount of carbidopa/levodopa as the patient was previously taking, then titrate to desired response. May need to reduce levodopa dose if not already taking entacapone. [Trade/generic: Tabs (carbidopa/levodopa/entacapone): Stalevo 50 (12.5/50/200 mg), Stalevo 75 (18.75/75/200 mg), Stalevo 100 (25/100/200 mg), Stalevo 125 (31.25/125/200 mg), Stalevo 150 (37.5/150/200 mg), Stalevo 200 (50/200/200 mg).] ▶L ♀C ▷– $$$$$

Parkinsonian Agents—Monoamine Oxidase Inhibitors (MAOIs)

RASAGILINE (*Azilect*) Parkinson's disease, or adjunctive when not taking levodopa: 1 mg PO q am. Parkinson's disease, adjunctive: 0.5 mg PO q am. Max 1 mg/day. Requires an MAOI diet that avoids foods very high in tyramine content. [Trade only: Tabs 0.5, 1 mg.] ▶L ♀C ▷? $$$$$

SELEGILINE (*Eldepryl, Zelapar*) Parkinson's disease: 5 mg PO every am and at noon, max 10 mg/day. Zelapar ODT: 1.25 to 2.5 mg every am, max 2.5 mg/day. [Generic/Trade: Caps 5 mg. Tabs 5 mg. Trade only: Orally disintegrating tabs (Zelapar ODT) 1.25 mg.] ▶LK ♀C ▷? $$$$

Other Agents

ABOBOTULINUM TOXIN A (*DYSPORT*) Cervical dystonia: 500 units IM total dose divided among affected muscles. May repeat every 12 weeks or longer. Max dose 1000 units per treatment. Glabellar lines (age younger than 65 yo): 50 units IM total dose divided into 10 unit injections at 5 sites (see prescribing information). May repeat every 12 weeks or longer. Risk of distant spread with symptoms of systemic botulism. Botulinum toxin products are not interchangeable. [Trade: Vials 300, 500 units for reconstitution.] ▶ ♀C ▷? ■

BOTULINUM TOXIN TYPE B (*Myobloc*) Start 2500 to 5000 units IM in affected muscles. Use lower initial dose if no prior history of botulinum toxin therapy. Benefits usually last for 12 to 16 weeks when a total dose of 5000 to 10,000 units has been administered. Titrate to effective dose. Give treatments at least 3 months apart to decrease the risk of producing neutralizing antibodies. ▶Not significantly absorbed ♀+ ▷? $$$$$

DEXTROMETHORPHAN/QUINIDINE (*Nuedexta*) Start 1 cap PO daily for 7 days, then increase to maintenance dose of 1 cap PO q 12 h. [Trade only: Caps 10 mg dextromethorphan plus 20 mg quinidine.] ▶LK – ♀C ▷? $$$$$

INCOBOTULINUMTOXIN A (*Xeomin*) Cervical dystonia: Total 120 units IM divided among appropriate muscle groups. May repeat at intervals of at least 12 weeks. Blepharospasm in patients previously treated with Botox: Use same dose as Botox. If dose unknown, start 1.25 to 2.5 units per injection site. Do not exceed initial dose of 35 units/eye. May repeat at intervals of at least 12 weeks. [Trade only: 50, 100 unit single-use vials.] ▶not absorbed ♀C ▶? ■

MANNITOL (*Osmitrol, Resectisol*) Intracranial HTN: 0.25 to 2 g/kg IV over 30 to 60 min. ▶K ♀C ▶? $$

MILNACIPRAN (*Savella*) Day 1: 12.5 mg PO once. Days 2 to 3: 12.5 mg two times per day. Days 4 to 7: 25 mg two times per day. After that: 50 mg two times per day. Max 200 mg/day. [Trade only: Tabs 12.5, 25, 50, 100 mg.] ▶KL ♀C ▶? $$$$

NIMODIPINE (*Nimotop, Nymalize*) Subarachnoid hemorrhage: 60 mg PO q 4 h for 21 days. [Generic only: Caps 30 mg. Trade only: 60 mg/20 mL oral solution (Nymalize)] ▶L ♀C ▶– $$$$$

ONABOTULINUM TOXIN TYPE A (*Botox, Botox Cosmetic*) Dose varies based on indication. Risk of distant spread with symptoms of systemic botulism. [Trade only: 100 unit single-use vials.] ▶Not absorbed ♀C ▶? $$$$$ ■

OXYBATE (*Xyrem, GHB*, gamma hydroxybutyrate) 2.25 g PO at bedtime. Repeat in 2.5 to 4 h. May increase by 1.5 g/day at 2-week intervals to max 9 g/day. From a centralized pharmacy. [Trade only: Soln 180 mL (500 mg/mL) supplied with measuring device and child-proof dosing cups.] ▶L ♀B ▶? ⊚III $$$$$ ■

RILUZOLE (*Rilutek*) 50 mg PO q 12 h. Monitor LFTs. [Generic/Trade: Tabs 50 mg.] ▶LK ♀C ▶– $$$$$

TETRABENAZINE (*Xenazine, ✦Nitoman*) Start 12.5 mg PO every am. Increase after 1 week to 12.5 mg PO two times per day. May increase by 12.5 mg/day weekly. Doses greater than 37.5 to 50 mg/day should be divided and given three times per day. For doses greater than 50 mg/day, genotype for CYP2D6. titrate by 12.5 mg/day weekly and divide in doses three times per day to max 37.5 mg/dose and 100 mg/day (extensive/intermediate metabolizers) or 25 mg/dose and 50 mg/day (poor metabolizers). Risk of depression, suicidality, and orthostatic hypotension. [Generic/Trade: Tabs 12.5, 25 mg.] ▶L ♀C ▶? ? $$$$$ ■

OB/GYN

EMERGENCY CONTRACEPTION

Emergency contraception within 72 h of unprotected sex.
Progestin-only methods (Causes less nausea and may be more effective. Available OTC with no age restriction): Fallback Solo, Plan B One-Step (levonorgestrel 1.5 mg tab): Take 1 pill. Next Choice (levonorgestrel 0.75 mg): Take 1 tab ASAP and 2nd dose 12 h later.
Progestin and estrogen method: Dose is defined as 2 pills of Ogestrel, 4 pills of Cryselle, Enpresse*, Jolessa, Levora, Lo/Ovral, Low-Ogestrel, Nordette, Portia, Quasense, Seasonale, Seasonique, Solia, or Trivora*, or 5 pills of Aviane, Lessina, LoSeasonique, Lutera, or Sronyx: Take 1 dose ASAP and 2nd dose 12 h later. If vomiting occurs within 1 h of taking dose, consider repeating that dose with an antiemetic 1 h prior.
Emergency contraception within 120 h of unprotected sex. Ella (ulipristal 30 mg): Take 1 pill. More info at: www.not-2-late.com.

*Use 0.125 mg levonorgestrel/30 mcg ethinyl estradiol tabs.

ORAL CONTRACEPTIVES* → L CX

	Estrogen (mcg)	Progestin (mg)
Monophasic		
Lo Loestrin Fe, Lo Minastrin Fe	10 ethinyl estradiol	1 norethindrone
Beyaz, Gianvi, Loryna, Nikki, *Yaz*	20 ethinyl estradiol	3 drospirenone
Aviane, Falmina, Lessina, Lutera, Orsythia, Sronyx		0.1 levonorgestrel
Gildess Fe 1/20, Junel 1/20, Junel Fe 1/20, Larin Fe 1/20, *Loestrin-21* 1/20, Loestrin Fe 1/20, Loestrin-24 Fe, Lo Media 1/20, Microgestin 1/20, Microgestin Fe 1/20, Minastrin 24 Fe		1 norethindrone
Generess Fe chewable (generic only)	25 ethinyl estradiol	0.8 norethindrone

(cont.)

ORAL CONTRACEPTIVES* → L CX (*continued*)

Apri, Desogen, Emoquette, *Enskyce, Ortho-Cept, Reclipsen*	30 ethinyl estradiol	0.15 desogestrel
Ocella, Safyral, Syeda, *Yasmin, Zarah*		3 drospirenone
Altavera, Kurvelo, Levora, Marlissa, *Nordette*, Portia		0.15 levonorgestrel
Gildess Fe 1.5/30, 1.5/30, Junel 1.5/30, Junel 1.5/30 Fe, Larin Fe 1.5/30, *Loestrin 1.5/30, Loestrin Fe 1.5/30*, Microgestin 1.5/30, Microgestin Fe 1.5/30		1.5 norethindrone
Cryselle, Elinest, Lo/Ovral		0.3 norgestrel
Kelnor 1/35, *Zovia 1/35E*	35 ethinyl estradiol	1 ethynodiol
Balziva, Briellyn, Femcon Fe, Gildagia, *Ovcon-35*, Philith, Vyfemla, Logestrel		0.4 norethindrone
Brevicon, *Modicon*, Nortrel 0.5/35, Wera		0.5 norethindrone
Alyacen 1/35, Cyclafem 1/35, Dasetta 1/35, Necon 1/35, Norinyl 1+35, Nortrel 1/35, Norethin 1/35, *Ortho-Novum 1/35*, Pirmella 1/35		1 norethindrone
Estarylla, Mono-Linyah, *Ortho-Cyclen*, Previfem, Sprintec		0.25 norgestimate
Zovia 1/50E	50 ethinyl estradiol	1 ethynodiol
Ogestrel		0.5 norgestrel
Necon 1/50, Norinyl 1+50	50 mestranol	1 norethindrone
Progestin only		
Camila, Errin, Heather, Jencycla, Jolivette, *Micronor*, Nora BE, Nor-Q.D.	None	0.35 norethindrone
Biphasic (estrogen and progestin contents vary)		
Azurette, Kariva, *Mircette*, Pimtrea, Viorele	20/10 ethinyl estradiol	0.15 desogestrel
Triphasic (estrogen and progestin contents vary)		
Estrostep Fe, Tri-Legest, Tri-Legest Fe	20/30/35 ethinyl estradiol	1 norethindrone

(cont.)

OB/GYN 183

OB/GYN

ORAL CONTRACEPTIVES* → L CX (continued)

Caziant, Cyclessa, Velivet	25 ethinyl estradiol	0.1/0.125/0.150 desogestrel
Ortho Tri-Cyclen Lo		0.18/0.215/0.25 norgestimate
Enpresse, Levonest, Myzilra, *Trivora-28*	30/40/30 ethinyl estradiol	0.5/0.75/0.125 levonorgestrel
Alyacen 7/7/7, Cyclafem 7/7/7, Dasetta 7/7/7, Necon 7/7/7, Nortrel 7/7/7, Ortho-Novum *7/7/7*, Primella 7/7/7	35 ethinyl estradiol	0.5/0.75/1 norethindrone
Aranelle, Leena, *Tri-Norinyi*		0.5/1/0.5 norethindrone
Ortho Tri-Cyclen, Tri-Estarylla, Tri-Linyah, Tri-Previfem, Tri-Sprintec		0.18/0.215/0.25 norgestimate
Quadphasic		
Natazia	3 mg/2 mg estradiol valerate	2/3/1 dienogest
Extended Cycle		
Lybrel†	20 ethinyl estradiol	0.09 levonorgestrel
Amethyst, LoSeasonique††	20/10 ethinyl estradiol	0.1 levonorgestrel
Quartette††	20/25/30/10 ethinyl estradiol	0.15 levonorgestrel
Introvale, Quasense, *Seasonale*	30 ethinyl estradiol	
Amethia, Camrese, Daysee, Seasonique††	30/10 ethinyl estradiol	

*All: Not recommended in smokers. Increases risk of thromboembolism, CVA, MI, hepatic neoplasia, and gallbladder disease. Nausea, breast tenderness, headache and breakthrough bleeding are common transient side effects. Effectiveness reduced by hepatic enzyme-inducing drugs such as certain anticonvulsants and barbiturates, rifampin, rifabutin, griseofulvin, and protease inhibitors. Coadministration with St. John's wort may decrease efficacy. Vomiting or diarrhea may also increase the risk of contraceptive failure. Consider an additional form of birth control in above circumstances. See product insert for instructions on missing doses.

Progestin only: Must be taken at the same time every day. Because much of the literature regarding OC adverse effects pertains mainly to estrogen/progestin combinations, the extent to which progestin-only contraceptives cause these effects is unclear. No significant interaction has been found with broad-spectrum antibiotics. The effect of St. John's wort is unclear. No placebo days, start new pack immediately after finishing current one. Available in 28-day packs. Readers may find the following website useful: www.managingcontraception.com.

†Approved for continuous use without a "pill-free" period.
††84 active pills and 7 ethinyl estradiol only pills.

DRUGS GENERALLY ACCEPTED AS SAFE IN PREGNANCY (SELECTED)

Analgesics	acetaminophen, codeine*, meperidine*, methadone*, oxycodone*
Antimicrobials	azithromycin, cephalosporins, clotrimazole, erythromycins (not estolate), metronidazole, penicillins, permethrin, nitrofurantoin***, nystatin
Antivirals	acyclovir, famciclovir, valacyclovir
CV	hydralazine*, labetalol, methyldopa, nifedipine
Derm	benzoyl peroxide, clindamycin, erythromycin
Endo	insulin, levothyroxine, liothyronine
ENT	chlorpheniramine, diphenhydramine, dextromethorphan, guaifenesin, nasal steroids, nasal cromolyn
GI	antacids*, bisacodyl, cimetidine, docusate, doxylamine, famotidine, lactulose, loperamide, meclizine, metoclopramide, nizatidine, ondansetron, psyllium, ranitidine, simethicone, trimethobenzamide
Heme	Heparin, low molecular wt heparins
Psych	bupropion, buspirone, desipramine, doxepin
Pulmonary	beclomethasone, budesonide, cromolyn, montelukast, nedocromil, prednisone**, short-acting inhaled beta-2 agonists, theophylline

*Except if used long-term or in high dose at term.

**Except 1st trimester.

***Contraindicated at term and during labor and delivery.

Contraceptives—Oral Monophasic

AVIANE (ethinyl estradiol + levonorgestrel, *Falmina, Lessina, Orsythia, ✦Alesse*) [Generic/Trade: Tabs 20 mcg ethinyl estradiol/0.1 mg levonorgestrel.] ▶L ♀X▶– $$

LOESTRIN FE (ethinyl estradiol + norethindrone + ferrous fumarate, *Larin Fe 1/20, Gildess Fe 1/20, Junel Fe 1/20, Microgestin Fe 1/20*) [Generic/Trade: Tabs 1 mg norethindrone/20 mcg ethinyl estradiol with 7 days 75 mg ferrous fumarate (1/20); 1.5 mg norethindrone/30 mcg ethinyl estradiol with 7 days 75 mg ferrous fumarate (1.5/30).] ▶L ♀X▶– $$$

LOSEASONIQUE (ethinyl estradiol + levonorgestrel, *Amethia Lo, Camrese Lo*) [Generic/Trade: Tabs 20 mcg ethinyl estradiol/0.1 mg levonorgestrel. 84 orange active pills followed by 7 yellow pills with 10 mcg ethinyl estradiol.] ▶L ♀X▶– $$$

NORDETTE (ethinyl estradiol + levonorgestrel, *Altavera, Kurvelo, Levora, Marlissa, Portia, ✦Min-Ovral*) [Generic/Trade: Tabs 30 mcg ethinyl estradiol/0.15 mg levonorgestrel.] ▶L ♀X▶– $$$

NORETHINDRONE (*Micronor, Camila, Errin, Heather, Jencycla, Jolivette, Nora BE, Nor-Q.D.*) 1 tab daily. [Generic/Trade: Tabs 0.35 mg.] ▶L ♀C ▶+

ORTHO CYCLEN (ethinyl estradiol + norgestimate, *Estarylla, Mono-Linyah, Previfem, Sprintec, ✦Cyclen*) [Generic/Trade: Tabs 35 mcg ethinyl estradiol/0.25 mg norgestimate.] ▶L ♀X▶– $$

ORTHO-CEPT (ethinyl estradiol + desogestrel, *Apri, Desogen, Emoquette, Enskyce, Reclipsen, ✦Marvelon*) [Generic/Trade: Tabs 30 mcg ethinyl estradiol/0.15 mg desogestrel.] ▶L ♀X▶– $$$

ORTHO-NOVUM 1/35 (ethinyl estradiol + norethindrone, *Alyacen 1/35, Cyclafem 1/35, Dasetta 1/35, Necon 1/35, Norinyl 1+35, Nortrel 1/35, Pirmella 1/35*) [Generic/Trade: Tabs 1 mg norethindrone/35 mcg ethinyl estradiol.] ▶L ♀X▶– $$$

OVCON-35 (ethinyl estradiol + norethindrone, *Balziva, Briellyn, Gildagia, Philith, Vyfemla, Zenchent*) [Generic/Trade: Tabs 35 mcg ethinyl estradiol/0.4 mg norethindrone.] ▶L ♀X▶– $$$

SEASONALE (ethinyl estradiol + levonorgestrel, *Introvale, Quasense*) [Generic/Trade: Tabs 30 mcg ethinyl estradiol/0.15 mg levonorgestrel. 84 pink active pills followed by 7 white placebo pills.] ▶L ♀X▶– $$$

YASMIN (ethinyl estradiol + drospirenone, *Ocella, Syeda, Zarah*) [Generic/Trade: Tabs 30 mcg ethinyl estradiol/3 mg drospirenone.] ▶L ♀X▶– $$$

YAZ (ethinyl estradiol + drospirenone, *Gianvi, Loryna,, Nikki*) [Generic/Trade: Tabs 20 mcg ethinyl estradiol/3 mg drospirenone. 24 active pills are followed by 4 inert pills.] ▶L ♀X▶– $$$

Contraceptives—Oral Biphasic

MIRCETTE (ethinyl estradiol + desogestrel, *Azurette, Kariva, Pimtrea, Viorele*) [Generic/Branded generics only: Tabs 20 mcg ethinyl estradiol/0.15 mg desogestrel (21), 10 mcg ethinyl estradiol (5).] ▶L ♀X▶– $$$

Contraceptives—Oral Triphasic

ESTROSTEP FE (ethinyl estradiol + norethindrone + ferrous fumarate, *Tilia Fe-28, Tri-Legest Fe*) [Generic/Trade: Tabs 20, 30, 35 mcg ethinyl estradiol/1 mg norethindrone + "placebo" tabs with 75 mg ferrous fumarate. Packs of 28 only.] ▶L ♀X▶– $$$

ORTHO TRI-CYCLEN LO (ethinyl estradiol + norgestimate) [Generic/Trade: Tabs 25 mcg ethinyl estradiol/0.18 (7), 0.215 (7), 0.25 mg norgestimate (7).] ▶L ♀X▶– $$$

ORTHO TRI-CYCLEN (ethinyl estradiol + norgestimate, *Tri-Estarylla, Tri-Linyah, Tri-Previfem, Tri-Sprintec, ✦Tri-Cyclen*) [Generic/Trade: Tabs 35 mcg ethinyl estradiol/0.18 (7), 0.215 (7), 0.25 mg norgestimate (7).] ▶L ♀X▶– $$

ORTHO-NOVUM 7/7/7 (ethinyl estradiol + norethindrone, *Alyacen 7/7/7, Cyclafem 7/7/7, Dasetta 7/7/7, Necon 7/7/7, Nortrel 7/7/7, Pirmella 7/7/7*) [Generic/Trade: Tabs 35 mcg ethinyl estradiol/0.5, 0.75, 1 mg norethindrone.] ▶L ♀X▶– $$

TRIVORA-28 (ethinyl estradiol + levonorgestrel, *Enpresse, Levonest, Myzilra*) [Generic/Trade: Tabs 30, 40, 30 mcg ethinyl estradiol/0.05, 0.075, 0.125 mg levonorgestrel.] ▶L ♀X▶– $$

Contraceptives—Oral Four-phasic

NATAZIA (estradiol valerate and estradiol valerate + dienogest) Contraception: 1 tab PO daily, start on day 1 of menstrual cycle. Heavy menstrual bleeding: 1 tab PO daily. [Trade only: Tabs 3 mg estradiol valerate (2), 2 mg estradiol valerate/2 mg dienogest (5), 2 mg estradiol valerate/3 mg dienogest (17), 1 mg estradiol valerate (2), inert (2).] ▶L – stomach ♀X ▶– ■

Contraceptives—Other

LEVONORGESTREL—INTRAUTERINE (*Mirena*) Contraception: 1 intrauterine system q 5 years. [Trade only: Single intrauterine implant. 25 mg levonorgestrel.] ▶L – ♀X ▶+
LEVONORGESTREL—SINGLE DOSE (*Plan B One-Step, Next Choice One-Step, Fallback Solo*) Emergency contraception: 1 tab PO ASAP but within 72 h of intercourse. [OTC Trade only: Tabs 1.5 mg.] ▶L ♀X ▶– $$
NUVARING (ethinyl estradiol + etonogestrel vaginal ring) Contraception: 1 ring intravaginally for 3 weeks each month. [Trade only: Flexible intravaginal ring, 15 mcg ethinyl estradiol/0.120 mg etonogestrel/day in 1, 3 rings/box.] ▶L ♀X ▶– $$$
ORTHO EVRA (ethinyl estradiol + norelgestromin, *Xulane, ✦Evra*) Contraception: 1 patch q week for 3 weeks, then 1 week patch-free. [Trade only: Transdermal patch: 150 mcg norelgestromin/20 mcg ethinyl estradiol/day in 1, 3 patches/box.] ▶L ♀X ▶– $$$ ■

Estrogens

NOTE: *See also Hormone Combinations.*

ESTERIFIED ESTROGENS (*Menest*) 0.3 to 1.25 mg PO daily. [Trade only: Tabs 0.3, 0.625, 1.25, 2.5 mg.] ▶L ♀X ▶– $$ ■
ESTRADIOL 1 to 2 mg PO daily. [Generic only: Tabs, micronized 0.5, 1, 2 mg, scored.] ▶L ♀X ▶– $ ■
ESTRADIOL ACETATE VAGINAL RING (*Femring*) Insert and replace after 90 days. [Trade only: 0.05 mg/day and 0.1 mg/day.] ▶L ♀X ▶– $$$ ■
ESTRADIOL CYPIONATE (*Depo-Estradiol*) 1 to 5 mg IM q 3 to 4 weeks. [Trade only: Injection 5 mg/mL in 5 mL vials.] ▶L ♀X ▶– – $ ■
ESTRADIOL GEL (*Divigel, Estrogel, Elestrin*) Thinly apply contents of 1 complete pump depression to one entire arm (Estrogel) or upper arm (Elestrin) or contents of 1 foil packet (Divigel) to one upper thigh. [Trade only: Gel 0.06% in nonaerosol, metered-dose pump with #64 or #32 1.25 g doses (Estrogel), #100 0.87 g doses (Elestrin). Gel 0.1% in single-dose foil packets of 0.25, 0.5, 1.0 g, carton of 30 (Divigel).] ▶L ♀X ▶– $$$ ■
ESTRADIOL TRANSDERMAL PATCH (*Alora, Climara, Menostar, Vivelle Dot, Minivelle, ✦Estradot, Oesclim*) Apply 1 patch weekly (Climara, Estradiol, Menostar) or twice per week (Minivelle, Vivelle Dot, Alora). [Generic/Trade: Transdermal patches doses in mg/day: Climara (once a week) 0.025, 0.0375,

(cont.)

0.05, 0.06, 0.075, 0.1. Trade only: Vivelle Dot (twice per week) 0.025, 0.0375, 0.05, 0.075, 0.1. Alora (twice per week) 0.025, 0.05, 0.075, 0.1. Minivelle (twice per week) 0.0375, 0.05, 0.075, 0.1. Menostar (once a week) 0.014.] ▶L ♀X ▶– $$$ ■

ESTRADIOL TRANSDERMAL SPRAY (*Evamist*) 1 to 3 sprays daily to forearm. [Trade only: 1.53 mg estradiol per 90 mcL spray, 56 sprays per metered-dose pump.] ▶L ♀X ▶– $$$ ■

ESTRADIOL VAGINAL RING (*Estring*) Insert and replace after 90 days. [Trade only: 2 mg ring single pack.] ▶L ♀X ▶– $$$ ■

ESTRADIOL VAGINAL TAB (*Vagifem*) 1 tab vaginally daily for 2 weeks, then 1 tab vaginally two times per week. [Trade only: Vaginal tab: 10 mcg in disposable single-use applicators, 8 or 18/pack.] ▶L ♀X ▶– $$$ ■

ESTROGEN VAGINAL CREAM (*Premarin, Estrace*) Menopausal atrophic vaginitis: Premarin: 0.5 to 2 g daily. Estrace: 2 to 4 g daily for 2 weeks, then reduce. Moderate to severe menopausal dyspareunia: Premarin: 0.5 g daily, then reduce to two times per week. [Trade only: Premarin: 0.625 mg conjugated estrogens/g in 42.5 g with or without calibrated applicator. Estrace: 0.1 mg estradiol/g in 42.5 g with calibrated applicator. Generic only: Cream 0.625 mg synthetic conjugated estrogens/g in 30 g with calibrated applicator.] ▶L ♀X ▶? $$$$ ■

ESTROGENS CONJUGATED (*Premarin, C.E.S., Congest*) 0.3 to 1.25 mg PO daily. Abnormal uterine bleeding: 25 mg IV/IM. Repeat in 6 to 12 h if needed. [Trade only: Tabs 0.3, 0.45, 0.625, 0.9, 1.25 mg.] ▶L ♀X ▶– $$$ ■

GnRH Agents

NOTE: *Anaphylaxis has occurred with synthetic GnRH agents.*

GANIRELIX (+*Orgalutran*) Inhibition of premature LH surges in women undergoing controlled ovarian hyperstimulation. [Generic only: Injection 250 mcg/0.5 mL in prefilled, disposable syringe.] ▶plasma ♀X ▶? $$$$$

LUPANETA PACK (leuprolide + norethindrone) Endometriosis: Leuprolide 3.75 mg IM injection q month. Norethindrone 5 mg PO daily. [Trade only: 3.75 mg leuprolide acetate IM injection + norethindrone acetate 5 mg PO tabs #30 (1 month kit). 11.25 mg leuprolide acetate IM injection and norethindrone acetate 5 mg PO tabs #90 (3-month kit).] ▶L ♀X ▶– $$$$$

Hormone Combinations

NOTE: *See also Estrogens.*

ACTIVELLA (estradiol + norethindrone) 1 tab PO daily. [Trade only: Tabs 1/0.5 mg and 0.5/0.1 mg estradiol/norethindrone acetate in calendar dial pack dispenser.] ▶L ♀X ▶– $$$ ■

ANGELIQ (estradiol + drospirenone) 1 tab PO daily. [Trade only: Tabs 1 mg estradiol/0.5 mg drospirenone.] ▶L ♀X ▶– $$$ ■

CLIMARA PRO (estradiol + levonorgestrel) 1 patch weekly. [Trade only: Transdermal 0.045/0.015 estradiol/levonorgestrel in mg/day, 4 patches/box.] ▶L ♀X ▶– $$$ ■

COMBIPATCH (estradiol + norethindrone acetate, *✦Estalis*) 1 patch twice per week. [Trade only: Transdermal patch 0.05 estradiol/0.14 norethindrone and 0.05 estradiol/0.25 norethindrone in mg/day, 8 patches/box.] ▶L ♀X ▶– $$$ ■

DUAVEE (conjugated estrogens/bazedoxifene) 1 tab daily. [Trade only: Conjugated estrogens 0.45 mg/bazedoxifene 20 mg tabs.] ▶glucuronidation ♀X ▶– ■

PREFEST (estradiol + norgestimate) 1 pink tab PO daily for 3 days followed by 1 white tab PO daily for 3 days, sequentially throughout the month. [Generic only: Tabs in 30-day blister packs 1 mg estradiol (15 pink), 1 mg estradiol/0.09 mg norgestimate (15 white).] ▶L ♀X ▶– $$$ ■

PREMPHASE (estrogens conjugated + medroxyprogesterone) 1 tab PO daily. [Trade only: Tabs in 28-day EZ-Dial dispensers: 0.625 mg conjugated estrogens (14), 0.625 mg/5 mg conjugated estrogens/medroxyprogesterone (14).] ▶L ♀X ▶– $$$ ■

PREMPRO (estrogens conjugated + medroxyprogesterone, *✦PremPlus*) 1 tab PO daily. [Trade only: Tabs in 28-day EZ-Dial dispensers: 0.625 mg/5 mg, 0.625 mg/2.5 mg, 0.45 mg/1.5 mg (Prempro low dose), or 0.3 mg/1.5 mg conjugated estrogens/medroxyprogesterone.] ▶L ♀X ▶– $$$ ■

Labor Induction / Cervical Ripening

DINOPROSTONE (*PGE2, Prepidil, Cervidil, Prostin E2*) Cervical ripening: 1 syringe of gel placed directly into the cervical os for cervical ripening or 1 insert in the posterior fornix of the vagina. [Trade only: Gel (Prepidil) 0.5 mg/3 g syringe. Vaginal insert (Cervidil) 10 mg. Vaginal supps (Prostin E2) 20 mg.] ▶Lung ♀C ▶? $$$$$

MISOPROSTOL—OB (*PGE1, Cytotec*) Cervical ripening: 25 mcg intravaginally q 3 to 6 h (or 50 mcg q 6 h). First trimester pregnancy failure: 800 mcg intravaginally, repeat on day 3 if expulsion incomplete. Postpartum hemorrhage: 800 mcg PR. [Generic/Trade: Oral tabs 100, 200 mcg.] ▶LK ♀X ▶– $$ ■

OXYTOCIN (*Pitocin*) Labor induction: 10 units in 1000 mL NS (10 milliunits/mL), start at 6 to 12 mL/h (1 to 2 milliunits/min). Postpartum bleeding: 10 units IM or 10 to 40 units in 1000 mL NS IV, infuse 20 to 40 milliunits/min. ▶LK ♀? ▶– $

Ovulation Stimulants

NOTE: *Potentially serious adverse effects include DVT/PE, ovarian hyperstimulation syndrome, adnexal torsion, ovarian enlargement and cysts, and febrile reactions.*

CHORIOGONADOTROPIN ALFA (*Ovidrel*) Specialized dosing for ovulation induction as part of ART. [Trade only: Prefilled syringe 250 mcg.] ▶L ♀X ▶? $$$

CLOMIPHENE CITRATE (*Clomid, Serophene*) Specialized dosing. [Generic/Trade: Tabs 50 mg, scored.] ▶L ♀D ▶? $$$$$

GONADOTROPINS (menotropins, FSH and LH, *Menopur, Pergonal, Repronex*) [Trade only: Powder for injection, 75 units FSH and 75 units LH activity.] ▶L ♀X ▶– $$$$$

Progestins

MEDROXYPROGESTERONE (*Provera*) 10 mg PO daily for last 10 to 12 days of month, or 2.5 to 5 mg PO daily. Secondary amenorrhea, abnormal uterine bleeding: 5 to 10 mg PO daily for 5 to 10 days. Endometrial hyperplasia: 10 to 30 mg PO daily for 12 to 14 days per month. [Generic/Trade: Tabs 2.5, 5, 10 mg, scored.] ▶L ♀X ▶– $

MEDROXYPROGESTERONE—INJECTABLE (*Depo-Provera, Depo-SubQ Provera 104*) Contraception/endometriosis: 150 mg IM in deltoid or gluteus maximus or 104 mg SC in anterior thigh or abdomen q 13 weeks. ▶L ♀X ▶– $ ■

MEGESTROL (*Megace, Megace ES*) Endometrial hyperplasia: 40 to 160 mg PO daily for 3 to 4 months. AIDS anorexia, cachexia, or unexplained weight loss: 800 mg (20 mL) susp PO daily or 625 mg (5 mL) ES daily. [Generic/Trade: Tabs 20, 40 mg. Susp 40 mg/mL in 240 mL. Trade only: Megace ES susp 125 mg/mL (150 mL).] ▶L ♀D ▶? $$$$$

NORETHINDRONE ACETATE (*Aygestin, ✦Norlutate*) Amenorrhea, abnormal uterine bleeding: 2.5 to 10 mg PO daily for 5 to 10 days during the 2nd half of the menstrual cycle. Endometriosis: 5 mg PO daily for 2 weeks. Increase by 2.5 mg q 2 weeks to 15 mg. [Generic/Trade: Tabs 5 mg, scored.] ▶L ♀X ▶– $$

PROGESTERONE MICRONIZED (*Prometrium*) 200 mg PO at bedtime 10 to 12 days per month or 100 mg at bedtime daily. Secondary amenorrhea: 400 mg PO at bedtime for 10 days. Contraindicated in peanut allergy. [Generic/Trade: Caps 100, 200 mg.] ▶L ♀B ▶+ $$

Selective Estrogen Receptor Modulators

OSPEMIFENE (*Osphena*) Dyspareunia: 1 tab PO daily with food. [Trade only: Tabs 60 mg.] ▶L ♀X ▶– $$$$ ■

RALOXIFENE (*Evista*) Osteoporosis prevention/treatment, breast cancer prevention: 60 mg PO daily. [Generic/Trade: Tabs 60 mg.] ▶L ♀X ▶– $$$$$ ■

TAMOXIFEN (*Soltamox, Tamone, ✦Tamofen*) Breast cancer prevention: 20 mg PO daily for 5 years. Breast cancer: 10 to 20 mg PO two times per day. [Generic/Trade: Tabs 10, 20 mg. Trade only (Soltamox): Sugar-free soln 10 mg/5 mL (150 mL).] ▶L ♀D ▶– $$ ■

Uterotonics

CARBOPROST (*Hemabate*, 15-methyl-prostaglandin F2 alpha) Refractory postpartum uterine bleeding: 250 mcg deep IM. ▶LK ♀C ▶? $$$

METHYLERGONOVINE (*Methergine*) Refractory postpartum uterine bleeding: 0.2 mg IM/PO three to four times per day prn. [Trade only: Tabs 0.2 mg.] ▶LK ♀C ▶– $$

Vaginitis Preparations

NOTE: *See also STD/vaginitis table in antimicrobial section.*

BORIC ACID Resistant vulvovaginal candidiasis: 1 vaginal suppository at bedtime for 2 weeks. [No commercial preparation; must be compounded by pharmacist. Vaginal supps 600 mg in gelatin caps.] ▶Not absorbed ♀? ▶– $

CLINDAMYCIN—VAGINAL (*Cleocin, Clindesse, ✦Dalacin*) Bacterial vaginosis: Cleocin: 1 applicatorful cream at bedtime for 7 days or 1 vaginal suppository at bedtime for 3 days. Clindesse: 1 applicatorful once. [Generic/Trade: 2% vaginal cream in 40 g tube with 7 disposable applicators (Cleocin). Vaginal supp (Cleocin Ovules) 100 mg (3) with applicator. 2% vaginal cream in a single-dose prefilled applicator (Clindesse).] ▶L ♀– ▶– $$

CLOTRIMAZOLE—VAGINAL (*Mycelex 7, Gyne-Lotrimin, ✦Canesten, Clotrimaderm*) Vulvovaginal candidiasis: 1 applicatorful 1% cream at bedtime for 7 days. 1 applicatorful 2% cream at bedtime for 3 days. 1 vaginal suppository 100 mg at bedtime for 7 days. 200 mg suppository at bedtime for 3 days. [OTC Generic/Trade: 1% vaginal cream with applicator (some prefilled). 2% vaginal cream with applicator and 1% topical cream in some combination packs. OTC Trade only (Gyne-Lotrimin): Vaginal supp 100 mg (7), 200 mg (3) with applicators.] ▶LK ♀B ▶? $

METRONIDAZOLE—VAGINAL (*MetroGel-Vaginal, Nuvessa, Vandazole, ✦Nidagel*) Bacterial vaginosis: 1 applicatorful at bedtime or two times per day for 5 days. [Generic/Trade: 0.75% gel in 70 g tube with applicator (MetroGel, Vandazole). Trade only: 1.3% gel in single 5 g pre-filled applicator (Nuvessa).] ▶LK ♀B ▶? $$

MICONAZOLE (*Monistat, Femizol-M, M-Zole, Micozole, Monazole*) Vulvovaginal candidiasis: 1 applicatorful at bedtime for 3 (4%) or 7 (2%) days. 100 mg vaginal supp at bedtime for 7 days. 400 mg vaginal suppository at bedtime for 3 days. 1200 mg vaginal supp once. [OTC Generic/Trade: 2% vaginal cream in 45 g with 1 applicator or 7 disposable applicators. Vaginal supp 100 mg (7). OTC Trade only: 400 mg (3), 1200 mg (1) with applicator. Generic/Trade: 4% vaginal cream in 25 g tubes or 3 prefilled applicators. Some in combination packs with 2% miconazole cream for external use.] ▶LK ♀+ ▶? $

TERCONAZOLE (*Terazol*) Vulvovaginal candidiasis: 1 applicatorful of 0.4% cream at bedtime for 7 days, or 1 applicatorful of 0.8% cream at bedtime for 3 days, or 80 mg vaginal suppository at bedtime for 3 days. [All forms supplied with applicators: Generic/Trade: Vaginal cream 0.4% (Terazol 7) in 45 g tube, 0.8% (Terazol 3) in 20 g tube. Vaginal supp (Terazol 3) 80 mg (#3).] ▶LK ♀C ▶– $$

Other OB/GYN Agents

HYDROXYPROGESTERONE CAPROATE (*Makena*) Specialized dosing (1 mL IM weekly) to reduce risk of preterm birth. [Trade only: 5 mL MDV (250 mg/mL) hydroxyprogesterone caproate in castor oil soln.] ▶L + glucuronidation ♀B ▶? $$$$$

PREMESIS-RX (pyridoxine + folic acid + cyanocobalamin + calcium carbonate) Pregnancy-induced nausea: 1 tab PO daily. [Trade only: Tabs 75 mg vitamin B6 (pyridoxine), sustained-release, 12 mcg vitamin B12 (cyanocobalamin), 1 mg folic acid, and 200 mg calcium carbonate.] ▶L ♀A ▶+ $

RHO IMMUNE GLOBULIN (*HyperRHO S/D, MICRhoGAM, RhoGAM, Rhophylac, WinRho SDF*) Prevention of hemolytic disease of the newborn if mother Rh– and baby is or might be Rh+: 300 mcg vial IM to mother at 28 weeks' gestation followed by a 2nd dose within 72 h of delivery. Microdose (50 mcg, MICRhoGAM) is appropriate if spontaneous abortion less than 12 weeks' gestation. ▶L ♀C ▶? $$$$$

ONCOLOGY

ONCOLOGY

ONCOLOGY

ALKYLATING AGENTS: altretamine (*Hexalen*), bendamustine (*Treanda*), busulfan (*Myleran, Busulfex*), carmustine (*BCNU, BiCNU, Gliadel*), chlorambucil (*Leukeran*), cyclophosphamide (*Neosar*), dacarbazine (*DTIC-Dome*), ifosfamide (*Ifex*), lomustine/gleostine (*CeeNu, CCNU*), mechlorethamine (*Mustargen*), melphalan (*Alkeran*), procarbazine (*Matulane*), streptozocin (*Zanosar*), temozolomide (*Temodar*, ✚ *Temodal*), thiotepa (*Thioplex*). **ANTIBIOTICS:** bleomycin (*Blenoxane-Canada only*), dactinomycin (*Cosmegen*), daunorubicin (*Cerubidine*), doxorubicin liposomal (*Doxil*, ✚ *Caelyx, Myocet*), doxorubicin, non-liposomal (*Adriamycin, Rubex*), epirubicin (*Ellence*, ✚ *Pharmorubicin*), idarubicin (*Idamycin*), mitomycin (*Mutamycin, Mitomycin-C*), mitoxantrone (*Novantrone*), valrubicin (*Valstar*, ✚ *Valtaxin*). **ANTIMETABOLITES:** azacitidine (*Vidaza*), capecitabine (*Xeloda*), cladribine (*Leustatin, chlorodeoxyadenosine*), clofarabine (*Clolar*), cytarabine (*Cytosar, AraC*), cytarabine liposomal (*Depo-Cyt*),decitabine (*Dacogen*), floxuridine (*FUDR*), fludarabine (*Fludara*), fluorouracil (*Adrucil, 5-FU*), gemcitabine (*Gemzar*), hydroxyurea (*Hydrea, Droxia*), mercaptopurine (*6-MP, Purinethol*), methotrexate, nelarabine (*Arranon*), pemetrexed (*Alimta*), pentostatin (*Nipent*), Pralatrexate (*Folotyn*), thioguanine (*Tabloid*, ✚ *Lanvis*). **CYTOPROTECTIVE AGENTS:** amifostine (*Ethyol*), dexrazoxane (*Zinecard, Totect*), mesna (*Mesnex*, ✚ *Uromitexan*), palifermin (*Kepivance*). **HORMONES:** anastrozole (*Arimidex*), bicalutamide (*Casodex*), cyproterone, (k *Androcur, Androcur Depot*), degarelix (*Firmagon*), estramustine (*Emcyt*), exemestane (*Aromasin*), flutamide (*Eulexin*, ✚ *Euflex*), fulvestrant (*Faslodex*), goserelin (*Zoladex*), histrelin (*Vantas, Supprelin LA*), letrozole (*Femara*), leuprolide (*Eligard, Lupron, Lupron Depot, Lupron Depot-Ped*), nilutamide (*Nilandron*),raloxifene (*Evista*) toremifene (*Fareston*), triptorelin (*Trelstar Depot*). **IMMUNOMODULATORS:** aldesleukin (*Proleukin, interleukin-2*), ✚ BCG (*Bacillus of Calmette & Guerin, Pacis, TheraCys, Tice BCG*, ✚ *Oncotice*, ✚ *Immucyst*), denileukin (*Ontak*), everolimus (*Afinitor*), interferon alfa-2b (*Intron-A*), lenalidomide (*Revlimid*), temsirolimus (*Torisel*), thalidomide (*Thalomid*). **MITOTIC INHIBITORS:** cabazitaxel (*Jevtana*), docetaxel (*Taxotere*), ixabepilone (*Ixempra*), paclitaxel (*Taxol, Abraxane, Onxol*), vinblastine (*Velban, VLB*), vincristine (*Oncovin, Vincasar, VCR*), vinorelbine (*Navelbine*). **MONOCLONAL ANTIBODIES:** alemtuzumab (Campath, ✚ *MabCampath*), bevacizumab (*Avastin*), cetuximab (*Erbitux*), ibritumomab (*Zevalin*), ofatumumab (*Arzerra*), panitumumab (*Vectibix*), rituximab (*Rituxan*), trastuzumab (*Herceptin*). **PLATINUM-CONTAINING AGENTS:** carboplatin (*Paraplatin*), cisplatin (*Platinol-AQ*), oxaliplatin (*Eloxatin*). **RADIOPHARMACEUTICALS:** samarium 153 (*Quadramet*), strontium-89 (*Metastron*). **TOPOISOMERASE INHIBITORS:** etoposide (*VP-16, Etopophos, Toposar, VePesid*), teniposide (*Vumon, VM-26*), topotecan (*Hycamtin*) **TYROSINE KINASE INHIBITORS:** dasatinib (*Sprycel*), erlotinib (*Tarceva*) gefitinib (*Iressa*), imatinib (*Gleevec*), lapatinib (*Tykerb*), nilotinib (*Tasigna*), pazopanib (*Votrient*), sorafenib (*Nexavar*), sunitinib (*Sutent*). **MISCELLANEOUS:** arsenic

(cont.)

ONCOLOGY (*continued*)

ONCOLOGY
trioxide (*Trisenox*), asparaginase (*Elspar*, ♦ *Kidrolase*), bexarotene (*Targretin*), bortezomib (*Velcade*), leucovorin, *(folinic acid)*, levoleucovorin (*Fusilev*), mitotane (*Lysodren*), pegaspargase (*Oncaspar*), porfimer (*Photofrin*), rasburicase (*Elitek*), romidepsin (*Istodax*), tretinoin (*Vesanoid*), vorinostat (*Zolinza*).

OPHTHALMOLOGY

Antiallergy—Decongestants & Combinations

NOTE: *Most eye medications can be administered 1 gtt at a time despite common manufacturer recommendations of 1 to 2 gtts concurrently. Even a single gtt is typically more than the eye can hold, and thus a second gtt is wasteful and increases the possibility of systemic toxicity. If 2 gtts of the medication are desired, separate single gtt by at least 5 min.*

NAPHAZOLINE (*Albalon, All Clear, Naphcon, Clear Eyes*) 1 to 2 gtts in each affected eye four times per day for up to 3 days. [OTC Generic/Trade: Soln 0.012, 0.025% (15, 30 mL). Rx Generic/Trade: 0.1% (15 mL).] ▶? ♀C ▶? $

NAPHCON-A (**naphazoline + pheniramine**) 1 gtt in each affected eye four times per day prn for up to 3 days. [OTC Trade only: Soln 0.025% + 0.3% (15 mL).] ▶L ♀C ▶? $

VASOCON-A (**naphazoline + antazoline**) 1 gtt in each affected eye four times per day prn for up to 3 days. [OTC Trade only: Soln 0.05% + 0.5% (15 mL).] ▶L ♀C ▶? $

Antiallergy—Dual Antihistamine & Mast Cell Stabilizer

AZELASTINE—OPHTHALMIC (*Optivar*) 1 gtt in each affected eye two times per day. [Trade/generic: Soln 0.05% (6 mL).] ▶L ♀C ▶? $$$

EPINASTINE (*Elestat*) 1 gtt in each affected eye two times per day. [Trade only: Soln 0.05% (5 mL).] ▶K ♀C ▶? $$$$

KETOTIFEN—OPHTHALMIC (*Alaway, Zaditor*) 1 gtt in each affected eye q 8 to 12 h. [OTC Generic/Trade: Soln 0.025% (5 mL, 10 mL).] ▶minimal absorption ♀C ▶? $

OLOPATADINE—OPHTHALMIC (*Pataday, Patanol*) 1 gtt of 0.1% soln in each affected eye two times per day (Patanol) or 1 gtt of 0.2% soln in each affected eye daily (Pataday). [Trade only: Soln 0.1% (5 mL, Patanol), 0.2% (2.5 mL, Pataday).] ▶K ♀C ▶? $$$$

Antiallergy—Pure Antihistamines

ALCAFTADINE (*Lastacaft*) 1gtt in each eye daily. [Trade: Soln 0.25%, 3 mL.] ▶not absorbed ♀B ▶? $$$

BEPOTASTINE (*Bepreve*) 1 gtt in each affected eye two times per day. [Trade only: Soln 1.5% (2.5, 5, 10 mL).] ▶L (but minimal absorption) – ♀C ▶? $$$

EMEDASTINE (*Emadine*) 1 gtt in each affected eye daily to four times per day. [Trade only: Soln 0.05% (5 mL).] ▶L ♀B ▶? $$$

Antiallergy—Pure Mast Cell Stabilizers

OLOPATADINE (*Pazeo*) 1 gtt in each affected eye once a day. [Trade only: Soln 0.7% (4 mL).] ▶minimal absorption ♀? ▶? $$$

CROMOLYN—OPHTHALMIC (*Crolom, Opticrom*) 1 to 2 gtts in each affected eye 4 to 6 times per day. [Generic/Trade: Soln 4% (10 mL).] ▶LK ♀B ▶? $$

LODOXAMIDE (*Alomide*) 1 to 2 gtts in each affected eye four times per day. [Trade only: Soln 0.1% (10 mL).] ▶K ♀B ▷? $$$

NEDOCROMIL—OPHTHALMIC (*Alocril*) 1 to 2 gtts in each affected eye two times per day. [Trade only: Soln 2% (5 mL).] ▶L ♀B ▷? $$$

Antibacterials—Aminoglycosides

GENTAMICIN—OPHTHALMIC (*Garamycin, Genoptic, Gentak, ✦Diogent*) 1 to 2 gtts in each affected eye q 2 to 4 h; ½ inch ribbon of ointment two to three times per day. [Generic/Trade: Soln 0.3% (5, 15 mL). Oint 0.3% (3.5 g tube).] ▶K ♀C ▷? $

TOBRAMYCIN—OPHTHALMIC (*Tobrex*) 1 to 2 gtts in each affected eye q 1 to 4 h or ½ inch ribbon of ointment q 3 to 4 h or two or three times per day. [Generic/Trade: Soln 0.3% (5 mL). Trade only: Oint 0.3% (3.5 g tube).] ▶K ♀B ▷– $

Antibacterials—Fluoroquinolones

BESIFLOXACIN (*Besivance*) 1 gtt in each affected eye three times per day for 7 days. [Trade: Soln 0.6% (5 mL).] ▶LK ♀C ▷? $$$

CIPROFLOXACIN—OPHTHALMIC (*Ciloxan*) 1 to 2 gtts in each affected eye q 1 to 6 h or ½ inch ribbon ointment two to three times per day. [Generic/Trade: Soln 0.3% (2.5, 5, 10 mL). Trade only: Oint 0.3% (3.5 g tube).] ▶LK ♀C ▷? $$

LEVOFLOXACIN—OPHTHALMIC (*Iquix, Quixin*) Quixin: 1 to 2 gtts in each affected eye q 2 h while awake (up to 8 times per day) on days 1 and 2, then 1 to 2 gtts q 4 h (up to four times per day) on days 3 to 7. Iquix: 1 to 2 gtts q 30 min to 2 h while awake and q 4 to 6 h overnight on days 1 to 3, then 1 to 2 gtts q 1 to 4 h while awake on day 4 to completion of therapy. [Trade/Generic: Soln 0.5% (5 mL).] ▶KL ♀C ▷? $$$

MOXIFLOXACIN—OPHTHALMIC (*Vigamox, Moxeza*) 1 gtt in each affected eye three times per day for 7 days (Vigamox) or 1 gtt in each affected eye two times per day for 7 days (Moxeza). [Trade only: Soln 0.5% (3 mL, Vigamox and Moxeza).] ▶LK ♀C ▷? $$$

OFLOXACIN—OPHTHALMIC (*Ocuflox*) 1 to 2 gtts in each affected eye q 1 to 6 h for 7 to 10 days. [Generic/Trade: Soln 0.3% (5, 10 mL).] ▶LK ♀C ▷? $$

Antibacterials—Other

AZITHROMYCIN—OPHTHALMIC (*AzaSite*) 1 gtt in each affected eye two times per day for 2 days, then 1 gtt once daily for 5 more days. [Trade only: Soln 1% (2.5 mL).] ▶L ♀B ▷? $$$

BACITRACIN—OPHTHALMIC (*AK Tracin*) ¼ to ½ inch ribbon of ointment in each affected eye q 3 to 4 h or two to four times per day for 7 to 10 days. [Generic/Trade: Oint 500 units/g (3.5 g tube).] ▶minimal absorption ♀C ▷? $

ERYTHROMYCIN—OPHTHALMIC (*Ilotycin, AK-Mycin*) ½ inch ribbon of ointment in each affected eye q 3 to 4 h or two to six times per day. [Generic only: Oint 0.5% (1, 3.5 g tube).] ▶L ♀B ▷+ $

FUSIDIC ACID—OPHTHALMIC (*✦Fucithalmic*) 1 gtt in both eyes twice daily for 7 days. [Canada trade only: gtts 1%. Multidose tubes of 3, 5 g. Single-dose, preservative-free tubes of 0.2 g in a box of 12.] ▶L ♀? ▷? $

NEOSPORIN OINTMENT—OPHTHALMIC (neomycin—ophthalmic + bacitracin—ophthalmic + polymyxin—ophthalmic) ½ inch ribbon of ointment in each affected eye q 3 to 4 h for 7 to 10 days or 1 inch ribbon two to three times per day for mild to moderate infection. [Generic only: Oint. (3.5 g tube).] ▶KL ♀C ▶? $

NEOSPORIN SOLUTION—OPHTHALMIC (neomycin—ophthalmic + polymyxin—ophthalmic + gramicidin) 1 to 2 gtts in each affected eye q 4 to 6 h for 7 to 10 days. [Generic/Trade: Soln (10 mL).] ▶KL ♀C ▶? $$

POLYSPORIN—OPHTHALMIC (polymyxin—ophthalmic + bacitracin—ophthalmic) ½ inch ribbon of ointment in each affected eye q 3 to 4 h for 7 to 10 days or ½ inch ribbon two to three times per day for mild to moderate infection. [Generic only: Oint (3.5 g tube).] ▶K ♀C ▶? $$

POLYTRIM—OPHTHALMIC (polymyxin—ophthalmic + trimethoprim—ophthalmic) 1 to 2 gtts in each affected eye q 4 to 6 h (up to 6 gtts per day) for 7 to 10 days. [Generic/Trade: Soln (10 mL).] ▶KL ♀C ▶? $$$$

SULFACETAMIDE—OPHTHALMIC (*Bleph-10, Sulf-10*) 1 to 2 gtts in each affected eye q 2 to 6 h for 7 to 10 days or ½ inch ribbon of ointment q 3 to 8 h for 7 to 10 days. [Generic/Trade: Soln 10% (15 mL), Oint 10% (3.5 g tube). Generic only: Soln 30% (15 mL).] ▶K ♀C ▶– $

Antiviral Agents

GANCICLOVIR—OPHTHALMIC (*Zirgan*) Herpetic keratitis: 1 gtt five times per day (approximately q 3 h) until ulcer heals, then 1 gtt 3 times per day for 7 days. [Trade only: Gel 0.15% (5g).] ▶minimal absorption ♀C ▶? $$$

TRIFLURIDINE (*Viroptic*) Herpetic keratitis: 1 gtt q 2 to 4 h for 7 to 14 days, max 9 gtts per day and max of 21 days of therapy. [Generic/Trade: Soln 1% (7.5 mL).] ▶minimal absorption ♀C ▶– $$$

Corticosteroid & Antibacterial Combinations

NOTE: *Recommend that only ophthalmologists or optometrists prescribe due to infection, cataract, corneal/scleral perforation, and glaucoma risk from prolonged use. Monitor intraocular pressure.*

BLEPHAMIDE (prednisolone—ophthalmic + sulfacetamide—ophthalmic) 2 gtts in each affected eye q 4 h and at bedtime or ½ inch ribbon to lower conjunctival sac 3 to 4 times per day and at bedtime. [Generic/Trade: Soln/Susp (5, 10 mL). Trade only: Oint (3.5 g tube).] ▶KL ♀C ▶? $

CORTISPORIN—OPHTHALMIC (neomycin—ophthalmic + polymyxin—ophthalmic + hydrocortisone—ophthalmic) 1 to 2 gtts or ½ inch ribbon of ointment in each affected eye q 3 to 4 h or more frequently prn. [Generic only: Susp (7.5 mL). Oint (3.5 g tube).] ▶LK ♀C ▶? $$

FML-S LIQUIFILM (prednisolone—ophthalmic + sulfacetamide—ophthalmic) 1 to 2 gtts in each affected eye q 1 to 8 h. [Trade only: Susp (10 mL).] ▶KL ♀C ▶? $$

MAXITROI (dexamethasone—ophthalmic + neomycin—ophthalmic + polymyxin—ophthalmic) Small amount (about ½ inch) ointment in affected eye

(cont.)

three to four times per day or at bedtime as an adjunct with gtts. 1 to 2 gtts susp into affected eye four to six times daily; in severe disease, gtts may be used hourly and tapered to discontinuation. [Generic/Trade: Susp (5 mL). Oint (3.5 g tube).] ▶KL ♀C ▶? $

PRED G (prednisolone—ophthalmic + gentamicin—ophthalmic) 1 to 2 gtts in each affected eye two to four times per day during and ½ inch ribbon of ointment one to three times per day. [Trade only: Susp (2, 5, 10 mL). Oint (3.5 g tube).] ▶KL ♀C ▶? $$

TOBRADEX (tobramycin—ophthalmic + dexamethasone—ophthalmic) 1 to 2 gtts in each affected eye q 2 to 6 h or ½ inch ribbon of ointment three to four times per day. [Trade/generic: Susp (tobramycin 0.3%/dexamethasone 0.1%, 2.5, 5, 10 mL). Trade: Oint (tobramycin 0.3%/dexamethasone 0.1%, 3.5 g tube).] ▶L ♀C ▶? $$$

TOBRADEX ST (tobramycin—ophthalmic + dexamethasone—ophthalmic) 1 gtt in each affected eye q 2 to 6 h. [Trade only: Tobramycin 0.3%/dexamethasone 0.05% susp (2.5, 5, 10 mL).] ▶L ♀C ▶? $$$

VASOCIDIN (prednisolone—ophthalmic + sulfacetamide—ophthalmic) 1 to 2 gtts in each affected eye q 1 to 8 h or ½ inch ribbon of ointment one to four times per day. [Generic only: Soln (5, 10 mL).] ▶KL ♀C ▶? $

ZYLET (loteprednol + tobramycin—ophthalmic) 1 to 2 gtts in each affected eye q 1 to 2 h for 1 to 2 days then 1 to 2 gtts q 4 to 6 h. [Trade only: Susp 0.5% loteprednol + 0.3% tobramycin (2.5, 5, 10 mL).] ▶LK ♀C ▶? $$$

Corticosteroids

NOTE: *Recommend that only ophthalmologists or optometrists prescribe due to infection, cataract, corneal/scleral perforation, and glaucoma risk from prolonged use. Monitor intraocular pressure.*

DIFLUPREDNATE (*Durezol*) Inflammation and pain associated with ocular surgery: 1 gtt in each affected eye four times per day, beginning 24 h after surgery for 2 weeks, then 1 gtt in each affected eye two times per day for 1 week, then taper based on response. Endogenous anterior uveitis: 1 gtt in each affected eye four times daily for 14 days followed by tapering as indicated. [Trade only: Ophthalmic emulsion 0.05% (2.5, 5 mL).] ▶not absorbed ♀C ▶? $$$$

FLUOROMETHOLONE (*FML, FML Forte, Flarex*) 1 to 2 gtts in each affected eye q 1 to 12 h or ½ inch ribbon of ointment q 4 to 24 h. [Trade only: Susp 0.1% (5, 10, 15 mL), 0.25% (2, 5, 10, 15 mL). Oint 0.1% (3.5 g tube).] ▶L ♀C ▶? $$

LOTEPREDNOL (*Alrex, Lotemax*) 1 to 2 gtts in each affected eye four times per day or ½ inch ointment four times daily beginning 24 h after surgery. [Trade only: Susp 0.2% (Alrex 5, 10 mL), 0.5% (Lotemax 2.5, 5, 10, 15 mL). Oint 0.5% 3.5 g, Gel drop 0.5% (Lotemax 10 mL).] ▶L ♀C ▶? $$$

PREDNISOLONE—OPHTHALMIC (*Pred Forte, Pred Mild, Inflamase Forte, Econopred Plus*) Soln: 1 to 2 gtts in each affected eye (up to q 1 h during day and q 2 h at night); when response observed, then 1 gtt in each affected eye q 4 h, then 1 gtt three to four times per day. Susp: 1 to 2 gtts in each affected

(cont.)

eye two to four times per day. [Generic/Trade: Soln, Susp 1% (5, 10, 15 mL). Trade only (Pred Mild): Susp 0.12% (5, 10 mL), Susp (Pred Forte) 1% (1 mL).] ▶L ♀C ▶? $$

RIMEXOLONE (*Vexol*) 1 to 2 gtts in each affected eye q 1 to 6 h. [Trade only: Susp 1% (5, 10 mL).] ▶L ♀C ▶? $$

Glaucoma Agents—Beta-Blockers

NOTE: *Use caution in cardiac conditions and asthma.*

BETAXOLOL—OPHTHALMIC (*Betoptic, Betoptic S*) 1 to 2 gtts in each affected eye two times per day. [Trade only: Susp 0.25% (10, 15 mL). Generic only: Soln 0.5% (5, 10, 15 mL).] ▶LK ♀C ▶? $$

CARTEOLOL—OPHTHALMIC (*Ocupress*) 1 gtt in each affected eye two times per day. [Generic only: Soln 1% (5, 10, 15 mL).] ▶KL ♀C ▶? $

LEVOBUNOLOL (*Betagan*) 1 to 2 gtts in each affected eye one to two times per day. [Generic/Trade: Soln 0.25% (5, 10 mL), 0.5% (5, 10, 15 mL).] ▶? ♀C ▶– $$

METIPRANOLOL (*Optipranolol*) 1 gtt in each affected eye two times per day. [Generic/Trade: Soln 0.3% (5, 10 mL).] ▶? ♀C ▶? $

TIMOLOL—OPHTHALMIC (*Betimol, Timoptic, Timoptic XE, Istalol, Timoptic Ocudose*) 1 gtt in each affected eye two times per day. Timoptic XE, Istalol: 1 gtt in each affected eye daily. [Generic/Trade: Soln 0.25, 0.5% (5, 10, 15 mL). Preservative-free soln (Timoptic Ocudose) 0.25% (0.2 mL). Gel-forming soln (Timoptic XE) 0.25, 0.5% (5 mL).] ▶LK ♀C ▶+ $$

Glaucoma Agents—Carbonic Anhydrase Inhibitors

NOTE: *Sulfonamide derivatives; verify absence of sulfa allergy before prescribing.*

ACETAZOLAMIDE (*Diamox, Diamox Sequels*) Glaucoma: 250 mg PO up to four times per day (immediate-release) or 500 mg PO up to two times per day (sustained-release). Max 1 g/day. Acute glaucoma: 250 mg IV q 4 h or 500 mg IV initially with 125 to 250 mg q 4 h, followed by oral therapy. Mountain sickness prophylaxis: 125 to 250 mg PO two to three times per day, beginning 1 to 2 days prior to ascent and continuing at least 5 days at higher altitude. Edema: Rarely used, start 250 to 375 mg IV/PO q am given intermittently (every other day or 2 consecutive days followed by none for 1 to 2 days) to avoid loss of diuretic effect. Urinary alkalinization: 5 mg/kg IV, may repeat two or three times daily prn to maintain an alkaline diuresis. [Generic only: Tabs 125, 250 mg. Generic/Trade: Caps extended-release 500 mg.] ▶LK ♀C ▶+ $$

BRINZOLAMIDE (*Azopt*) 1 gtt in each affected eye three times per day. [Trade only: Susp 1% (10, 15 mL).] ▶LK ♀C ▶? $$$

DORZOLAMIDE (*Trusopt*) 1 gtt in each affected eye three times per day. [Generic/Trade: Soln 2% (10 mL).] ▶KL ♀C ▶– $$$

METHAZOLAMIDE 25 to 50 mg PO daily (up to three times per day). [Generic only: Tabs 25, 50 mg.] ▶LK ♀C ▶? $$

Glaucoma Agents—Combinations and Other

COMBIGAN (*brimonidine + timolol—ophthalmic*) 1 gtt in each affected eye twice a day. Contraindicated in children younger than 2 yo. [Trade only: Soln brimonidine 0.2% + timolol 0.5% (5, 10 mL).] ▶LK ♀C ▶– $$$

COSOPT (*dorzolamide + timolol—ophthalmic*) 1 gtt in each affected eye two times per day. [Generic/Trade: Soln dorzolamide 2% + timolol 0.5% (5, 10 mL). Trade only: Soln, preservative-free dorzolamide 2% + timolol 0.5% (30 single use containers).] ▶LK ♀D ▶– $$$

SIMBRINZA (*brinzolamide + brimonidine*) 1 gtt in each affected eye three times per day. [Trade: brinzolamide 1% and brimonidine 0.2% 8 mL.] ▶LK – ♀C ▶? $$$$

Glaucoma Agents—Miotics

CARBACHOL (*Isopto Carbachol, Miostat*) [Trade only: Soln (Isopto Carbachol) 1.5, 3% (15 mL). Intraocular soln (Miostat) 0.01%.] ▶? ♀C ▶? $$

PILOCARPINE—OPHTHALMIC (*Isopto Carpine, ✦Diocarpine, Akarpine*) 1 gtt in each affected eye up to four times per day. [Generic/Trade: Soln 0.5% (15 mL), 1% (2 mL, 15 mL), 2% (2 mL, 15 mL), 4% (2 mL, 15 mL), 6% (15 mL).] ▶plasma ♀C ▶? $

Glaucoma Agents—Prostaglandin Analogs

BIMATOPROST (*Lumigan, Latisse*) Glaucoma (Lumigan): 1 gtt in each affected eye at bedtime. Hypotrichosis of the eyelashes (Latisse): 1 gtt to eyelashes at bedtime. [Generic only: Soln 0.03% 2.5, 5, 7.5 mL. Trade only: Soln 0.01% (Lumigan), 2.5, 5, 7.5 mL. Soln 0.03%(Latisse) 3 mL with 70 disposable applicators, 5 mL with 140 disposable applicators.] ▶LK ♀C ▶? $$$$

LATANOPROST (*Xalatan*) 1 gtt in each affected eye at bedtime. [Generic/Trade: Soln 0.005% (2.5 mL).] ▶LK ♀C ▶? $

TAFLUPROST (*Zioptan*) 1 gtt in each affected eye q pm. [Trade: Soln 0.0015%] ▶L ♀C ▶? $$$

TRAVOPROST (*Travatan Z*) 1 gtt in each affected eye at bedtime. [Trade only: Benzalkonium chloride-free (Travatan Z) 0.004% (2.5, 5 mL). Generic only: Travoprost 0.004% (2.5 mL, 5 mL).] ▶L ♀C ▶? $$$$

Glaucoma Agents—Sympathomimetics

NOTE: *Do not administer while wearing soft contact lenses. Wait 10 min after use before inserting contact lenses. On average, each mL of eye drop soln contains approximately 20 gtts. Reserve ointment formulations for bedtime use due to severe vision blurring. Most eye medications can be administered 1 gtt at a time despite common manufacturer recommendations of 1 to 2 gtts concurrently. Even a single gtt is typically more than the eye can hold and thus a second gtt is both wasteful and increases the possibility of systemic toxicity. If 2 gtts of the medication are desired, separate single gtts by at least 5 min.*

BRIMONIDINE (*Alphagan P, ✦Alphagan*) 1 gtt in each affected eye three times per day. [Trade only: Soln 0.1% (5, 10, 15 mL). Generic/Trade: Soln 0.15% (5, 10, 15 mL). Generic only: Soln 0.2% (5, 10, 15 mL).] ▶L ♀B ▶? $$

Mydriatics & Cycloplegics

ATROPINE—OPHTHALMIC (*Isopto Atropine, Atropine Care*) 1 to 2 gtts in each affected eye before procedure or daily to four times per day or 1/8 to 1/4 inch ointment before procedure or one to three times per day. Cycloplegia may last up to 5 to 10 days and mydriasis may last up to 7 to 14 days. [Generic/Trade: Soln 1% (2, 5, 15 mL). Generic only: Oint 1% (3.5 g tube).] ▶L ♀C ▶+ $

CYCLOPENTOLATE (*AK-Pentolate, Cyclogyl, Pentolair*) 1 to 2 gtts in each affected eye for 1 to 2 doses before procedure. Cycloplegia may last 6 to 24 h; mydriasis may last 1 day. [Generic/Trade: Soln 1% (2, 15 mL). Trade only (Cyclogyl): 0.5% (15 mL), 1% (5 mL), 2% (2, 5, 15 mL).] ▶? ♀C ▶? $

HOMATROPINE—OPHTHALMIC (*Isopto Homatropine*) 1 to 2 gtts in each affected eye before procedure or two to three times per day. Cycloplegia and mydriasis last 1 to 3 days. [Trade only: Soln 2% (5 mL), 5% (5 mL). Generic/Trade: Soln 5% (5 mL).] ▶? ♀C ▶? $

PHENYLEPHRINE—OPHTHALMIC 1 to 2 gtts in each affected eye before procedure or three to four times per day. No cycloplegia; mydriasis may last up to 5 h. Red eyes: 1 or 2 gtts (0.12%) in each affected eye up to four times daily. [Rx Generic: Soln 2.5% (2, 3, 5, 15 mL), 10% (5 mL).] ▶plasma L ♀C ▶? $

TROPICAMIDE (*Mydriacyl, Tropicacyl*) 1 to 2 gtts in each affected eye before procedure. Mydriasis may last 6 h. [Generic/Trade: Soln 0.5% (15 mL), 1% (3, 15 mL). Generic only: Soln 1% (2 mL).] ▶? ♀C ▶? $

Non-Steroidal Anti-Inflammatories

BROMFENAC—OPHTHALMIC (*Bromday, Prolensa*) 1 gtt in each affected eye once daily beginning 1 day prior to surgery and continuing for 14 days after surgery (Bromday, Prolensa) or twice daily (generic). [Trade only: Soln 0.09% (Bromday) 1.7 mL, 3.4 mL (two 1.7-mL twin packs). Soln 0.07% (Prolensa) 1.6, 3 mL. Generic only: Soln 0.09% (twice-daily soln 2.5 mL, 5 mL)] ▶minimal absorption ♀C, D (3rd trimester) ▶? $$$$$

DICLOFENAC—OPHTHALMIC (*Voltaren, ✦Voltaren Ophtha*) 1 gtt in each affected eye one to four times per day. [Generic/Trade: Soln 0.1% (2.5, 5 mL).] ▶L ♀C ▶? $$$

FLURBIPROFEN—OPHTHALMIC (*Ocufen*) Inhibition of intraoperative miosis: 1 gtt q 30 min beginning 2 h prior to surgery (total of 4 gtts). [Generic/Trade: Soln 0.03% (2.5 mL).] ▶L ♀C ▶? $

KETOROLAC—OPHTHALMIC (*Acular, Acular LS, Acuvail*) 1 gtt in each affected eye four times per day (Acular, Acular LS). 1 gtt in each affected eye twice daily (Acuvail). [Generic/Trade: Soln (Acular LS) 0.4% (5 mL). Trade only: Acular 0.5% (3, 5, 10 mL), preservative-free Acuvail 0.45% unit dose (0.4 mL).] ▶L ♀C ▶? $$$$

NEPAFENAC (*Nevanac, Ilevro*) 1 gtt in each affected eye three times per day for 2 weeks. [Trade only: Susp 0.1% (Nevanac-3 mL). Susp 0.3% (Ilevro-1.7 mL).] ▶minimal absorption ♀C C, D in 3rd trimester ▶? $$$$

Other Ophthalmologic Agents

AFLIBERCEPT (*Eylea*) Wet macular degeneration, macular edema after central retinal vein occlusion, diabetic retinopathy with diabetic macular edema, macular edema following retinal vein occlusion: 2 mg (0.05 mL) intravitreal injection, frequency varies by indication. [Sterile powder for reconstitution.] ▶minimal absorption ♀C ▶– $$$$$

ARTIFICIAL TEARS (*Tears Naturale, Hypotears, Refresh Tears, GenTeal, Systane*) 1 to 2 gtts prn. [OTC Generic/Trade: Soln (15, 30 mL, among others).] ▶minimal absorption ♀A ▶+ $

CYCLOSPORINE—OPHTHALMIC (*Restasis*) 1 gtt in each eye q 12 h. [Trade only: Emulsion 0.05% (0.4 mL single-use vials).] ▶minimal absorption ♀C ▶? $$$$

HYDROXYPROPYL CELLULOSE (*Lacrisert*) Moderate to severe dry eyes: 1 insert in each eye daily. Some patients may require twice-daily use. [Trade only: Ocular insert 5 mg.] ▶minimal absorption ♀+ ▶+ $$$

LIDOCAINE—OPHTHALMIC Do not prescribe for unsupervised or prolonged use. Corneal toxicity and ocular infections may occur with repeated use. 2 gtts before procedure, repeat prn. [Generic only: Gel 3.5% (5 mL).] ▶L ♀B ▶? $

PETROLATUM (*Lacri-lube, Dry Eyes, Refresh PM, ✦DuoLube*) Apply ¼ to ½ inch ointment to inside of lower lid prn. [OTC Trade only: Oint (3.5, 7 g) tube.] ▶minimal absorption ♀A ▶+ $

PROPARACAINE (*Ophthaine, Ophthetic, ✦Alcaine*) Do not prescribe for unsupervised or prolonged use. Corneal toxicity and ocular infections may occur with repeated use. 1 to 2 gtts into affected eye before procedure. [Generic/Trade: Soln 0.5% (15 mL).] ▶L ♀C ▶? $

TETRACAINE—OPHTHALMIC (*Pontocaine*) Do not prescribe for unsupervised or prolonged use. Corneal toxicity and ocular infections may occur with repeated use. 1 to 2 gtts in each affected eye before procedure. [Generic only: Soln 0.5% (15 mL), unit-dose vials (0.7, 2 mL).] ▶plasma ♀C ▶? $

PSYCHIATRY

BODY MASS INDEX

BMI	Class	4' 10"	5' 0"	5' 4"	5' 8"	6' 0"	6' 4"
< 19	Underweight	< 91	< 97	< 110	< 125	< 140	< 156
19–24	Healthy weight	91–119	97–127	110–144	125–163	140–183	156–204
25–29	Overweight	120–143	128–152	145–173	164–196	184–220	205–245
30–40	Obese	144–191	153–204	174–233	197–262	221–293	246–328
> 40	Very Obese	> 191	> 204	174–233	> 262	> 293	> 328

*BMI = kg/m^2 = (wt in pounds)(703)/(height in inches)^2. Anorectants appropriate if BMI ≥30 (with comorbidities ≥27); surgery an option if BMI > 40 (with comorbidities 35–40). www.nhlbi.nih.gov

Antidepressants—Heterocyclic Compounds

NOTE: *Gradually taper when discontinuing cyclic antidepressants to avoid withdrawal symptoms. Seizures, orthostatic hypotension, arrhythmias, and anticholinergic side effects may occur. Don't use with MAOIs. Antidepressants increase the risk of suicidal thinking and behavior in children, adolescents, and young adults; carefully weigh the risks and benefits before starting and monitor patients closely. Use of serotonergic drugs in late third trimester of pregnancy can lead to prolonged hospitalizations, need for respiratory support, and tube feeding.*

AMITRIPTYLINE Start 25 to 100 mg PO at bedtime; gradually increase to usual effective dose of 50 to 300 mg/day. Primarily inhibits serotonin reuptake. Demethylated to nortriptyline, which primarily inhibits norepinephrine reuptake. Suicidality. [Generic: Tabs 10, 25, 50, 75, 100, 150 mg. Elavil brand name no longer available.] ▶L ♀D ▶– $$ ■

CLOMIPRAMINE (*Anafranil*) Start 25 mg PO at bedtime; gradually increase to usual effective dose of 150 to 250 mg/day. Max 250 mg/day. Primarily inhibits serotonin reuptake. Suicidality. [Generic/Trade: Caps 25, 50, 75 mg.] ▶L ♀C ▶+ $$$ ■

DESIPRAMINE (*Norpramin*) Start 25 to 100 mg PO given once daily or in divided doses. Gradually increase to usual effective dose of 100 to 200 mg/day, max 300 mg/day. Primarily inhibits norepinephrine reuptake. Suicidality. [Generic/Trade: Tabs 10, 25, 50, 75, 100, 150 mg.] ▶L ♀C ▶– $$ ■

DOXEPIN (*Silenor*) Depression: Start 75 mg PO at bedtime. Gradually increase to usual effective dose of 75 to 150 mg/day, max 300 mg/day. Insomnia (Silenor): 6 mg PO 30 min before bed, 3 mg in age 65 yo or older. Suicidality. [Generic only: Caps 10, 25, 50, 75, 100, 150 mg. Oral concentrate 10 mg/mL. Trade only: Tabs 3, 6 mg (Silenor).] ▶L ♀C ▶– $$ ■

IMIPRAMINE (*Tofranil, Tofranil PM*) Depression: Start 75 to 100 mg PO at bedtime or in divided doses; gradually increase to max 300 mg/day. Enuresis: 25 to 75

(cont.)

mg PO at bedtime. Suicidality. [Generic/Trade: Tabs 10, 25, 50 mg. Caps 75, 100, 125, 150 mg (as pamoate salt).] ▶L ♀D ▶– $$$ ■

NORTRIPTYLINE (***Aventyl, Pamelor***) Start 25 mg PO given once daily or divided two to four times per day. Usual effective dose is 75 to 100 mg/day, max 150 mg/day. Primarily inhibits norepinephrine reuptake. Suicidality. [Generic/Trade: Caps 10, 25, 50, 75 mg. Oral soln 10 mg/5 mL.] ▶L ♀D ▶+ $$$

PROTRIPTYLINE (***Vivactil***) 15 to 40 mg/day PO divided three to four times per day. Max 60 mg/day. Suicidality. [Generic/Trade: Tabs 5, 10 mg.] ▶L ♀C ▶+ $$$$ ■

Antidepressants—Monoamine Oxidase Inhibitors (MAOIs)

NOTE: *Must be on tyramine-free diet throughout treatment and for 2 weeks after discontinuation. Numerous drug interactions; risk of hypertensive crisis and serotonin syndrome with many medications, including OTC. Allow at least 2 weeks wash-out when converting from an MAOI to an SSRI (6 weeks after fluoxetine), TCA, or other antidepressant.*

ISOCARBOXAZID (***Marplan***) Start 10 mg PO two times per day; increase by 10 mg every 2 to 4 days. Usual effective dose is 20 to 40 mg/day. MAOI diet. Suicidality. [Trade only: Tabs 10 mg.] ▶L ♀C ▶? $$$ ■

PHENELZINE (***Nardil***) Start 15 mg PO three times per day. Usual effective dose is 60 to 90 mg/day in divided doses. MAOI diet. Suicidality. [Trade only: Tabs 15 mg.] ▶L ♀C ▶? $$$ ■

SELEGILINE—TRANSDERMAL (***Emsam***) Start 6 mg/24 h patch, change daily. Max 12 mg/24 h. MAOI diet for doses 9 mg/day or higher. Suicidality. [Trade only: Transdermal patch 6 mg/day, 9 mg/24 h, 12 mg/24 h.] ▶L ♀C ▶? $$$$$ ■

TRANYLCYPROMINE (***Parnate***) Start 10 mg PO q am; increase by 10 mg/day at 1- to 3-week intervals to usual effective dose of 10 to 40 mg/day divided two times per day. MAOI diet. Suicidality. [Generic/Trade: Tabs 10 mg.] ▶L ♀C ▶– $$ ■

Antidepressants—Selective Serotonin Reuptake Inhibitors (SSRIs)

CITALOPRAM (***Celexa***) Start 20 mg PO daily. May increase after 1 or more weeks to max 40 mg daily or 20 mg daily if older than 60 yo. Suicidality. [Generic/Trade: Tabs 10, 20, 40 mg. Generic only: Oral disintegrating tab 10, 20, 40 mg, oral soln 10 mg/5 mL.] ▶LK ♀C Use in 3rd trimester is associated with complications at birth. ▶– $$$ ■

ESCITALOPRAM (***Lexapro, ✦Cipralex***) Depression, generalized anxiety disorder, adults, and age 12 yo or older: Start 10 mg PO daily; max 20 mg/day. Suicidality. [Generic/Trade: Tabs 5, 10, 20 mg. Oral soln 1 mg/mL.] ▶LK ♀C Use in 3rd trimester is associated with complications at birth. ▶– $$$$ ■

FLUOXETINE (***Prozac, Prozac Weekly, Sarafem***) Depression, OCD: Start 20 mg PO q am; usual effective dose is 20 to 40 mg/day, max 80 mg/day. Depression, maintenance: 20 to 40 mg/day (standard-release) or 90 mg PO once a week (Prozac Weekly) starting 7 days after last standard-release dose. Bulimia: 60 mg PO daily; may need to titrate slowly, over several days. Panic disorder: Start 10 mg PO q am; titrate to 20 mg/day after 1 week, max 60 mg/day. Premenstrual dysphoric disorder (Sarafem): 20 mg PO daily, given either throughout the

(cont.)

menstrual cycle or for 14 days prior to menses; max 80 mg/day. Doses greater than 20 mg/day can be divided two times per day (in morning and at noon). Bipolar depression, olanzapine + fluoxetine: Start 5 mg olanzapine + 20 mg fluoxetine daily in the evening. Increase to usual range of 5 to 12.5 mg olanzapine + 20 to 50 mg fluoxetine as tolerated. Treatment-resistant depression, olanzapine + fluoxetine: Start 5 mg olanzapine + 20 mg fluoxetine daily in the evening. Increase to usual range of 5 to 20 mg olanzapine + 20 to 50 mg fluoxetine as tolerated. Suicidality, many drug interactions. [Generic/Trade: Tabs 10 mg. Caps 10, 20, 40 mg. Oral soln 20 mg/5 mL. Caps (Sarafem) 10, 20 mg. Trade only: Tabs (Sarafem) 10, 15, 20 mg. Caps, delayed-release (Prozac Weekly) 90 mg. Generic only: Tabs 20, 40 mg.] ▶L ♀C Use in 3rd trimester is associated with complications at birth. ▶– $$$ ■

FLUVOXAMINE (*Luvox, Luvox CR*) Immediate-release: Start 50 mg PO at bedtime; usual effective dose is 100 to 300 mg/day divided two times per day, max 300 mg/day. Controlled-release: Start 100 mg PO at bedtime and increase by 50 mg/day weekly as tolerated to max 300 mg/day. Children age 8 yo or older: Start 25 mg PO at bedtime; usual effective dose is 50 to 200 mg/day divided two times per day, max 200 mg/day. Do not use with thioridazine, pimozide, alosetron, cisapride, tizanidine, tryptophan, or MAOIs; use caution with benzodiazepines, TCAs, theophylline, and warfarin. Suicidality. [Generic/Trade: Tabs 25, 50, 100 mg. Caps, extended-release 100, 150 mg.] ▶L ♀C Use in 3rd trimester is associated with complications at birth. ▶– $$$ ■

PAROXETINE (*Paxil, Paxil CR, Pexeva*) Depression: Start 20 mg PO q am, max 50 mg/day. Controlled-release: Start 25 mg PO q am, max 62.5 mg/day. OCD: Start 10 to 20 mg PO q am, max 60 mg/day. Social anxiety disorder: Start 10 to 20 mg PO q am, max 60 mg/day. Controlled-release: Start 12.5 mg PO q am, max 37.5 mg/day. Generalized anxiety disorder: Start 20 mg PO q am, max 50 mg/day. Panic disorder: Start 10 mg PO q am, increase by 10 mg/day at intervals of 1 week or more to usual effective dose of 10 to 60 mg/day; max 60 mg/day. Controlled-release: Start 12.5 mg PO q am, max 75 mg/day. Post-traumatic stress disorder: Start 20 mg PO q am, max 50 mg/day. Premenstrual dysphoric disorder (PMDD), continuous dosing: Start 12.5 mg PO q am (controlled-release); may increase dose after 1 week to max 25 mg q am. Intermittent dosing (given for 2 weeks prior to menses): 12.5 mg PO q am (controlled-release), max 25 mg/day. Suicidality, many drug interactions. [Generic/Trade: Tabs 10, 20, 30, 40 mg. Oral susp 10 mg/5 mL. Controlled-release tabs 12.5, 25 mg. Trade only: (Paxil CR) 37.5 mg.] ▶LK ♀D ▶? $$$

SERTRALINE (*Zoloft*) Depression, OCD: Start 50 mg PO daily; usual effective dose is 50 to 200 mg/day, max 200 mg/day. Panic disorder, post-traumatic stress disorder, social anxiety disorder: Start 25 mg PO daily, max 200 mg/day. PMDD, continuous dosing: Start 50 mg PO daily, max 150 mg/day. Intermittent dosing: (given for 14 days prior to menses): Start 50 mg PO daily for 3 days, then increase to 100 mg/day. Suicidality. [Generic/Trade: Tabs 25, 50, 100 mg. Oral concentrate 20 mg/mL (60 mL).] ▶LK ♀C Use in 3rd trimester is associated with complications at birth. ▶+ $$$

VORTIOXETINE (*Brintellix, ✦Trintellix*) Start 10 mg PO daily. Max 20 mg/day. Reduce dose if given with strong CYP2D6 inhibitors. [Trade only: Tabs 5, 10, 15, 20 mg] ▶L ♀C Use in 3rd trimester is associated with complications at birth. ▶? $$$$$ ■

Antidepressants—Serotonin-Norepinephrine Reuptake Inhibitors (SNRIs)

DESVENLAFAXINE (*Pristiq, Khedezla*) 50 mg PO daily. Max 400 mg/day. [Trade only: Tabs (Pristiq), extended-release 25 mg. Tabs (Pristiq, Khedezla) extended-release 50, 100 mg. Generic only: Extended-release tabs 50, 100 mg .] ▶LK ♀C ▶? $$$$ ■

DULOXETINE (*Cymbalta*) Depression: Start: 20 mg PO two times per day. May start 30 mg PO once daily in some patients to improve tolerability. Increase as tolerated to 60 mg/day given once daily or divided twice daily. Max 120 mg/day. Doses of 120 mg/day have been used but have not been shown to be more effective than 60 mg/day. Generalized anxiety disorder: Start 30 to 60 mg PO daily, max 120 mg/day. Elderly: Start 30 mg PO daily for 2 weeks. Then increase to target dose of 60 mg/day, max 120 mg/day. Diabetic peripheral neuropathic pain: 60 mg PO daily. Fibromyalgia: Start 30 mg PO daily for one week then increase to 60 mg/day if needed and tolerated. Max 60 mg/day. Suicidality, hepatotoxicity, many drug interactions. [Generic/Trade: Caps 20, 30, 60 mg.] ▶L ♀C ▶? $$$$ ■

LEVOMILNACIPRAN (*Fetzima*) Start 20 mg PO once daily. Increase after 2 days to 40 mg/day. May increase by 40 mg/day at intervals of 2 or more days to max 120 mg/day. [Trade only: Caps 20, 40, 80, 120 mg.] ▶KL ♀C ▶? ■

VENLAFAXINE (*Effexor XR*) Depression/anxiety: Start 37.5 to 75 mg PO daily (Effexor XR) or 75 mg/day divided two to three times per day (Effexor). Usual effective dose is 150 to 225 mg/day, max 225 mg/day (Effexor XR) or 375 mg/day (Effexor). Generalized anxiety disorder: Start 37.5 to 75 mg PO daily (Effexor XR), max 225 mg/day (Effexor XR). Social anxiety disorder: Start 75 mg PO daily (Effexor XR). Panic disorder: Start 37.5 mg PO daily (Effexor XR), may titrate by 75 mg/day at weekly intervals to max 225 mg/day. Suicidality, seizures, HTN. [Generic/Trade: Caps, extended-release 37.5, 75, 150 mg. Tabs 25, 37.5, 50, 75, 100 mg. Generic only: Tabs, extended-release 37.5, 75, 150, 225 mg.] ▶LK ♀C ▶? $$$$

Antidepressants—Other

BUPROPION (*Wellbutrin, Wellbutrin SR, Wellbutrin XL, Aplenzin, Zyban, Buproban, Forfivo XL*) Depression: Start 100 mg PO two times per day (immediate-release tabs); can increase to 100 mg three times per day after 4 to 7 days. Usual effective dose is 300 to 450 mg/day, max 150 mg/dose and 450 mg/day. Sustained-release: Start 150 mg PO q am; may increase to 150 mg two times per day after 4 to 7 days, max 400 mg/day. Give last dose no later than 5 pm. Extended-release: Start 150 mg PO q am; may increase to 300 mg q am after 4 days, max 450 mg q am. Extended-release (Aplenzin): Start 174 mg PO q am; increase to target dose of 348 mg/day after 4 days or more. May increase to max dose of 522 mg/day after 4 weeks or more. Extended-release (Forfivo XL): Do not use to initiate therapy. If standard tabs tolerated and patient requires more than 300 mg/day, may use 450 mg PO daily, max 450 mg/day. Seasonal affective disorder: Start 150 mg of extended-release PO q am in autumn; can increase to 300 mg q am after 1 week, max 300 mg/day. In the spring, decrease to 150 mg/day for 2 weeks and then discontinue. Extended-release (Aplenzin): Start 174 mg PO each morning. Increase to 348

(cont.)

mg/day after 7 days. Smoking cessation (Zyban, Buproban): Start 150 mg PO q am for 3 days, then increase to 150 mg PO two times per day for 7 to 12 weeks. Max 150 mg PO two times per day. Give last dose no later than 5 pm. Seizures, suicidality. [Generic/Trade (for depression, bupropion HCl): Tabs 75, 100 mg. Sustained-release tabs 100, 150, 200 mg. Extended-release tabs 150, 300 mg (Wellbutrin XL). Generic/Trade (Smoking cessation): Sustained-release tabs 150 mg (Zyban, Buproban). Trade only: Extended-release (Aplenzin, bupropion hydrobromide) tabs 174, 348, 522 mg. Extended-release (Forfivo XL) tab 450 mg.] ▶LK ♀C ▶– $$ ■

MIRTAZAPINE (Remeron, Remeron SolTab) Start 15 mg PO at bedtime. Usual effective dose is 15 to 45 mg/day. Agranulocytosis in 0.1% of patients. Suicidality. [Generic/Trade: Tabs 15, 30, 45 mg. Tabs orally disintegrating (SolTab) 15, 30, 45 mg. Generic only: Tabs 7.5 mg.] ▶LK ♀C ▶? $$ ■

TRAZODONE (Oleptro) Depression: Start 50 to 150 mg/day PO in divided doses; usual effective dose is 400 to 600 mg/day. Extended-release: Start 150 mg PO at bedtime. May increase by 75 mg/day q 3 days to max 375 mg/day. Insomnia: 50 to 150 mg PO at bedtime. [Trade only: Extended-release tabs (Oleptro) 150, 300 mg. Generic only: Tabs 50, 100, 150, 300 mg.] ▶L ♀C ▶– $

VILAZODONE (Viibryd) Start 10 mg PO once daily for 7 days, then increase to 20 mg once daily. May increase to max 40 mg/day if needed. [Trade only: Tabs 10, 20, 40 mg.] ▶L ♀C ▶? ■

Antimanic (Bipolar) Agents

LAMOTRIGINE (Lamictal, Lamictal CD, Lamictal ODT, Lamictal XR) Bipolar disorder (maintenance): Start 25 mg PO daily, 50 mg PO daily if on enzyme-inducing drugs, or 25 mg PO every other day if on valproate; titrate to 200 mg/day, up to 400 mg/day divided two times per day if on enzyme-inducing drugs, or 100 mg/day if on valproate. Potentially life-threatening rashes in 0.3% of adults and 0.8% of children; discontinue at 1st sign of rash. Drug interaction with valproic acid; see prescribing information for adjusted dosing guidelines. [Generic/Trade: Chewable dispersible tabs (Lamictal CD) 5, 25 mg. Tabs 25, 100, 150, 200 mg. Extended-release tabs (XR) 25, 50, 100, 200, 250, 300 mg. Trade only: Orally disintegrating tabs (ODT) 25, 50, 100, 200 mg. Chewable dispersible tabs 2 mg.] ▶LK ♀C ▶– $$$$ ■

LITHIUM (Lithobid, ✦Lithane) Acute mania: Start 300 to 600 mg PO two to three times per day; usual effective dose is 900 to 1800 mg/day. May start 300 mg PO two or three times daily to improve tolerability. Steady state is achieved in 5 days. Bipolar maintenance: Usually 900 to 1200 mg/day titrated to therapeutic trough level of 0.6 to 1.2 mEq/L. [Generic/Trade: Caps 300, Extended-release tabs 300, 450 mg. Generic only: Caps 150, 600 mg, Tabs 300 mg, Syrup 300 mg/5 mL.] ▶K ♀D ▶– $ ■

TOPIRAMATE (Topamax) Bipolar disorder (unapproved): Start 25 to 50 mg/day PO. Titrate prn to max 400 mg/day divided two times per day. [Generic/Trade: Tabs 25, 50, 100, 200 mg. Sprinkle Caps 15, 25 mg.] ▶K ♀D ▶? $$$$$ ■

VALPROIC ACID (Depakote, Depakote ER, Stavzor, divalproex, ✦Epival) Mania: 250 mg PO three times per day (Depakote) or 25 mg/kg once daily (Depakote ER);

(cont.)

PSYCHIATRY

max 60 mg/kg/day. Hepatotoxicity, drug interactions, reduce dose in the elderly. [Generic only: Syrup (Valproic acid) 250 mg/5 mL. Generic/Trade: Delayed-release tabs (Depakote) 125, 250, 500 mg. Extended-release tabs (Depakote ER) 250, 500 mg. Delayed-release sprinkle caps (Depakote) 125 mg. Trade only (Stavzor): Delayed-release caps 125, 250, 500 mg.] ▶L ♀D ▶+ $$$$

ANTIPSYCHOTIC RELATIVE ADVERSE EFFECTS[a]

Generation	Antipsychotic	Anticholinergic	Sedation	Hypotension	EPS	Weight Gain	Diabetes/Hyperglycemia	Dyslipidemia
1st	chlorpromazine	+++	+++	++	++	+++	+++	+++
1st	fluphenazine	++	+	+	++++	+	+	+
1st	haloperidol	+	+	+	++++	+	+	+
1st	loxapine	++	+	+	++	++	++	?
1st	molindone	++	++	+	++	+	?	?
1st	perphenazine	++	++	+	++	++	++	?
1st	pimozide	+	+	+	+++	+	+	?
1st	thioridazine	++++	+++	+++	+	++	++	?
1st	thiothixene	+	++	+	+++	++	++	?
1st	trifluoperazine	++	+	+	+++	++	++	?
2nd	aripiprazole	++	+	0	0	0/+	0/+	0
2nd	asenapine	+	+	++	++	++	++	0
2nd	brexipiprazole	+	+	0/+	+	+	?	?
2nd	cariprazine	+	+	+	++	+	?	?
2nd	clozapine	++++	+++	+++	0	++++	++++	++++
2nd	lurasidone	+	+	+	+	+	+	0
2nd	iloperidone	++	+	+++	+	++	++	++
2nd	olanzapine	+++	++	+	0[b]	++++	++++	++++
2nd	paliperidone	+	+	++	++	+++	+++	+
2nd	risperidone	+	++	+	+[b]	+++	+++	+
2nd	quetiapine	+	+++	++	0	+++	+++	+++
2nd	ziprasidone	+	+	0	0	0/+	0	0

Crismon M, Argo T, Bickley P. Schizophrenia. In: DiPiro J, Talbert R, Yee G, et al. ed. Pharmacotherapy. A pathophysiologic approach, 9th ed. New York: McGraw Hill Education, 2014 and Jibson M. Second generation antipsychotic medications: pharmacology, administration, and comparative side effects. UpToDate, 2015 (www.uptodate.com), and Muench J, Hamer A. Adverse effects of antipsychotic medications, Am Fam Physician 2010;81(5):617-22.

[a] Risk of specific adverse effects is graded from 0 (absent) to ++++ (high). ? = Limited or inconsistent comparative data.

[b] Extrapyramidal symptoms (EPS) are dose-related and are more likely for risperidone greater than 6 to 8 mg/day, olanzapine greater than 20 mg/day. Akathisia risk remains unclear and may not be reflected in these ratings. There are limited comparative data for aripiprazole iloperidone, paliperidone, and asenapine relative to other 2nd-generation antipsychotics.

Antipsychotics—First Generation (Typical)

CHLORPROMAZINE Start 10 to 50 mg PO/IM two to three times per day, usual dose 300 to 800 mg/day. [Generic only: Tabs 10, 25, 50, 100, 200 mg. Generic/Trade: Oral concentrate 30 mg/mL, 100 mg/mL. Trade only: Syrup 10 mg/5 mL, Supps 25, 100 mg.] ▶LK ♀C ▷– $$$ ■

FLUPHENAZINE (✦*Modecate*) 1.25 to 10 mg/day IM divided q 6 to 8 h. Start 0.5 to 10 mg/day PO divided q 6 to 8 h. Usual effective dose 1 to 20 mg/day. Depot (fluphenazine decanoate/enanthate): 12.5 to 25 mg IM/SC q 3 to 6 weeks is equivalent to 10 to 20 mg/day PO fluphenazine. [Generic/Trade: Tabs 1, 2.5, 5, 10 mg. Elixir 2.5 mg/5 mL. Oral concentrate 5 mg/mL.] ▶LK ♀C ▷– $$$ ■

HALOPERIDOL (*Haldol*) 2 to 5 mg IM to max 20 mg/day IM. Start 0.5 to 5 mg PO two to three times per day, usual effective dose 6 to 20 mg/day. Max PO dose 100 mg/day. Therapeutic range 2 to 15 ng/mL. Depot haloperidol (haloperidol decanoate): 100 to 200 mg IM q 4 weeks is equivalent to 10 mg/day oral haloperidol. [Generic only: Tabs 0.5, 1, 2, 5, 10, 20 mg. Oral concentrate 2 mg/mL.] ▶LK ♀C ▷– $$ ■

PERPHENAZINE Start 4 to 8 mg PO three times per day or 8 to 16 mg PO two to four times per day (hospitalized patients), max 64 mg/day PO. Can give 5 to 10 mg IM q 6 h, max 30 mg/day IM. [Generic only: Tabs 2, 4, 8, 16 mg. Oral concentrate 16 mg/5 mL.] ▶LK ♀C ▷? $$$

PIMOZIDE (*Orap*) Start 1 to 2 mg/day PO in divided doses, increase every 2 days to usual effective dose of 1 to 10 mg/day. [Trade only: Tabs 1, 2 mg.] ▶L ♀C ▷? $$$ ■

THIORIDAZINE Start 50 to 100 mg PO three times per day, usual dose 200 to 800 mg/day. Not 1st-line therapy. Causes QTc prolongation, torsades de pointes, and sudden death. Contraindicated with SSRIs, propranolol, pindolol. Monitor baseline ECG and potassium. Pigmentary retinopathy with doses greater than 800 mg/day. [Generic only: Tabs 10, 15, 25, 50, 100, 150, 200 mg. Oral concentrate 30, 100 mg/mL.] ▶LK ♀C ▷? $$ ■

THIOTHIXENE Start 2 mg PO three times per day. Usual effective dose is 20 to 30 mg/day, max 60 mg/day PO. [Generic/Trade: Caps 1, 2, 5, 10. Oral concentrate 5 mg/mL. Trade only: Caps 20 mg.] ▶LK ♀C ▷? $$$ ■

TRIFLUOPERAZINE Start 2 to 5 mg PO two times per day. Usual effective dose is 15 to 20 mg/day. [Generic/Trade: Tabs 1, 2, 5, 10 mg. Trade only: Oral concentrate 10 mg/mL.] ▶LK ♀C ▷– $$$ ■

Antipsychotics—Second Generation (Atypical)

ARIPIPRAZOLE (*Abilify, Abilify Maintena*) Schizophrenia: Start 10 to 15 mg PO daily. Max 30 mg daily. Schizophrenia, maintenance (Maintena): 400 mg IM monthly. May reduce to 300 mg IM monthly if adverse reactions to higher dose. Bipolar disorder: Start 15 mg PO daily. Max 30 mg/day. Agitation associated with schizophrenia or bipolar disorder: 9.75 mg IM recommended. May consider 5.25 to 15 mg if indicated. May repeat in 2 h up to max 30 mg/day. Depression, adjunctive therapy: Start 2 to 5 mg PO daily. Max 15 mg/day. [Generic/Trade: Tabs 2, 5, 10, 15, 20, 30 mg. Susp, extended-release for injection (Abilify Maintena) 300 mg and 400 mg/vial.] ▶L ♀C ▷? $$$$$ ■

ASENAPINE (*Saphris*) Schizophrenia: Acute and maintenance: Start 5 mg SL twice per day. Max 10 mg twice per day. Bipolar disorder, acute manic or mixed episodes, monotherapy: Start 5 mg SL two times per day (adjunctive) or 10 mg SL two times per day (monotherapy). Max 20 mg/day. [Trade: SL tabs 5, 10 mg.] ▶L ♀C ▶— ■

BREXPIPRAZOLE (*Rexulti*) Major depressive disorder, adjunctive: Start 0.5 mg to 1 mg PO once daily. Increase weekly by 1 mg/day to max 3 mg/day. Schizophrenia: Start 1 mg PO daily for days 1-4. Then increase to 2 mg once daily for days 5-7. Then increase to 4 mg/day as needed and tolerated. Reduce dose with hepatic or severe renal impairment. [Trade only: Tabs 0.25, 0.5, 1, 2, 3, 4 mg.] ▶L ♀? Withdrawal and extrapyramidal symptoms for neonate at birth ▶? ■

CARIPRAZINE (*Vraylar*) Schizophrenia: Start 1.5 mg PO once daily. The dose can be increased to 3 mg/day on day 2. May increase by 1.5 mg/day to 3 mg/day as needed and tolerated to max 6 mg/day. Manic or mixed episodes of bipolar I disorder: Start 1.5 mg PO once daily. May increase to 3 mg/day on day 2. May increase by 1.5 mg/day to 3 mg/day to recommended range of 3-6 mg/day. [Trade only: Caps 1.5, 3, 4.5, 6 mg.] ▶L ♀? Neonates who have been exposed in the third trimester are at increased risk for extrapyramidal or withdrawal reactions at delivery. ▶? ■

CLOZAPINE (*Clozaril, FazaClo ODT, Versacloz*) Start 12.5 mg PO one to two times per day. Usual effective dose is 300 to 450 mg/day divided two times per day, max 900 mg/day. Agranulocytosis 1 to 2%; check ANC weekly for 6 months, then every 2 weeks for another 6 months and then monthly. Seizures, myocarditis, cardiopulmonary arrest. [Generic/Trade: Tabs 25, 100 mg. Generic only: Tabs 12.5, 50, 200 mg. Orally disintegrating tabs 12.5, 25, 100 mg Trade only: Orally disintegrating tab (Fazaclo ODT) 12.5, 25, 100, 150, 200 mg (scored). Susp (Versacloz): 50 mg/mL.] ▶L ♀B ▶— $$$$$ ■

ILOPERIDONE (*Fanapt*) Start 1 mg PO two times per day. Increase to 2 mg PO two times per day on day 2, then by 2 mg per dose each day to usual effective range of 6 to 12 mg PO two times per day. Max 24 mg/day. [Trade: Tabs 1, 2, 4, 6, 8, 10, 12 mg.] ▶L ♀C ▶— ? ■

LURASIDONE (*Latuda*) Schizophrenia: Start 40 mg PO daily. Effective dose range 40 to 160 mg/day, max 160 mg/day. Take with food. Reduce starting dose to 20 mg PO daily if moderate to severe renal or hepatic insufficiency or use with moderate CYP3A4 inhibitors, max 80 mg/day unless severe hepatic insufficiency which is 40 mg/day. Depression associated with bipolar I disorder (monotherapy or adjunctive with lithium or valproate): Start 20 mg PO daily. Usual range 20 to 120 mg/day. Doses greater than 20 to 60 mg/day did not provide further efficacy as monotherapy. [Trade only: Tabs 20, 40, 60, 80, 120 mg.] ▶K – ♀B ▶— ■

OLANZAPINE (*Zyprexa, Zyprexa Zydis, Zyprexa Relprevv*) Agitation in acute bipolar mania or schizophrenia: Start 10 mg IM (2.5 to 5 mg in elderly or debilitated patients); may repeat in 2 h to max 30 mg/day. Schizophrenia, oral therapy: Start 5 to 10 mg PO daily; usual effective dose is 10 to 15 mg/day. Schizophrenia, long-acting injection: dose based on prior oral dose and ranges from 150 mg to 300 mg deep IM (gluteal) q 2 weeks or 300 mg to 405 mg q 4 weeks. See prescribing information. Bipolar disorder, maintenance treatment, or monotherapy for acute manic or mixed episodes: Start 10 to 15 mg PO daily.

(cont.)

Increase by 5 mg/day at intervals after 24 h to usual effective dose of 5 to 20 mg/day, max 20 mg/day. Bipolar disorder, adjunctive for acute manic or mixed episodes: Start 10 mg PO daily; usual effective dose is 5 to 20 mg/day, max 20 mg/day. Bipolar depression, olanzapine + fluoxetine: Start 5 mg olanzapine + 20 mg fluoxetine daily in the evening. Increase to usual range of 5 to 12.5 mg olanzapine plus 20 to 50 mg fluoxetine as tolerated. Treatment-resistant depression, olanzapine + fluoxetine: Start 5 mg olanzapine + 20 mg fluoxetine daily in the evening. Increase to usual range of 5 to 20 mg olanzapine plus 20 to 50 mg fluoxetine as tolerated. [Generic/Trade: Tabs 2.5, 5, 7.5, 10, 15, 20 mg. Tabs, orally disintegrating (Zyprexa Zydis) 5, 10, 15, 20 mg. Trade only: Long-acting injection (Zyprexa Relprevv) 210, 300, 405 mg/vial.] ▶L ♀C ▶– $$$$$ ■

PALIPERIDONE (*Invega Trinza, Invega, Invega Sustenna*) Schizophrenia and schizoaffective disorder (adjunctive and monotherapy): Start 6 mg PO q am. 3 mg/day may be sufficient in some. Max 12 mg/day. Extended-release injection: Schizophrenia (Invega Sustenna): Start 234 mg IM (deltoid) and then 156 mg IM 1 week later. Recommended monthly dose 117 mg IM (deltoid or gluteal) or within range of 39 to 234 mg, based on response. Patient must be able to tolerate oral paliperidone or risperidone prior to starting Sustenna. Schizophrenia (Invega Trinza): Use only after tolerability to Invega Sustenna has been established for at least 4 months. The dose of Trinza is given IM q 3 months based on the prior dose of Sustenna. For Sustenna 78, use Trinza 273 mg; Sustenna 117 mg, use Trinza 410 mg; Sustenna 156 mg, use Trinza 546 mg; and Sustenna 234 mg, use Trinza 819 mg. Adjust dose at intervals of 3 months. Schizoaffective disorder (Invega Sustenna): Start 234 mg IM (deltoid) and then 156 mg IM on day 8. Usual dose range 78 to 234 mg, max 234 mg. [Trade only: Extended-release tabs 1.5, 3, 6, 9 mg. Depot formulation (Sustenna): 39, 78, 117, 156, 234 mg. Depot formulation (Trinza) 273, 410, 546, 819 mg.] ▶KL ♀C ▶– $$$$$ ■

QUETIAPINE (*Seroquel, Seroquel XR*) Schizophrenia: Start 25 mg PO two times per day (regular tabs); increase by 25 to 50 mg two to three times per day on days 2 and 3, and then to target dose of 300 to 400 mg/day divided two to three times per day on day 4. Usual effective dose is 150 to 750 mg/day, max 800 mg/day. Extended-release tabs: Start 300 mg PO daily in evening, increase by up to 300 mg/day at intervals of more than 1 day to usual effective range of 400 to 800 mg/day. Acute bipolar mania, monotherapy, or adjunctive: Start 50 mg PO two times per day on day 1, then increase to no higher than 100 mg two times per day on day 2, 150 mg two times per day on day 3, and 200 mg two times per day on day 4. May increase prn to 300 mg two times per day on day 5 and 400 mg two times per day thereafter. Usual effective dose is 400 to 800 mg/day. Extended-release: Start 300 mg PO evening of day 1, 600 mg day 2, and 400 to 800 mg/day thereafter. Bipolar depression, regular and extended-release: 50 mg PO at bedtime on day 1, 100 mg at bedtime day 2, 200 mg at bedtime day 3, and 300 mg at bedtime day 4. Bipolar maintenance: Continue dose required to maintain remission. Major depressive disorder, adjunctive to antidepressants, extended-release: Start 50 mg evening of day 1, may increase to 150 mg on day 3. Max 300 mg/day. Eye exam for cataracts recommended q 6 months. [Generic/Trade: Tabs 25, 50, 100, 200, 300, 400 mg. Trade only: Extended-release tabs 50, 150, 200, 300, 400 mg.] ▶LK ♀C ▶– $$$$

RISPERIDONE (*Risperdal, Risperdal Consta, Risperdal M-Tab*) Schizophrenia: Start 2 mg/day PO given once daily or divided two times per day (0.5 mg two times per day in the elderly, debilitated, or with hypotension, severe renal or hepatic disease); increase by 1 to 2 mg/day (no more than 0.5 mg two times per day in elderly and debilitated) at intervals of 24 h or more to usual effective dose of 4 to 8 mg/day given once daily or divided two times per day, max 16 mg/day. Schizophrenia, bipolar type 1 maintenance: Long-acting injection (Consta): Start 25 mg IM q 2 weeks while continuing oral dose for 3 weeks. May increase at 4-week intervals to max 50 mg q 2 weeks. Schizophrenia (13 to 17 yo): Start 0.5 mg PO daily; increase by 0.5 to 1 mg/day at intervals of 24 h or more to target dose of 3 mg/day. Max 6 mg/day. Bipolar mania (adults): Start 2 to 3 mg PO daily; may increase by 1 mg/day at 24 h intervals to max 6 mg/day. Bipolar mania (10 to 17 yo): Start 0.5 mg PO daily; increase by 0.5 to 1 mg/day at intervals of 24 h to recommended dose of 2.5 mg/day. Max 6 mg/day. Autistic disorder irritability (age 5 to 16 yo): Start 0.25 mg (for wt less than 20 kg) or 0.5 mg (wt 20 kg or greater) PO daily. May increase after 4 days to 0.5 mg/day (for wt less than 20 kg) or 1.0 mg/day (wt 20 kg or greater). Maintain at least 14 days. May then increase at 14-day intervals or more by increments of 0.25 mg/day (for wt less than 20 kg) or 0.5 mg/day (wt 20 kg or greater) to max 1.0 mg/day (for wt less than 20 kg), 2.5 mg/day (20 to 44 kg), or 3.0 mg/day (wt more than 45 kg). [Generic/Trade: Tabs 0.25, 0.5, 1, 2, 3, 4 mg. Oral soln 1 mg/mL (30 mL). Orally disintegrating tabs 0.5, 1, 2, 3, 4 mg. Generic only: Orally disintegrating tabs 0.25 mg. Trade only: IM Injection (Risperdal Consta) 12.5, 25, 37.5, 50 mg] ▶LK ♀C ▶— $$$$ ■

ZIPRASIDONE (*Geodon, ✦Zeldox*) Schizophrenia: Start 20 mg PO two times per day with food; may adjust at more than 2-day intervals to max 80 mg PO two times per day. Acute agitation: 10 to 20 mg IM, max 40 mg/day. Bipolar mania: Start 40 mg PO two times per day with food; may increase to 60 to 80 mg two times per day on day 2. Usual effective dose is 40 to 80 mg two times per day. Must be taken with a meal of at least 500 Cal for adequate absorption. [Trade/Generic: Caps 20, 40, 60, 80 mg. Trade only: 20 mg/mL injection.] ▶L ♀C ▶— $$$$$ ■

Anxiolytics/Hypnotics—Benzodiazepines—Long Half-Life (25-100 h)

BROMAZEPAM (*✦Lectopam*) Canada only. 6 to 18 mg/day PO in divided doses. [Generic/Trade: Tabs 1.5, 3, 6 mg.] ▶L ♀D ▶— $

CHLORDIAZEPOXIDE Anxiety: 5 to 25 mg PO three to four times per day. Acute alcohol withdrawal: 50 to 100 mg PO, repeat q 3 to 4 h prn up to 300 mg/day. Half-life 5 to 30 h. [Generic/Trade: Caps 5, 10, 25 mg.] ▶LK ♀D ▶—©IV $$

CLONAZEPAM (*Klonopin, Klonopin Wafer, ✦Rivotril, Clonapam*) Panic disorder: Start 0.25 to 0.5 mg PO two to three times per day, max 4 mg/day. Half-life 18 to 50 h. Epilepsy: Start 0.5 mg PO three times per day. Max 20 mg/day. [Generic/Trade: Tabs 0.5, 1, 2 mg. Orally disintegrating tabs (approved for panic disorder only) 0.125, 0.25, 0.5, 1, 2 mg.] ▶LK ♀D ▶—©IV $

CLORAZEPATE (*Tranxene*) Anxiety: Start 7.5 to 15 mg PO at bedtime or two to three times per day, usual effective dose is 15 to 60 mg/day. Acute alcohol withdrawal: 60 to 90 mg/day on 1st day divided two to three times per day, reduce dose to 7.5

(cont.)

to 15 mg/day over 5 days. Partial seizures, adjunctive: 13 yo and older, start no higher than 7.5 mg PO three times daily. May increase by no more than 7.5 mg per week to max 90 mg/day. Age 9 to 12 yo: Start 7.5 mg PO twice daily. May increase by no more than 7.5 mg per week to max of 60 mg/day. [Generic/Trade: Tabs 3.75, 7.5, 15 mg.] ▶LK ♀D ▶— ©IV $$$$

DIAZEPAM (*Valium, Diastat, Diastat AcuDial, Diazemuls*) Active seizures: 5 to 10 mg IV q 10 to 15 min to max 30 mg, or 0.2 to 0.5 mg/kg rectal gel PR. Skeletal muscle spasm, spasticity related to cerebral palsy, paraplegia, athetosis, "stiff man syndrome": 2 to 10 mg PO/PR three to four times per day. Anxiety: 2 to 10 mg PO two to four times per day. Half-life 20 to 80 h. Alcohol withdrawal: 10 mg PO three to four times per day for 24 h then 5 mg PO three to four times per day prn. [Generic/Trade: Tabs 2, 5, 10 mg. Rectal gel 2.5 mg ($$$$$). Generic only: Oral soln 5 mg/5 mL. Oral concentrate (Intensol) 5 mg/mL. Rectal gel 10, 20 mg ($$$$$). Trade only: Rectal gel (Diastat AcuDial–$$$$$) 10, 20 mg syringes. Available doses from 10 mg AcuDial syringe 5, 7.5, 10 mg. Available doses from 20 mg AcuDial syringe 12.5, 15, 17.5, 20 mg.] ▶LK ♀D ▶— ©IV $

FLURAZEPAM 15 to 30 mg PO at bedtime. Half-life 70 to 90 h. [Generic/Trade: Caps 15, 30 mg.] ▶LK ♀X ▶— ©IV $

Anxiolytics/Hypnotics—Benzodiazepines—Medium Half-Life (10 to 15 h)

NOTE: *To avoid withdrawal, gradually taper when discontinuing after prolonged use. Sedative-hypnotics have been associated with severe allergic reactions and complex sleep behaviors including sleep driving. Use caution and discuss with patients.*

ESTAZOLAM (*ProSom*) 1 to 2 mg PO at bedtime. [Generic/Trade: Tabs 1, 2 mg.] ▶LK ♀X ▶— ©IV $$

LORAZEPAM (*Ativan*) Anxiety: 0.5 to 2 mg IV/IM/PO q 6 to 8 h, max 10 mg/day. Half-life 10 to 20 h. Status epilepticus: Adult: 4 mg IV over 2 min; may repeat in 10 to 15 min. Status epilepticus: Peds: 0.05 to 0.1 mg/kg (max 4 mg) IV over 2 to 5 min; may repeat 0.05 mg/kg once in 10 to 15 min. [Generic/Trade: Tabs 0.5, 1, 2 mg. Generic only: Oral concentrate 2 mg/mL.] ▶LK ♀D ▶— ©IV $

TEMAZEPAM (*Restoril*) 7.5 to 30 mg PO at bedtime. Half-life 8 to 25 h. [Generic/Trade: Caps 7.5, 15, 22.5, 30 mg.] ▶LK ♀X ▶— ©IV $

Anxiolytics/Hypnotics—Benzodiazepines—Short Half-Life (< 12 h)

NOTE: *To avoid withdrawal, gradually taper when discontinuing after prolonged use. Sedative-hypnotics have been associated with severe allergic reactions and complex sleep behaviors including sleep driving. Use caution and discuss with patients.*

ALPRAZOLAM (*Xanax, Xanax XR, Niravam*) 0.25 to 0.5 mg PO two to three times per day. Half-life 12 h. Multiple drug interactions. [Generic/Trade: Tabs 0.25, 0.5, 1, 2 mg. Tabs, extended-release 0.5, 1, 2, 3 mg. Orally disintegrating tab (Niravam) 0.25, 0.5, 1, 2 mg. Generic only: Oral concentrate (Intensol) 1 mg/mL.] ▶LK ♀D ▶— ©IV $

OXAZEPAM 10 to 30 mg PO three to four times per day. Half-life 8 h. [Generic/Trade: Caps 10, 15, 30 mg. Trade only: Tabs 15 mg.] ▶LK ♀D ▶— ©IV $$$

TRIAZOLAM (*Halcion*) 0.125 to 0.5 PO at bedtime. 0.125 mg/day in elderly. Half-life 2 to 3 h. [Generic/Trade: Tabs 0.25 mg. Generic only: Tabs 0.125 mg.] ▶LK ♀X ▶— ⊚IV $

Anxiolytics/Hypnotics—Other

BUSPIRONE Start 15 mg "dividose" daily (7.5 mg PO two times per day), usual effective dose 30 mg/day. Max 60 mg/day. [Generic/Trade: Tabs 5, 10 mg. Dividose Tabs 15, 30 mg (scored to be easily bisected or trisected). Generic only: Tabs 7.5 mg.] ▶K ♀B ▶— $$$

ESZOPICLONE (*Lunesta*) 2 mg PO at bedtime prn. Max 3 mg. Elderly: 1 mg PO at bedtime prn, max 2 mg. [Generic/Trade: Tabs 1, 2, 3 mg.] ▶L ♀C ▶? ⊚IV $$$$$

RAMELTEON (*Rozerem*) 8 mg PO at bedtime. [Trade only: Tabs 8 mg.] ▶L ♀C ▶? $$$$

SUVOREXANT (*Belsomra*) Start 10 mg PO once nightly 30 minutes before bedtime. May increase if needed to max 20 mg once nightly. [Trade: Tabs 5, 10, 15, 20 mg.] ▶L ♀C ▶? ⊚IV

ZALEPLON (*Sonata*) 5 to 10 mg PO at bedtime prn, max 20 mg. Do not use for benzodiazepine or alcohol withdrawal. [Generic/Trade: Caps 5, 10 mg.] ▶L ♀C ▶— $$$$

ZOPICLONE (✱*Imovane*) Canada only. 5 to 7.5 mg PO at bedtime. Reduce dose in elderly. [Generic/Trade: Tabs 5, 7.5 mg. Generic only: Tabs 3.75 mg.] ▶L ♀D ▶— $

Combination Drugs

SYMBYAX (olanzapine + fluoxetine) Bipolar type 1 with depression and treatment-resistant depression: Start 6/25 mg PO at bedtime. Max 18/75 mg/day. [Generic/Trade: Caps (olanzapine/fluoxetine) 3/25, 6/25, 6/50, 12/25, 12/50 mg.] ▶LK ♀C ▶— $$$$$ ■

Drug Dependence Therapy

ACAMPROSATE (*Campral*) Maintenance of abstinence from alcohol: 666 mg (2 tabs) PO three times per day. Start after alcohol withdrawal and when patient is abstinent. [Generic/Trade: Tabs, delayed-release 333 mg.] ▶K ♀C ▶? $$$$$

DISULFIRAM (*Antabuse*) Maintenance of abstinence from alcohol: 125 to 500 mg PO daily. Patient must abstain from any alcohol for at least 12 h before using. Metronidazole and alcohol in any form (cough syrups, tonics, etc.) contraindicated. [Generic/Trade: Tabs 250, 500 mg.] ▶L ♀C ▶? $$

NALTREXONE (*ReVia, Depade, Vivitrol*) Alcohol/opioid dependence: 25 to 50 mg PO daily. Extended-release injectable susp: 380 mg IM q 4 weeks or monthly. Avoid if recent ingestion of opioids (past 7 to 10 days). Hepatotoxicity with higher than approved doses. [Generic/Trade: Tabs 50 mg. Trade only (Vivitrol): Extended-release injectable susp kits 380 mg.] ▶LK ♀C ▶? $$$$

NICOTINE GUM (*Nicorette, Nicorette DS*) Smoking cessation: Gradually taper: 1 piece q 1 to 2 h for 6 weeks, 1 piece q 2 to 4 h for 3 weeks, then 1 piece q 4 to 8 h for 3 weeks, max 30 pieces/day of 2 mg or 24 pieces/day of 4 mg. Use Nicorette

(cont.)

DS 4 mg/piece in high cigarette use (more than 24 cigarettes/day). [OTC/Generic/Trade: Gum 2, 4 mg.] ▶LK ♀C ▶– $$$$

NICOTINE INHALATION SYSTEM (*Nicotrol Inhaler*, ✦*Nicorette Inhaler*) Smoking cessation: 6 to 16 cartridges/day for 12 weeks. [Trade only: Oral inhaler 10 mg/cartridge (4 mg nicotine delivered), 42 cartridges/box.] ▶LK ♀D ▶– $$$$$

NICOTINE LOZENGE (*Commit, Nicorette*) Smoking cessation: In those who smoke within 30 min of waking, use 4 mg lozenge; others use 2 mg. Take 1 to 2 lozenges q 1 to 2 h for 6 weeks, then q 2 to 4 h in weeks 7 to 9, then q 4 to 8 h weeks 10 to 12. Length of therapy 12 weeks. [OTC Generic/Trade: Lozenge 2, 4 mg.] ▶LK ♀D ▶– $$$$$

NICOTINE NASAL SPRAY (*Nicotrol NS*) Smoking cessation: 1 to 2 doses q 1 h, each dose is 2 sprays, 1 in each nostril (1 spray contains 0.5 mg nicotine). Minimum recommended: 8 doses/day, max 40 doses/day. [Trade only: Nasal soln 10 mg/mL (0.5 mg/inhalation); 10 mL bottles.] ▶LK ♀D ▶– $$$$$

NICOTINE PATCHES (*Habitrol, NicoDerm CQ, Nicotrol*) Smoking cessation: Start 1 patch (14 to 22 mg) daily, taper after 6 weeks. Patients who slip up while using the patch may continue to use it but suggest curbing use. OTC/Trade: 15 mg/16 h (Nicotrol). ▶LK ♀D ▶– $$$$

SUBOXONE (buprenorphine + naloxone, *Bunavail, Zubsolv*) Treatment of opioid dependence: Induction (Suboxone SL film): Day 1 start with 2 mg/0.5 mg SL or 4 mg/1 mg SL and titrate upward in increments of 2 or 4 mg of buprenorphine at approximately 2 h intervals to 8 mg/2 mg total dose. Day 2 a dose of up to 16 mg/4 mg is recommended. Maintenance (SL tabs and film): Target dose 16 mg SL daily. Can individualize to range of 4 to 24 mg SL daily. Induction (Zubsolv): Day 1 start with 1.4mg/0.36 mg and titrate upward in increments of 1 or 2 of these tablets every 1.5-2 hours to a dose of 5.7 mg/1.4 mg. Some patients may tolerate three of the tablets as the second dose depending upon recent narcotic exposure. Day 2 a dose of 11.4 mg/2.9 mg is recommended. Maintenance (Zubsolv): 11.4 mg/2.8 mg SL daily. Can individualize to range of 2.8/0.72 to 17.1/4.2 mg SL daily. [Generic only: SL tabs 2/0.5 mg and 8/2 mg buprenorphine/naloxone. Trade only: SL film 2/0.5, 4/1, 8/2, 12/3 mg buprenorphine/naloxone, SL tabs (Zubsolv) 1.4/0.36, 5.7/1.4 mg.] ▶L ♀C ▶– ©III $$$$$

VARENICLINE (*Chantix*, ✦*Champix*) Smoking cessation: Start 0.5 mg PO daily for days 1 to 3, then 0.5 mg two times per day days 4 to 7, then 1 mg two times per day thereafter. Take after meals with full glass of water. Start 1 week prior to cessation and continue for 12 weeks, or patient may start the drug and stop smoking between days 8 and 35 of treatment. [Trade only: Tabs 0.5, 1 mg.] ▶K ♀C ▶? $$$$ ∎

Stimulants/ADHD/Anorexiants

NOTE: *Sudden cardiac death has been reported with stimulants and atomoxetine at usual ADHD doses; carefully assess prior to treatment and avoid if cardiac conditions or structural abnormalities. Amphetamines are associated with high abuse potential and dependence with prolonged administration. Stimulants may also cause or worsen underlying psychosis or induce a manic or mixed episode in bipolar disorder. Problems with visual accommodation have also been reported with stimulants.*

ADDERALL XR (**dextroamphetamine + amphetamine**, ***Adderall***) ADHD, standard-release tabs: Start 2.5 mg (3 to 5 yo) or 5 mg (age 6 yo or older) PO one to two times per day, increase by 2.5 to 5 mg every week, max 40 mg/day. Extended-release caps (Adderall XR): Age 6 to 12 yo, start 5 to 10 mg PO daily to a max of 30 mg/day. Age 13 to 17 yo, start 10 mg PO daily to a max of 20 mg/day. Adults: Give 20 mg PO daily. Narcolepsy, standard-release: Start 5 to 10 mg PO every morning, increase by 5 to 10 mg every week, max 60 mg/day. Avoid evening doses. Monitor growth and use drug holidays when appropriate. [Generic/Trade: Tabs 5, 7.5, 10, 12.5, 15, 20, 30 mg. Caps, extended-release (Adderall XR) 5, 10, 15, 20, 25, 30 mg.] ▶L ♀C ▶– ⊚II $$$$

ARMODAFINIL (***Nuvigil***) Obstructive sleep apnea/hypopnea syndrome and narcolepsy: 150 to 250 mg PO every am. Inconsistent evidence for improved efficacy of 250 mg/day dose. Shift work sleep disorder: 150 mg PO 1 h prior to start of shift. [Trade only: Tabs 50, 150, 200, 250 mg.] ▶L ♀C ▶? ⊚IV $$$$$

ATOMOXETINE (***Strattera***) All ages wt greater than 70 kg: Start 40 mg PO daily, then increase after more than 3 days to target of 80 mg/day divided one to two times per day. Max 100 mg/day. [Trade only: Caps 10, 18, 25, 40, 60, 80, 100 mg.] ▶K ♀C ▶? $$$$$ ■

CAFFEINE (***NoDoz, Vivarin, Caffedrine, Stay Awake, Quick-Pep, Cafcit***) 100 to 200 mg PO every 3 to 4 h prn. [OTC Generic/Trade: Tabs/Caps 200 mg. Oral soln caffeine citrate (Cafcit) 20 mg/mL. OTC Trade only: Tabs, extended-release 200 mg. Lozenges 75 mg.] ▶L ♀B/C ▶? $

DEXMETHYLPHENIDATE (***Focalin, Focalin XR***) Extended-release, not already on stimulants: Start 5 mg (children) or 10 mg (adults) PO every am. Max 30 mg/day (children) or 40 mg/day (Adults). Immediate-release, not already on stimulants: 2.5 mg PO two times per day. Max 20 mg/day. If taking racemic methylphenidate, use conversion of 2.5 mg for each 5 mg of methylphenidate. [Generic/Trade: Tabs, immediate-release 2.5, 5, 10 mg. Extended-release caps (generic) 10, 15, 20, 30, 40 mg. Trade only: Extended-release caps (Focalin XR–$$$$$) 5, 10, 15, 20, 25, 30, 35, 40 mg.] ▶L ♀C ▶– ⊚II $$$

DEXTROAMPHETAMINE (***Dexedrine, ProCentra, Zenzedi***) Narcolepsy: Age 6 to 12 yo: Start 5 mg PO every am, increase by 5 mg/day each week. Age older than 12 yo: Start 10 mg PO every am, increase by 10 mg/day each week. Usual dose range 5 to 60 mg/day in divided doses (tabs) or daily (extended-release). ADHD: 2.5 to 5 mg PO every am, usual max 40 mg/day. Avoid evening doses. Monitor growth and use drug holidays when appropriate. [Generic/Trade: Caps, extended-release 5, 10, 15 mg. Tabs 5, 10 mg. Oral soln 5 mg/5mL. Trade only: Tabs 2.5, 7.5 mg (Zenzedi)] ▶L ♀C ▶– ⊚II $$$$$

GUANFACINE (***Intuniv***) Start 1 mg PO once daily. Increase by 1 mg/week to max 7 mg/day based on weight. Refer to package insert. [Generic/Trade: Tabs, extended-release 1, 2, 3, 4 mg.] ▶LK – ♀B ▶?

LISDEXAMFETAMINE (***Vyvanse***) ADHD: Adults, adolescents, and children ages 6 yo and older: Start 30 mg PO every am. May increase weekly by 10 to 20 mg/day to max 70 mg/day. Avoid evening doses. Monitor growth and use drug holidays when appropriate. Binge eating disorder, mild to moderate: Start 30

(cont.)

mg PO once daily. May increase weekly by 20 mg/day to suggested range of 50 mg to 70 mg daily. Max 70 mg/day. [Trade: Caps 20, 30, 40, 50, 60, 70 mg.] ▶L ♀C ▶— ⊙II $$$$

METHYLPHENIDATE (*Aptensio XR, Ritalin, Ritalin LA, Ritalin SR, Methylin, Methylin ER, Metadate ER, Metadate CD, Concerta, Daytrana, Quillivant XR, ✦Biphentin*) ADHD/narcolepsy: 5 to 10 mg PO two to three times per day or 20 mg PO every am (sustained- and extended-release), max 60 mg/day. Or 18 to 36 mg PO every am (Concerta), max 72 mg/day. Extended-release (Aptensio XR): Start 10 mg PO once daily in the morning. May increase by 10 mg/day to max 60 mg/day. ADHD: Sustained-release suspension (6 yo and older): Start 20 mg PO in the morning. May increase weekly by 10 to 20 mg daily to max 60 mg/day. Avoid evening doses. Monitor growth and use drug holidays when appropriate. [Trade only: Tabs, extended-release 10, 20 mg (Methylin ER, Metadate ER). Tabs sustained-release 20 mg (Ritalin SR). Transdermal patch (Daytrana) 10 mg/9 h, 15 mg/9 h, 20 mg/9 h, 30 mg/9 h. Susp, extended-release 5 mg/mL (Quillivant XR). Generic/Trade: Tabs, chewable 2.5, 5, 10 mg (Methylin). Tabs, 5, 10, 20 mg (Ritalin). Tabs, extended-release 18, 27, 36, 54 mg (Concerta). Caps, extended-release 10, 20, 30, 40, 50, 60 mg (Metadate CD) may be sprinkled on food. Caps, extended-release 10, 20, 30, 40 mg (Ritalin LA). Caps, extended-release (Aptensio XR) 10, 15, 20, 30, 40, 50, 60 mg. Oral soln 5 mg/5 mL, 10 mg/5 mL. Generic only: Tabs 5, 10, 20 mg. Tabs, extended-release 10, 20 mg; tabs, sustained-release 20 mg.] ▶LK ♀C ▶? ⊙II $$

MODAFINIL (*Provigil, ✦Alertec*) Narcolepsy and sleep apnea/hypopnea: 200 mg PO q am. Shift work sleep disorder: 200 mg PO 1 h before shift. [Generic/Trade: Tabs 100, 200 mg.] ▶L ♀C ▶? ⊙II $$$$$

PHENTERMINE (*Adipex-P, Suprenza*) 15 mg to 37.5 mg/day every am before or 1 to 2 h after breakfast. Alternatively 18.75 mg PO two times daily. Avoid late evening dosing. For short-term use. [Generic/Trade: Caps 15, 30, 37.5 mg. Tabs 37.5 mg. Trade only: Orally disintegrating tables (Suprenza) 15, 30, 37.5 mg. Generic only: Caps, extended-release 15, 30 mg.] ▶KL ♀C ▶— ⊙IV $

PULMONARY

INHALER COLORS (Body then cap—Generics may differ)

Inhaler	Colors
Advair	purple
Advair HFA	purple/light purple
Aerobid-M	grey/green
Aerospan	purple/grey
Alupent	clear/blue
Alvesco 80 mcg 160 mcg	brown/red red/red
Asmanex	white/pink
Atrovent HFA	clear/green
Combivent	clear/orange
Flovent HFA	orange/peach
Foradil	grey/beige
Maxair Autohaler	white/white
ProAir HFA	red/white
Proventil HFA	yellow/orange
Pulmicort	white/brown
QVAR 40 mcg 80 mcg	beige/grey mauve/grey
Serevent Diskus	green
Spiriva	grey
Ventolin HFA	light blue/navy
Xopenex HFA	blue/red

PULMONARY

INHALED STEROIDS: ESTIMATED COMPARATIVE DAILY DOSES*

Adults and Children older than 12 yo				
Drug	Form	Low dose	Medium dose	High dose
beclomethasone HFA MDI	40 mcg/puff 80 mcg/puff	2–6 puffs/day 1–3 puffs/day	6–12 puffs/day 3–6 puffs/day	> 12 puffs/day > 6 puffs/day
budesonide DPI	90 mcg/dose 180 mcg/dose	2–6 inhalations/day 1–3 inhalations/day	6–13 inhalations/day 3–7 inhalations/day	> 13 inhalations/day > 7 inhalations/day
budesonide	soln for nebs	—	—	—
flunisolide HFA MDI	80 mcg/puff	4 puffs/day	5–8 puffs/day	> 8 puffs/day
fluticasone HFA MDI	44 mcg/puff 110 mcg/puff 220 mcg/puff	2–6 puffs/day 1–2 puffs/day 1 puff/day	6–10 puffs/day 2–4 puffs/day 1–2 puffs/day	> 10 puffs/day > 4 puffs/day > 2 puffs/day
fluticasone DPI	50 mcg/dose 100 mcg/dose 250 mcg/dose	2–6 inhalations/day 1–3 inhalations/day 1 inhalation/day	6–10 inhalations/day 3–5 inhalations/day 2 inhalations/day	> 10 inhalations/day > 5 inhalations/day > 2 inhalations/day
mometasone DPI	220 mcg/dose	1 inhalation/day	2 inhalations/day	> 2 inhalations/day

CHILDREN (age 5 to 11 yo)				
Drug	Form	Low dose	Medium dose	High dose
beclomethasone HFA MDI	40 mcg/puff 80 mcg/puff	2–4 puffs/day 1–2 puffs/day	4–8 puffs/day 2–4 puffs/day	> 8 puffs/day > 4 puffs/day
budesonide DPI	90 mcg/dose 180 mcg/dose	2–4 inhalations/day 1–2 inhalations/day	4–9 inhalations/day 2–4 inhalations/day	> 9 inhalations/day > 4 inhalations/day
budesonide	soln for nebs	0.5 mg 0.25–0.5 mg (0–4 yo)	1 mg > 0.5–1 mg (0–4 yo)	2 mg > 1 mg (0–4 yo)
flunisolide HFA MDI	80 mcg/puff	2 puffs/day	4 puffs/day	≥ 8 puffs/day
fluticasone HFA MDI (0–11 yo)	44 mcg/puff 110 mcg/puff 220 mcg/puff	2–4 puffs/day 1–2 puff/day n/a	4–8 puffs/day 2–3 puffs/day 1–2 puffs/day	> 8 puffs/day > 4 puffs/day > 2 puffs/day
fluticasone DPI	50 mcg/dose 100 mcg/dose 250 mcg/dose	2–4 inhalations/day 1–2 inhalations/day n/a	4–8 inhalations/day 2–4 inhalations/day 1 inhalation/day	> 8 inhalations/day > 4 inhalations/day > 1 inhalation/day
mometasone DPI	220 mcg/dose	n/a	n/a	n/a

http://www.nhlbi.nih.gov/guidelines/asthma/asthsumm.pdf

*HFA = Hydrofluoroalkane (propellant). MDI = metered dose inhaler. DPI = dry powder inhaler.

PREDICTED PEAK EXPIRATORY FLOW (liters/min)

Age (yo)	Women (height in inches)					Men (height in inches)					Child (height in inches)
	55"	60"	65"	70"	75"	60"	65"	70"	75"	80"	
20	390	423	460	496	529	554	602	649	693	740	44–160"
30	380	413	448	483	516	532	577	622	664	710	46–187"
40	370	402	436	470	502	509	552	596	636	680	48–214"
50	360	391	424	457	488	486	527	569	607	649	50–240"
60	350	380	412	445	475	463	502	542	578	618	52–267"
70	340	369	400	432	461	440	477	515	550	587	54–293"

Am Rev Resp Dis 1963;88:644.

Beta Agonists—Long-Acting

ARFORMOTEROL (*Brovana*) COPD: 15 mcg nebulized two times per day. [Trade only: Soln for inhalation 15 mcg in 2 mL vial.] ▶L ♀C ▷? $$$$$ ■

FORMOTEROL (*Foradil, Perforomist, ✦Oxeze Turbuhaler*) 1 puff two times per day. Nebulized: 20 mcg q 12 h. Not for acute bronchospasm. For asthma, use only in combination with corticosteroids. [Trade only: DPI 12 mcg, 12, 60 blisters/pack (Foradil). To be used only with Aerolizer device. Soln for inhalation: 20 mcg in 2 mL vial (Perforomist). Canada only (Oxeze): DPI 6, 12 mcg 60 blisters/pack.] ▶L ♀C ▷? $$$ ■

INDACATEROL (*Arcapta, ✦Onbrez Breezhaler*) COPD: DPI: 75 mcg inhaled once daily. [Trade only: DPI: 75 mcg caps for inhalation, 30 blisters. To be used only with Neohaler device. Contains lactose.] ▶L – ♀C ▷? ■

OLODATEROL (*Striverdi Respimat*) COPD: 2 inhalations once daily. [Trade only: Carton with canister containing 28 or 60 metered actuations for use with provided Striverdi Respimat device. Each actuation delivers 2.5 mcg olodaterol.] ▶LK ♀C ▷? ■

SALMETEROL (*Serevent Diskus*) 1 puff two times per day. Not for acute bronchospasm. For asthma, use only in combination with corticosteroids. [Trade only: DPI (Diskus): 50 mcg, 60 blisters.] ▶L ♀C ▷? $$$$ ■

Beta Agonists—Short-Acting

ALBUTEROL (*ProAir RespiClick, AccuNeb, Ventolin HFA, Proventil HFA, ProAir HFA, VoSpire ER, ✦Airomir, salbutamol, Apo-Salvent*) MDI: 2 puffs q 4 to 6 h prn. Soln: 0.5 mL of 0.5% soln (2.5 mg) nebulized three to four times per day. One 3 mL unit dose (0.083%) nebulized three to four times per day. Caps for

(cont.)

PULMONARY

inhalation: 200 to 400 mcg q 4 to 6 h. Tabs: 2 to 4 mg PO three to four times per day or extended-release 4 to 8 mg PO q 12 h up to 16 mg PO q 12 h. Peds: 0.1 to 0.2 mg/kg/dose PO three times per day up to 4 mg three times per day for age 2 to 5 yo, 2 to 4 mg or extended-release 4 mg PO q 12 h for age 6 to 12 yo. Prevention of exercise-induced bronchospasm: MDI: 2 puffs 10 to 30 min before exercise. [Trade only: MDI 90 mcg/actuation, 200 metered doses/canister. "HFA" inhalers use hydrofluoroalkane propellant instead of CFCs but are otherwise equivalent. "RespiClick" is a breath-actuated dry powder inhaler. Generic/Trade: Soln for inhalation 0.021% (AccuNeb), 0.042% (AccuNeb), and 0.083% in 3 mL vials, 0.5% (5 mg/mL) in 20 mL with dropper. Tabs, extended-release 4, 8 mg (VoSpire ER). Generic only: Syrup 2 mg/5 mL. Tabs, immediate-release 2, 4 mg.] ▶L ♀C ▷? $$

LEVALBUTEROL (*Xopenex Concentrate, Xopenex, Xopenex HFA*) MDI 2 puffs q 4 to 6 h prn. Nebulizer 0.63 to 1.25 mg q 6 to 8 h. Peds: 0.31 mg nebulized three times per day for age 6 to 11 yo. [Generic/Trade: Soln for inhalation 0.31, 0.63, 1.25 mg in 3 mL and 1.25 mg in 0.5 mL unit-dose vials. Trade only: HFA MDI 45 mcg/actuation, 15 g 200/canister. "HFA" inhalers use hydrofluoroalkane propellant.] ▶L ♀C ▷? $$$

METAPROTERENOL (*Alupent, ◆orciprenaline*) MDI: 2 to 3 puffs q 3 to 4 h. Soln: 0.2 to 0.3 mL 5% soln nebulized q 4 h. Peds: Tabs: 20 mg PO three to four times per day age older than 9 yo, 10 mg PO three to four times per day if age 6 to 9 yo, 1.3 to 2.6 mg/kg/day divided three to four times per day if age 2 to 5 yo. [Trade only: MDI 0.65 mg/actuation, 14 g 200/canister. Generic/Trade: Soln for inhalation 0.4%, 0.6% in 2.5 mL unit-dose vials. Generic only: Syrup 10 mg/5 mL, Tabs 10, 20 mg.] ▶L ♀C ▷? $$

PIRBUTEROL (*Maxair Autohaler*) MDI: 1 to 2 puffs q 4 to 6 h. [Trade only: MDI 200 mcg/actuation, 14 g 400/canister.] ▶L ♀C ▷? $$$$

Combinations

ADVAIR (fluticasone—inhaled + salmeterol) Asthma: DPI: 1 puff two times per day (all strengths). MDI: 2 puffs two times per day (all strengths). COPD: DPI: 1 puff two times per day (250/50 only). [Trade only: DPI: 100/50, 250/50, 500/50 mcg fluticasone/salmeterol per actuation; 60 doses/DPI. Trade only (Advair HFA): MDI 45/21, 115/21, 230/21 mcg fluticasone/salmeterol per actuation; 120 doses/canister.] ▶L ♀C ▷? $$$$$ ■

BREO ELLIPTA (fluticasone—inhaled + vilanterol) Chronic asthma, COPD: 1 inhalation once daily. 200/25 mcg fluticasone/vilanterol strength only approved for asthma. [Trade only: DPI: 100/25 mcg, 200/25 mcg fluticasone/vilanterol per actuation; 30 doses/DPI.] ▶L – ♀C ▷? $$$$$ ■

COMBIVENT (albuterol—inhaled + ipratropium—inhaled, *Combivent Respimat*) MDI: 2 puffs four times per day, max 12 puffs/day. Contraindicated with soy or peanut allergy. Respimat: 1 inhalation four times per day, max 6 inhalations/day. [Trade only: MDI: 90 mcg albuterol/18 mcg ipratropium per actuation, 200/canister. Respimat: 100 mcg albuterol/20 mcg ipratropium per inhalation, 120/canister.] ▶L ♀C ▷? $$$$

DULERA **(mometasone—inhaled + formoterol, ✦*Zenhale*)** Chronic asthma: 2 puffs two times per day (all strengths). [Trade only: MDI 100/5, 200/5 mcg mometasone/formoterol per actuation, 120 doses/canister.] ▶L – ♀C ▶? $$$$$ ■

DUONEB **(albuterol—inhaled + ipratropium—inhaled, ✦*Combivent inhalation soln*)** 1 unit dose four times per day. [Generic/Trade: Unit dose: 2.5 mg albuterol/0.5 mg ipratropium per 3 mL vial, premixed; 30, 60 vials/carton.] ▶L ♀C ▶? $$$$$

SYMBICORT **(budesonide—inhaled + formoterol, ✦*Symbicort Turbuhaler*)** Asthma: 2 puffs two times per day (both strengths). COPD: 2 puffs two times per day (160/4.5). [Trade only: MDI: 80/4.5, 160/4.5 mcg budesonide/formoterol per actuation; 120 doses/canister.] ▶L ♀C ▶? $$$$ ■

Inhaled Steroids

NOTE: *See Endocrine-Corticosteroids when oral steroids necessary.*

BECLOMETHASONE—INHALED (*QVAR*) 1 to 4 puffs two times per day (40 mcg). 1 to 2 puffs two times per day (80 mcg). [Trade only: HFA MDI: 40, 80 mcg/actuation, 7.3 g 100 actuations/canister.] ▶L ♀C ▶? $$$

BUDESONIDE—INHALED (*Pulmicort Respules, Pulmicort Flexhaler, ✦Pulmicort Turbuhaler*) 1 to 2 puffs daily up to 4 puffs two times per day. Respules: 0.5 to 1 mg daily or divided two times per day. [Trade only: DPI (Flexhaler) 90, 180 mcg powder/actuation 60, 120 doses/canister, repsectively. Respules 1 mg/2 mL unit dose. Generic/Trade: Respules 0.25, 0.5 mg/2 mL unit dose.] ▶L ♀B ▶? $$$$

CICLESONIDE—INHALED (*Alvesco*) 80 mcg/puff: 1 to 4 puffs two times per day. 160 mcg/puff: 1 to 2 puffs two times per day. [Trade only: 80 mcg/actuation, 60 per canister. 160 mcg/actuation, 60, 120 per canister.] ▶L ♀C ▶? $$$$

FLUNISOLIDE—INHALED (*AeroBid, AeroBid-M, Aerospan*) 2 to 4 puffs two times per day. [Trade only: MDI: 250 mcg/actuation, 100 metered doses/canister. AeroBid-M (AeroBid + menthol flavor). Aerospan HFA MDI: 80 mcg/actuation, 60, 120 metered doses/canister.] ▶L ♀C ▶? $$$

FLUTICASONE FUROATE (*Arnuity Ellipta*) Chronic asthma: 1 inhalation once daily. [Trade only: Foil strip with 30 blisters each containing 100 or 200 mcg fluticasone furoate for use with Ellipta DPI device.] ▶L ♀C ▶?

FLUTICASONE—INHALED (*Arnuity Ellipta, Flovent HFA, Flovent Diskus*) 2 to 4 puffs two times per day. [Trade only: HFA MDI: 44, 110, 220 mcg/actuation 120/canister. DPI (Diskus): 50, 100, 250 mcg/actuation delivering 44, 88, 220 mcg respectively.] ▶L ♀C ▶? $$$$

MOMETASONE—INHALED (*Asmanex HFA, Asmanex Twisthaler*) 1 to 2 puffs in the evening or 1 puff two times per day. If prior oral corticosteroid therapy: 2 puffs two times per day. [Trade only: DPI: 110 mcg/actuation with #30 dosage units, 220 mcg/actuation with #30, 60, 120 dosage units.] ▶L ♀C ▶? $$$$

TRIAMCINOLONE—INHALED (*Azmacort*) 2 puffs three to four times per day or 4 puffs two times per day; max dose 16 puffs/day. [Trade only: MDI: 75 mcg/actuation, 240/canister. Built-in spacer.] ▶L ♀C ▶? $$$$

Leukotriene Inhibitors

MONTELUKAST (*Singulair*) Adults: 10 mg PO daily in the evening. Chronic asthma, allergic rhinitis: Give 4 mg (chew tab or oral granules) PO daily for age 2 to 5 yo, give 5 mg PO daily for age 6 to 14 yo. Asthma: Age 12 to 23 mo: 4 mg (oral granules) PO daily. Allergic rhinitis: Age 6 to 23 mo: 4 mg (oral granules) PO daily. Prevention of exercise-induced bronchoconstriction: 10 mg PO 2 h before exercise. [Generic/Trade only: Tabs 10 mg. Oral granules 4 mg packet, 30/box. Chewable tabs (cherry flavored) 4, 5 mg.] ▶L ♀B ▶? $$$$

ZAFIRLUKAST (*Accolate*) 20 mg PO two times per day. Peds age 5 to 11 yo, 10 mg PO two times per day. Take at least 1 h before or 2 h after meals. Potentiates warfarin and theophylline. [Trade only: Tabs 10, 20 mg.] ▶L ♀B ▶− − $$$$

ZILEUTON (*Zyflo CR*) 1200 mg PO two times per day. Take within 1 h after morning and evening meals. Hepatotoxicity, potentiates warfarin, theophylline, and propranolol. [Trade only: Tabs, extended-release 600 mg.] ▶L ♀C ▶? $$$$$

Other Pulmonary Medications

ACETYLCYSTEINE—INHALED (*Mucomyst*) Mucolytic: 3 to 5 mL of 20% or 6 to 10 mL of 10% soln nebulized three to four times per day. [Generic/Trade: Soln for inhalation 10, 20% in 4, 10, 30 mL vials.] ▶L ♀B ▶? $

ACLIDINIUM (*Tudorza Pressair*, ✦*Turdoza Genuair*) COPD: Pressair: 400 mcg two times per day. [Trade only: Sealed aluminum pouches 400 mcg per actuation. To be used with "Pressair" device only. Packages of 60 with Pressair device.] ▶L − ♀C ▶? $$$$$

CROMOLYN—INHALED (*Intal, Gastrocrom*, ✦*Nalcrom*) Asthma: 2 to 4 puffs four times per day or 20 mg nebs four times per day. Prevention of exercise-induced bronchospasm: 2 puffs 10 to 15 min prior to exercise. Mastocytosis: Oral concentrate 100 mg four times per day in children 2 to 12 yo, 200 mg PO four times per day for adults. [Generic only: Soln for nebs: 20 mg/2 mL. Generic/Trade: Oral concentrate 100 mg/5 mL in individual amps.] ▶LK ♀B ▶? $

DORNASE ALFA (*Pulmozyme*) Cystic fibrosis: 2.5 mg nebulized one to two times per day. [Trade only: Soln for inhalation: 1 mg/mL in 2.5 mL vials.] ▶L ♀B ▶? $$$$$

EPINEPHRINE RACEMIC (*S-2*, ✦*Vaponefrin*) Severe croup: 0.05 mL/kg/dose diluted to 3 mL w/NS. Max dose 0.5 mL. [Trade only: Soln for inhalation: 2.25% epinephrine in 15, 30 mL.] ▶plasma ♀C ▶− $

IPRATROPIUM—INHALED (*Atrovent, Atrovent HFA*) 2 puffs four times per day, or one 500 mcg vial neb three to four times per day. Contraindicated with soy or peanut allergy (Atrovent MDI only). [Trade only: Atrovent HFA MDI: 17 mcg/ actuation, 200/canister. Generic/Trade: Soln for nebulization: 0.02% (500 mcg/ vial) in unit dose vials.] ▶Lung ♀B ▶? $$$$

KETOTIFEN (✦*Zaditen*) Canada only. For age 6 mo to 3 yo: Give 0.05 mg/kg PO two times per day. Age older than 3 yo: Give 1 mg PO two times per day. [Generic/ Trade: Tabs 1 mg. Syrup 1 mg/5 mL.] ▶L ♀C ▶? $$

NINTEDANIB (*Ofev*) Idiopathic pulmonary fibrosis: 150 mg twice daily 12 h apart with food. [Trade only: Caps: 100, 150 mg.] ▶L ♀D ▶?

PIRFENIDONE (*Esbriet*) Idiopathic pulmonary fibrosis: 267 mg three times a day for 7 days, then 534 mg three times a day for 7 days, then 801 mg three times a day thereafter. Should be taken with meals. [Trade only: Caps 267 mg.] ▶LK ♀C ▶?

ROFLUMILAST (*Daliresp, ✦Daxas*) Severe COPD due to chronic bronchitis: 500 mcg PO daily with or without food. [Trade only: Tabs 500 mcg.] ▶L – ♀C ▶– $$$$$

THEOPHYLLINE (*Elixophyllin, Uniphyl, Theo-24, T-Phyl, ✦Theo-Dur, Theolair*) 5 to 13 mg/kg/day PO in divided doses. Max dose 900 mg/day. Peds dosing variable. [Generic/Trade: Elixir 80 mg/15 mL. Trade only: Caps: Theo-24: 100, 200, 300, 400 mg. T-Phyl: 12 h SR tabs 200 mg. Theolair: Tabs 125, 250 mg. Generic only: 12 h tabs 100, 200, 300, 450 mg, 12 h caps 125, 200, 300 mg.] ▶L ♀C ▶– $

TIOTROPIUM (*Spiriva HandiHaler, Spiriva Respimat, ✦Spiriva, Spiriva Respimat*) COPD: HandiHaler: 18 mcg inhaled daily. [Trade only: Caps for oral inhalation 18 mcg. To be used with "HandiHaler" device only. Packages of 5, 30, 90 caps with HandiHaler device.] ▶K ♀C ▶– $$$$

UMECLIDINIUM (*Incruse Ellipta*) COPD: 1 inhalation once daily. [Trade only: Foil blister strip with 30 blisters each containing 62.5 mcg for use with Ellipta device.] ▶L ♀C ▶?

PULMONARY

RHEUMATOLOGY

INITIAL TREATMENT OF RHEUMATOID ARTHRITIS (RA): AMERICAN COLLEGE OF RHEUMATOLOGY RECOMMENDATIONS

Disease activity	No poor prognostic factors*	Poor prognostic factors present*
Early disease (duration <6 months)		
Low	DMARD monotherapy†	DMARD monotherapy†
Moderate	DMARD monotherapy†	DMARD combination‡
High	DMARD monotherapy† OR MTX + HCQ	DMARD combination‡ OR TNF blocker ± MTX¶
Established disease (duration ≥6 months)		
Low	DMARD monotherapy†	MTX monotherapy OR DMARD combination‡
Moderate/High	MTX monotherapy OR DMARD combination‡	MTX monotherapy OR DMARD combination‡

Adapted from: Arthritis Care Res 2012;64:625–39. Available online at: http://www.rheumatology.org.

DMARD = disease-modifying anti-rheumatic drug; HCQ = hydroxychloroquine; LEF = leflunomide; MTX = methotrexate; TNF = tumor necrosis factor.

*Poor prognostic factors: Functional limitation; extra-articular disease (e.g. rheumatoid nodules; RA vasculitis; Felty's syndrome); positive rheumatoid factor or anti-cyclic citrullinated peptide antibodies; bony erosions by radiograph.

†DMARD monotherapy: HCQ, LEF, MTX, minocycline (usually only for early RA), or sulfasalazine. Reassess after 3 months of therapy.

‡DMARD combination: MTX + HCQ; MTX + LEF; MTX + sulfasalazine; sulfasalazine + HCQ; sulfasalazine + HCQ + MTX. Reassess after 3 months of therapy.

¶TNF blocker regimens include: adalimumab ± MTX; certolizumab ± MTX; etanercept ± MTX; golimumab ± MTX; infliximab ± MTX. Reassess after 3 months of therapy.

Biologic Response Modifiers—TNF-Blockers

NOTE: *TNF-blockers increase the risk of serious infections (e.g., TB, sepsis, invasive fungal, opportunistic infections); discontinue if serious infection. Test for latent TB, and treat if present, before starting a TNF-blocker. Monitor for signs and symptoms of active TB. Lymphoma and other malignancies have*

(cont.)

been reported in children and adolescents. Other adverse effects include new onset or exacerbation of demyelinating disorders and heart failure, reactivation of hepatitis B virus infection, a lupus-like syndrome, and serious hypersensitivity reactions. Avoid live vaccines. Do not coadminister with abatacept, anakinra, tofacitinib, or other biologic response modifiers. Refer to ACR RA guidelines (www.rheumatology.org) for advice on TB screening, vaccine administration, and other safety issues. Monitor CBC, hepatic transaminases, and serum creatinine.

ADALIMUMAB (*Humira*) RA, psoriatic arthritis, ankylosing spondylitis: 40 mg SC q 2 weeks, alone or in combination with methotrexate or other non-biologic DMARDs. May increase frequency to q week if not on methotrexate. Plaque psoriasis: 80 mg SC at week 0, 40 mg SC at week 1, then 40 mg SC q 2 weeks. Crohn's disease, ulcerative colitis: 160 mg SC at week 0, 80 mg at week 2, then 40 mg q 2 weeks starting at week 4. Peds. Polyarticular JIA, age 2 yo and older: 10 mg SC q 2 weeks for 10 to less than 15 kg; 20 mg SC q 2 weeks for 15 to less than 30 kg; 40 mg SC q 2 weeks for 30 kg and greater. Crohn's disease, age 6 yo and older. For wt 17 kg to less than 40 kg: 80 mg SC (two 40 mg injections) on day 1, then 40 mg SC 2 weeks later. Maintain with 20 mg SC q 2 weeks. For wt 40 kg and greater: 160 mg SC on day 1, then 80 mg SC (two 40 mg injections) 2 weeks later. Maintain with 40 mg SC q 2 weeks. Can give initial 160 mg dose as four 40 mg injections on day 1 or two 40 mg injections per day for 2 days. Inject SC into thigh or abdomen, rotating injection sites. [Trade only: Single-use injection pen or syringe (2 per pack): 40 mg/0.8 mL. Crohn's disease/ulcerative colitis starter pack: six 40 mg pens. Psoriasis starter pack: four 40 mg pens. Pediatric single-use syringe (2 per pack): 10 mg/0.2 mL, 20 mg/0.4 mL. Pediatric Crohn's disease starter pack: three or six 40 mL syringes.] ▶ proteolysis ♀B ▶? Caution advised, but no known risks $$$$$ ■

CERTOLIZUMAB (*Cimzia*) Crohn's disease: 400 mg SC at 0, 2, and 4 weeks. If response occurs, then 400 mg SC q 4 weeks. RA, psoriatic arthritis: 400 mg SC at 0, 2, and 4 weeks. Then maintain with 200 mg SC q 2 weeks; can consider 400 mg SC q 4 weeks. Ankylosing spondylitis: 400 mg at 0, 2, and 4 weeks, then 200 mg q 2 weeks or 400 mg q 4 weeks. Divide 400 mg dose into 2 separate 200 mg SC injections at different sites on thigh or abdomen. Rotate injection sites. [Trade only: Packs containing 2 vials for reconstitution or 2 prefilled syringes, 200 mg/1 mL each. Starter pack of 6 syringes.] ▶K proteolysis ♀B ▶? $$$$$ ■

ETANERCEPT (*Enbrel*) RA, psoriatic arthritis, ankylosing spondylitis: 50 mg SC q week. Plaque psoriasis: 50 mg SC 2 times per week for 3 months, then 50 mg SC q week. JIA, age 2 yo and older: 0.8 mg/kg SC q week for wt less than 63 kg; 50 mg SC for wt of 63 kg or greater. Inject into thigh, abdomen, or outer upper arm. Rotate injection sites. [Trade only: Single-use prefilled syringe or autoinjector 50 mg/1 mL. Single-use prefilled syringe 25 mg/0.5 mL. Multidose vial 25 mg.] ▶proteolysis ♀B ▶? $$$$$ ■

GOLIMUMAB (*Simponi, Simponi Aria*) RA, psoriatic arthritis, ankylosing spondylitis: 50 mg SC q month. IV regimen (Simponi Aria) for RA: 2 mg/kg IV infused over 30 minutes at weeks 0 and 4, then q 8 weeks thereafter. Use IV/SC golimumab with

(cont.)

methotrexate to treat RA. Ulcerative colitis: 200 mg SC at week 0, 100 mg SC at week 2, then 100 mg SC q 4 weeks. Give SC injection in thigh, abdomen, or upper outer arm. Rotate injection sites. Give at separate sites if a dose requires more than 1 injection. [Trade only: Single-dose autoinjector or prefilled syringe: 50 mg/0.5 mL, 100 mg/1 mL.] ▶? ♀B ▶− $$$$$ ■

INFLIXIMAB (*Remicade*) RA, with methotrexate: 3 mg/kg IV at weeks 0, 2, and 6 and q 8 weeks thereafter. Ankylosing spondylitis: 5 mg/kg IV at weeks 0, 2, and 6 and q 6 weeks thereafter. Plaque psoriasis, psoriatic arthritis, Crohn's disease, ulcerative colitis: 5 mg/kg IV at weeks 0, 2, and 6, and q 8 weeks thereafter. Peds, ulcerative colitis, Crohn's disease, age 6 yo or older: 5 mg/kg IV at weeks 0, 2, and 6, and q 8 weeks thereafter. Infuse over 2 h or more. ▶proteolysis ♀B ▶? $$$$$ ■

Biologic Response Modifiers—Other

ABATACEPT (*Orencia*, ✦*Orencia*) RA: IV regimen: Infuse IV over 30 minutes with wt-based doses of 500 mg for wt less than 60 kg, 750 mg for 60 to 100 kg, 1000 mg for greater than 100 kg. Give additional IV doses at weeks 2 and 4, and q 4 weeks thereafter. SC regimen: 125 mg SC q week with or without initial IV dose. If patient receives 1st dose IV, give 1st SC dose within 1 day of IV infusion. Give SC in thigh, abdomen, or upper outer arm. Rotate injection sites. Peds. JIA, age 6 yo or older: 10 mg/kg IV infused over 30 minutes. Give additional IV doses at weeks 2 and 4, and q 4 weeks thereafter. Use adult dose if weight 75 kg or greater (max 1000 mg per IV dose). [Trade only: Prefilled single-dose syringe 125 mg/1 mL.] ▶serum ♀C ▶− $$$$$

ANAKINRA (*Kineret*) RA: 100 mg SC daily, alone or in combination with non-biologic DMARDs. JIA: Initial dose of 1 to 2 mg/kg (max 100 mg) SC once daily. Inject SC into thigh, abdomen, outer upper arm, or upper outer area of buttocks. Rotate injection sites. [Trade only: Prefilled graduated syringe 100 mg/0.67 mL.] ▶K ♀B ▶? $$$$$

CANAKINUMAB (*Ilaris*) Systemic JIA, age 2 yo and older and wt 7.5 kg and greater: 4 mg/kg (max dose of 300 mg) SC q 4 weeks. Cryopyrin-associated periodic syndromes. Adults and children with wt greater than 40 kg: 150 mg SC q 8 weeks. For children age 4 yo and older and wt 15 to 40 kg: 2 mg/kg SC q 8 weeks, increasing to 3 mg/kg q 8 weeks if inadequate response. ▶? ♀C ▶? $$$$$

RITUXIMAB (*Rituxan*) RA, with methotrexate: 1000 mg IV infusion weekly for 2 doses q 24 weeks. Give methylprednisolone 100 mg IV 30 minutes before infusion. Granulomatosis with polyangiitis (Wegener's), microscopic polyangiitis, with corticosteroids: 375 mg/m^2 q week for 4 weeks. Non-Hodgkin's lymphoma, chronic lymphocytic leukemia: Doses vary by indication. Can cause life-threatening infusion reactions. Premedicate with acetaminophen and antihistamine. ▶? ♀C ▶− $$$$$

SECUKINUMAB (*Cosentyx*) Plaque psoriasis: 300 mg SC weekly for 5 weeks, then 300 mg SC q 4 weeks. Each 300 mg dose is two SC 150 mg injections at different sites. A dose of 150 mg may be adequate for some patients. [Trade only: 150 mg/mL prefilled syringe or pen. 150 mg vial for reconstitution by healthcare provider.] ▶proteolysis ♀B ▶? $$$$$

TOCILIZUMAB (*Actemra*) RA, moderate to severe: 162 mg SC q 2 weeks titrated to q week based on clinical response for wt less than 100 kg; 162 mg SC q week for wt 100 kg or greater. RA, IV regimen: 4 mg/kg IV q 4 weeks, increasing to 8 mg/kg IV q 4 weeks based on clinical response (max dose of 800 mg per infusion). Polyarticular JIA, age 2 yo or older: 10 mg/kg IV q 4 weeks for wt less than 30 kg; 8 mg/kg q 4 weeks for wt 30 kg or greater. Systemic JIA, age 2 yo or older: 12 mg/kg q 2 weeks for wt less than 30 kg; 8 mg/kg q 2 weeks for 30 kg or greater. IV infused over 1 h. [Trade only: 162 mg/0.9 mL prefilled single-use syringe.] ▶?
♀C ▶– $$$$$ ■

TOFACITINIB (*Xeljanz*) RA: 5 mg PO two times per day. Reduce to 5 mg PO once daily if given with fluconazole, strong CYP3A4 inhibitor, or combination of moderate CYP3A4 inhibitor and strong CYP2C19 inhibitor (see P450 isozyme table). Dosage adjustments for lymphopenia, neutropenia, and anemia in product labeling. Indicated for moderate to severe RA with inadequate response or intolerance to methotrexate. For use as monotherapy or in combination with methotrexate or another nonbiologic DMARD. [Trade only: Tabs 5 mg.] ▶LK
♀C ▶– $$$$$ ■

Disease-Modifying Antirheumatic Drugs (DMARDs)

AZATHIOPRINE (*Azasan, Imuran, AZA*) RA: Initial dose 1 mg/kg (50 to 100 mg) PO daily or divided two times per day. Increase after 6 to 8 weeks. Prevention of rejection after renal transplant: Individualized dosing. Azathioprine dosage reduction required if allopurinol coadministered. [Generic/Trade: Tabs 50 mg, scored. Trade only (Azasan): 75, 100 mg, scored.] ▶LK ♀D ▶– $$$ ■

HYDROXYCHLOROQUINE (*Plaquenil, HCQ*) RA: Start 400 to 600 mg PO daily, then taper to 200 to 400 mg daily. SLE: 400 PO one to two times per day to start, then taper to 200 to 400 mg daily. Take with food or milk to improve GI tolerability. [Generic/Trade: Tabs 200 mg hydroxychloroquine sulfate (200 mg sulfate equivalent to 155 mg base), scored.] ▶K ♀C ▶+ $ ■

LEFLUNOMIDE (*LEF, Arava*) RA: Loading dose: 100 mg PO daily for 3 days. Maintenance dose: 10 to 20 mg PO daily. [Generic/Trade: Tabs 10, 20 mg. Trade only: Tabs 100 mg.] ▶LK ♀X ▶– $$$$$ ■

METHOTREXATE—RHEUMATOLOGY (*Otrexup, Rasuvo, Rheumatrex, Trexall, MTX*) Severe RA: Initial dose of 7.5 mg PO/SC once weekly. Alternative regimen: 2.5 mg PO q 12 h for 3 doses given as a course once weekly. May increase dose gradually to max of 20 mg/week. After clinical response, reduce to lowest effective dose. Severe psoriasis: 10 to 25 mg PO/SC/IV/IM once weekly until response, then decrease to lowest effective dose. Max usual dose is 30 mg/week. Supplement with 1 mg/day of folic acid. Severe JIA: 10 mg/m² PO/SC q week. When converting between PO and SC administration, consider that SC administration has higher bioavailability. Give SC injection in abdomen or thigh. [Trade only (Trexall): Tabs 5, 7.5, 10, 15 mg. Dose Pak (Rheumatrex) 2.5 mg (# 8, 12, 16, 20, 24). Generic/Trade: Tabs 2.5 mg, scored. Trade only: Single-dose SC auto-injectors. Otrexup: 10, 15, 20, 25 mg/0.4 mL. Rasuvo: 7.5, 10, 12.5, 15, 17.5, 20, 22.5, 25, 27.5, 30 mg (volume ranges from 0.15 to 0.6 mL).)]
▶LK ♀X ▶– $$ ■

SULFASALAZINE—RHEUMATOLOGY (*Azulfidine, Azulfidine EN-tabs, ✦Salazopyrin EN-tabs*) RA: 500 mg PO two times per day after meals up to 1 g PO two times per day. May turn body fluids, contact lenses, or skin orange-yellow. [Generic/Trade: Tabs 500 mg, scored. Enteric-coated, delayed-release (EN-tabs) 500 mg.] ▶L ♀B ▷? $$

COLCHICINE: DOSAGE REDUCTIONS FOR COADMINISTRATION WITH INHIBITORS OF COLCHICINE METABOLISM

Usual colchicine dose	Colchicine dosage reduction for...		
	Strong CYP3A4 inhibitors*	Moderate CYP3A4 inhibitors†	P-glycoprotein inhibitors‡
Prevention of gout flares: 0.6 mg PO two times per day	0.3 mg PO once daily	0.3 mg PO two times per day or 0.6 mg PO once daily	0.3 mg PO once daily
Prevention of gout flares: 0.6 mg PO once daily	0.3 mg PO once every other day	0.3 mg PO once daily	0.3 mg PO once every other day
Treatment of gout flares: 1.2 mg PO followed by 0.6 mg 1 hour later	0.6 mg PO followed by 0.3 mg 1 hour later	1.2 mg PO in a single dose	0.6 mg PO in a single dose
Familial Mediterranean Fever: Up to 1.2 to 2.4 mg/day PO	Up to 0.6 mg/day PO (can be given as 0.3 mg two times per day)	Up to 1.2 mg/day PO (can be given as 0.6 mg two times per day)	Up to 0.6 mg/day PO (can be given as 0.3 mg two times per day)

Notes: Do not give colchicine to patients with renal or hepatic impairment who are taking a strong CYP3A4 or P-glycoprotein inhibitor. Do not treat gout flares with colchicine in patients already receiving colchicine for prevention of gout flares and who are also receiving a CYP3A4 inhibitor. Dosage reductions of colchicine are recommended for patients who are currently taking or have discontinued a CYP3A4 or P-glycoprotein inhibitor within the past 14 days. Be aware that this table may not list all possible CYP3A4 and P-glycoprotein inhibitors that increase the risk of colchicine toxicity via inhibition of colchicine metabolism.

* **Strong CYP 3A4 inhibitors:** atazanavir, boceprevir, clarithromycin, cobicistat (alone or in Stribild), conivaptan, darunavir-ritonavir, fosamprenavir-ritonavir, indinavir, itraconazole, ketoconazole, lopinavir-ritonavir, nefazodone, nelfinavir, posaconazole, ritonavir, saquinavir-ritonavir, telithromycin, tipranavir-ritonavir, voriconazole.

†**Moderate CYP 3A4 inhibitors:** aprepitant, ciprofloxacin, crizotinib, diltiazem, dronedarone, erythromycin, fluconazole, fosamprenavir (unboosted), grapefruit juice, imatinib, isavuconazole, netupitant (in Akynzeo), verapamil.

‡**P-glycoprotein inhibitors:** cyclosporine, ranolazine.

RHEUMATOLOGY

Gout-Related—Other

COLCHICINE (*Colcrys, Mitigare*) Treatment of gout flares: 1.2 mg PO at signs of attack then 0.6 mg 1 h after initial administration. Do not repeat this regimen earlier than 3 days. Prevention of gout flares: 0.6 mg PO one or two times per day. Max dose of 1.2 mg/day. Familial Mediterranean fever: 1.2 to 2.4 mg PO daily or divided two times per day. See table for dosage reductions when given with strong/moderate CYP3A4 inhibitors or P-glycoprotein inhibitors. [Trade only: Tabs 0.6 mg (Colcrys). Caps 0.6 mg (Mitigare).] ▶L ♀C ▶? $$$$

COLCHICINE + PROBENECID Gout: 1 tab PO daily for 1 week, then 1 tab two times per day. [Generic only: Tabs 0.5 mg colchicine + 500 mg probenecid.] ▶KL ♀C ▶? $

PEGLOTICASE (*Krystexxa*) Chronic gout (refractory): 8 mg IV infusion q 2 weeks. ▶? ♀C ▶? $$$$$ ■

PROBENECID Gout: 250 mg PO two times per day for 7 days, then 500 mg PO two times per day. Adjunct to penicillin/cephalosporin: 1 g PO single dose to 500 mg PO four times per day. [Generic only: Tabs 500 mg.] ▶KL ♀B ▶? $

Gout-Related—Xanthine Oxidase Inhibitors

ALLOPURINOL (*Aloprim, Zyloprim*) Prevention of recurrent gout: 100 mg PO daily initially, titrating upward q 1 to 5 weeks to achieve target serum urate level (usually <6 mg/dL, but may be <5 mg/dL). For CrCl less than 30 mL/min: initial dose is 50 mg/day. Maximum dose is 800 mg/day. Divide doses greater than 300 mg/day. To improve tolerability, take PO allopurinol after meals. [Generic/Trade: Tabs 100, 300 mg.] ▶K ♀C ▶+ $

FEBUXOSTAT (*Uloric*) Hyperuricemia with gout: Start 40 mg PO daily, max 80 mg daily. [Trade only: Tabs 40, 80 mg.] ▶LK ♀C ▶? $$$$

Rheumatology—Other

APREMILAST (*Otezla*) Psoriatic arthritis, moderate to severe plaque psoriasis: Give PO 10 mg in am on day 1, 10 mg two times per day on day 2, 10 mg in am and 20 mg in pm on day 3, 20 mg two times per day on day 4, 20 mg in am and 30 mg in pm on day 5, 30 mg two times per day on day 6 and thereafter. Do not crush, split, or chew tabs. [Trade only: Tabs 30 mg. Two-week starter pack of 10, 20, and 30 mg tabs.] ▶L ♀C ▶? $$$$$

TOXICOLOGY

ANTIDOTES

Toxin	Antidote/Treatment
acetaminophen	N-acetylcysteine
TCAs	sodium bicarbonate
arsenic, mercury	dimercprol (BAL)
benzodiazepine	flumazenil
beta-blockers	glucagon
calcium channel blockers	calcium chloride, glucagon
cyanide	cyanide antidote kit, Cyanokit (hydroxocobalamin)
digoxin	dig immune Fab
ethylene glycol	fomepizole
heparin	protamine
iron	deferoxamine
lead	BAL, EDTA, succimer
methanol	fomepizole
methemoglobin	methylene blue
opioids/opiates	naloxone
organophosphates	atropine + pralidoxime
warfarin	vitamin K, FFP

ACETYLCYSTEINE (*N-acetylcysteine, Mucomyst, Acetadote, ✦Parvolex*) Contrast nephropathy prophylaxis: 600 mg PO two times per day on the day before and on the day of contrast. Acetaminophen toxicity: Mucomyst (Oral): Loading dose 140 mg/kg PO or NG, then 70 mg/kg q 4 h for 17 doses. May be mixed in water or soft drink diluted to a 5% soln. Acetadote (IV): Loading dose 150 mg/kg in 200 mL of D5W infused over 60 min; maintenance dose 50 mg/kg in 500 mL of D5W infused over 4 h followed by 100 mg/kg in 1000 mL of D5W infused over 16 h. [Generic/Trade: Soln 10%, 20%. Intravenous (Acetadote).] ▶L ♀B ▶? $$$$

CHARCOAL (**activated charcoal**, *Actidose-Aqua, CharcoAid, EZ-Char, ✦Charcodate*) 25 to 100 g (1 to 2 g/kg) PO or NG as soon as possible. May repeat

(cont.)

q 1 to 4 h prn at doses equivalent to 12.5 g/h. When sorbitol is coadministered, use only with the 1st dose if repeated doses are to be given. [OTC/Generic/Trade: Powder 15, 30, 40, 120, 240 g. Soln 12.5 g/60 mL, 15 g/75 mL, 15 g/120 mL, 25 g/120 mL, 30 g/120 mL, 50 g/240 mL. Susp 15 g/120 mL, 25 g/120 mL, 30 g/150 mL, 50 g/240 mL. Granules 15 g/120 mL.] ▶Not absorbed ♀+ ▶+ $

DEFEROXAMINE (*Desferal*) Chronic iron overload: 500 to 1000 mg IM daily and 2 g IV infusion (no faster than 15 mg/kg/h) with each unit of blood or 1 to 2 g SC daily (20 to 40 mg/kg/day) over 8 to 24 h via continuous infusion pump. Acute iron toxicity: IV infusion up to 15 mg/kg/h (consult poison center). ▶K ♀C ▶? $$$$$

FLUMAZENIL (*Romazicon*) Benzodiazepine sedation reversal: 0.2 mg IV over 15 sec, then 0.2 mg q 1 min prn up to 1 mg total dose. Overdose reversal: 0.2 mg IV over 30 sec, then 0.3 to 0.5 mg q 30 sec prn up to 3 mg total dose. Contraindicated in mixed drug overdose or chronic benzodiazepine use. ▶LK ♀C ▶? $$$$

FOMEPIZOLE (*Antizol*) Consult poison center. Ethylene glycol or methanol toxicity: 15 mg/kg IV (load), then 10 mg/kg IV q 12 h for 4 doses, then 15 mg/kg IV q 12 h until ethylene glycol or methanol level is below 20 mg/dL. Administer doses as slow IV infusions over 30 min. Increase frequency to q 4 h during hemodialysis. ▶L ♀C ▶? $$$$$

HYDROXOCOBALAMIN (*Cyanokit*) Cyanide poisoning: 5 g IV over 15 min; may repeat prn. ▶K ♀C ▶? $$$$$

IPECAC SYRUP Emesis: 30 mL PO for adults, 15 mL age 1 to 12 yo. [OTC Generic only: Syrup 30 mL.] ▶Gut ♀C ▶? $

METHYLENE BLUE (*Urolene blue*) Methemoglobinemia: 1 to 2 mg/kg IV over 5 min. Dysuria: 65 to 130 mg PO three times per day after meals with liberal water. May turn urine/contact lenses blue. [Trade only: Tabs 65 mg.] ▶K ♀C ▶? $

PRALIDOXIME (*Protopam, 2-PAM*) Organophosphate poisoning: consult poison center: 1 to 2 g IV infusion over 15 to 30 min or slow IV injection over 5 min or longer (max rate 200 mg/min). May repeat dose after 1 h if muscle weakness persists. High-dose regimen (unapproved): 2 g over 30 min, followed by 1 g/h for 48 h, then 1 g/h q 4 h until improved. Peds: 20 to 50 mg/kg/dose IV over 15 to 30 min. ▶K ♀C ▶? $$$$

SUCCIMER (*Chemet*) Lead toxicity in children 1 yo or older: Start 10 mg/kg PO or 350 mg/m² q 8 h for 5 days, then reduce the frequency to q 12 h for 2 weeks. [Trade only: Caps 100 mg.] ▶K ♀C ▶? $$$$$

UROLOGY

Benign Prostatic Hyperplasia

ALFUZOSIN (*UroXatral*, *✦Xatral*) 10 mg PO daily after the same meal each day. [Generic/Trade: Tabs, extended-release 10 mg.] ▶KL ♀B ▶– $

COMBODART (dutasteride + tamsulosin, *Duodart, Jalyn*) 0.5 mg dutasteride + 0.4 mg tamsulosin daily 30 minutes after the same meal each day. [Trade only: Caps 0.5 mg dutasteride + 0.4 mg tamsulosin.] ▶LK - ♀X ▶– $$$$

DUTASTERIDE (*Avodart*) BPH: 0.5 mg PO daily. [Trade only: Caps 0.5 mg.] ▶L ♀X Capsules should not be touched by a woman who is pregnant or may become pregnant due to transdermal absorption resulting in fetal exposure. ▶– $$$$

FINASTERIDE (*Proscar, Propecia*) To reduce the risk of symptomatic progression of BPH: Proscar: 5 mg PO daily alone or in combination with doxazosin. Androgenetic alopecia in men: Propecia: 1 mg PO daily. [Generic/Trade: Tabs 1 mg (Propecia), 5 mg (Proscar).] ▶L ♀X ▶– $

SILODOSIN (*RAPAFLO*) 8 mg PO daily with a meal. [Trade: Caps 8 mg.] ▶LK - ♀B ▶– $$$$

TAMSULOSIN (*Flomax*) 0.4 mg PO daily, 30 min after a meal. Max 0.8 mg/day. [Generic/Trade: Caps 0.4 mg.] ▶LK ♀B ▶– $$$$

Bladder Agents—Anticholinergics and Combinations

DARIFENACIN (*Enablex*) Overactive bladder with symptoms of urinary urgency, frequency, and urge incontinence: 7.5 mg PO daily. May increase to max dose 15 mg PO daily in 2 weeks. Max dose 7.5 mg PO daily with moderate liver impairment or when coadministered with potent CYP3A4 inhibitors (ketoconazole, itraconazole, ritonavir, nelfinavir, clarithromycin, and nefazodone). [Trade only: Tabs, extended-release 7.5, 15 mg.] ▶LK ♀C ▶– $$$$

FESOTERODINE (*Toviaz*) Overactive bladder: 4 to 8 mg PO daily. [Trade only: Tabs, extended-release 4, 8 mg.] ▶plasma ♀C ▶– $$$$

OXYBUTYNIN (*Ditropan, Ditropan XL, Gelnique, Oxytrol,* *✦Oxybutyn, Uromax*) Bladder instability: 2.5 to 5 mg PO two to three times per day, max 5 mg PO four times per day. Extended-release tabs: 5 to 10 mg PO daily, increase 5 mg/day q week to 30 mg/day. Oxytrol: 1 patch twice a week on abdomen, hips, or buttocks. Gelnique: Apply gel once daily to abdomen, upper arms/shoulders, or thighs. [Generic/Trade: Tabs 5 mg. Syrup 5 mg/5 mL. Tabs, extended-release 5, 10, 15 mg. Trade only: OTC Transdermal patch (Oxytrol) 3.9 mg/day. Gelnique 3%, 10% gel, 1 g unit dose.] ▶LK ♀B ▶? $$$

PROSED/DS (methenamine + phenyl salicylate + methylene blue + benzoic acid + hyoscyamine) Bladder spasm: 1 tab PO four times per day with liberal fluids. May turn urine/contact lenses blue. [Trade only: Tabs (methenamine 81.6 mg/phenyl salicylate 36.2 mg/methylene blue 10.8 mg/benzoic acid 9.0 mg/ hyoscyamine sulfate 0.12 mg).] ▶KL ♀C ▶? $$

SOLIFENACIN (*VESIcare*) Overactive bladder with symptoms of urinary urgency, frequency, or urge incontinence: 5 mg PO daily. Max dose: 10 mg daily (5 mg

(cont.)

daily if CrCl less than 30 mL/min, moderate hepatic impairment, or concurrent ketoconazole or other potent CYP3A4 inhibitors). [Trade only: Tabs 5, 10 mg.] ▶LK ♀C▶– $$$$

TOLTERODINE (*Detrol, Detrol LA*) Overactive bladder: 1 to 2 mg PO two times per day (Detrol) or 4 mg PO daily; may be reduced to 2 mg PO daily based on response and tolerability (Detrol LA). [Generic/Trade: Tabs 1, 2 mg. Caps, extended-release 2, 4 mg.] ▶L ♀C▶– $$$$$

TROSPIUM (*Sanctura, Sanctura XR, ✦Trosec*) Overactive bladder with urge incontinence: 20 mg PO two times per day; give 20 mg at bedtime if CrCl less than 30 mL/min. If age 75 yo or older may taper down to 20 mg daily. Extended-release: 60 mg PO q am, 1 h before food. [Generic only: Tabs 20 mg. Caps, extended-release 60 mg.] ▶LK ♀C▶? $$$$

URISED (methenamine + phenyl salicylate + atropine + hyoscyamine + benzoic acid + methylene blue) Dysuria: 2 tabs PO four times per day. May turn urine/contact lenses blue. Do not use with sulfa. [Trade only: Tabs (methenamine 40.8 mg/phenyl salicylate 18.1 mg/atropine 0.03 mg/hyoscyamine 0.03 mg/4.5 mg benzoic acid/5.4 mg methylene blue).] ▶K ♀C▶? $

UTA (methenamine + sodium phosphate + phenyl salicylate + methylene blue + hyoscyamine) Bladder spasm: 1 cap PO four times per day with liberal fluids. [Trade only: Caps (methenamine 120 mg/sodium phosphate 40.8 mg/phenyl salicylate 36 mg/methylene blue 10 mg/hyoscyamine 0.12 mg).] ▶KL ♀C▶? $

UTIRA-C (methenamine + sodium phosphate + phenyl salicylate + methylene blue + hyoscyamine) Bladder spasm: 1 cap PO four times per day with liberal fluids. [Trade only: Tabs (methenamine 81.6 mg/sodium phosphate 40.8 mg/phenyl salicylate 36.2 mg/methylene blue 10.8 mg/hyoscyamine 0.12 mg).] ▶KL ♀C▶? $$

Bladder Agents—Other

BETHANECHOL (*Urecholine, Duvoid, ✦Myotonachol*) Urinary retention: 10 to 50 mg PO three to four times per day. [Generic/Trade: Tabs 5, 10, 25, 50 mg.] ▶L ♀C▶? $$$$

MIRABEGRON (*Myrbetriq*) Overactive bladder with symptoms of urge urinary incontinence, urgency, and urinary frequency: 25 mg PO daily. May increase to 50 mg unless severe renal impairment or moderate hepatic impairment. [Trade only: Extended-release tabs: 25, 50 mg.] ▶LK - ♀C▶?

PHENAZOPYRIDINE (*Pyridium, Azo-Standard, Urogesic, Prodium, Pyridiate, Urodol, Baridium, UTI Relief, Azourinary Pain Relief, Uristat, Azo-Gesic, Azo-Septic, Phenazo, Re-Azo, Uricalm*) Dysuria: 200 mg PO three times per day for 2 days. May turn urine/contact lenses orange. [OTC Generic/Trade: Tabs 95, 97.2 mg. Rx Generic/Trade: Tabs 100, 200 mg.] ▶K ♀B▶? $

Erectile Dysfunction

ALPROSTADIL (*Muse, Caverject, Caverject Impulse, Edex, Prostin VR Pediatric, prostaglandin E1, ✦Prostin VR*) 1 intraurethral pellet (Muse) or intracavernosal injection (Caverject, Edex) at lowest dose that will produce erection. Onset

(cont.)

of effect is 5 to 20 min. [Trade only: Syringe system (Edex) 10, 20, 40 mcg; (Caverject) 5, 10, 20, 40 mcg; (Caverject Impulse) 10, 20 mcg. Pellet (Muse) 125, 250, 500, 1000 mcg. Intracorporeal injection of locally compounded combination agents (many variations): "Bi-mix" can be 30 mg/mL papaverine + 0.5 to 1 mg/mL phentolamine, or 30 mg/mL papaverine + 20 mcg/mL alprostadil in 10 mL vials. "Tri-mix" can be 30 mg/mL papaverine + 1 mg/mL phentolamine + 10 mcg/mL alprostadil in 5, 10, or 20 mL vials.] ▶L ♀– ▶– $$$$

AVANAFIL (Stendra) Start 100 mg PO as early as 15 min prior to sexual activity. Max 1 dose/day. May increase to 200 mg or decrease to 50 mg prn. Contraindicated with nitrates and strong CYP3A4 inhibitors. Start at 50 mg if concurrent alpha blocker or moderate CYP3A4 inhibitor. Contraindicated if severe renal or hepatic impairment. [Trade only (Stendra): Tabs 50, 100, 200 mg.] ▶L – ♀C ▶? $$$$

SILDENAFIL (Viagra) Start 50 mg PO 0.5 to 4 h prior to intercourse. Max 1 dose/day. Usual effective range 25 to 100 mg. Start at 25 mg if for age 65 yo or older or liver/renal impairment. Contraindicated with nitrates. [Trade only (Viagra): Tabs 25, 50, 100 mg. Unscored tab but can be cut in half.] ▶LK ♀B ▶– $$$$

TADALAFIL (Cialis) ED: 2.5 to 5 mg PO daily without regard to timing of sexual activity. Daily dosing should not exceed 2.5 mg if on concomitant CYP3A4 inhibitor. As-needed dosing: Start 10 mg PO at least 30 to 45 min prn prior to sexual activity. May increase to 20 mg or decrease to 5 mg prn. Max 1 dose/day. Start 5 mg (max 1 dose/day) if CrCl is 31 to 50 mL/min. Max 5 mg/day if CrCl less than 30 mL/min including patients on dialysis. Max 10 mg/day if mild to moderate hepatic impairment; avoid in severe hepatic impairment. Max 10 mg once in 72 h if concurrent potent CYP3A4 inhibitors. BPH with or without erectile dysfunction: 5 mg PO daily. Contraindicated with nitrates and alpha-blockers (except tamsulosin 0.4 mg daily). Not FDA approved for women. [Trade only (Cialis): Tabs 2.5, 5, 10, 20 mg.] ▶L ♀B ▶– $$$$

VARDENAFIL (Levitra, Staxyn) Start 10 mg PO 1 h before sexual activity. Usual effective dose range 5 to 20 mg. Max 1 dose/day. Use lower dose (5 mg) if age 65 yo or older or moderate hepatic impairment (max 10 mg). Contraindicated with nitrates and alpha-blockers. Not FDA approved in women. [Trade only: Tabs 2.5, 5, 10, 20 mg. Oral, disintegrating tab, 10 mg (Staxyn).] ▶LK ♀B ▶– $$$$$

YOHIMBINE (Yocon, Yohimex) 5.4 mg PO three times per day. Not FDA approved. [Generic/Trade: Tabs 5.4 mg.] ▶L ♀– ▶– $

Nephrolithiasis

CITRATE (Polycitra-K, Urocit-K, Bicitra, Oracit, Polycitra, Polycitra-LC) Urinary alkalinization: 1 packet in water/juice PO three to four times per day. [Generic/Trade: Polycitra-K packet 3300 mg potassium citrate/ea, Polycitra-K oral soln (1100 mg potassium citrate/5 mL, 480 mL). Oracit oral soln (490 mg sodium citrate/5 mL, 15, 30, 480 mL). Bicitra oral soln (500 mg sodium citrate/5 mL, 480 mL). Urocit-K wax (potassium citrate) Tabs 5, 10 mEq. Polycitra-LC oral soln (550 mg potassium citrate/500 mg sodium citrate per 5 mL, 480 mL). Polycitra oral syrup (550 mg potassium citrate/500 mg sodium citrate per 5 mL, 480 mL.] ▶K ♀C ▶? $$$

INDEX

A

A-spaz, 142–143
A/T/S, 97
abacavir, 39, 41
abatacept, 227
ABC, 41
abciximab, 79
Abelcet, 31
Abenol, 11
Abilify, 207
Abilify Maintena, 207
abobotulinum toxin A, 179
Abraxane, 191
Abreva, 102
Absorica, 97
Abstral, 6–7
acamprosate, 212
Acanya, 96
acarbose, 113
Accolate, 222
Accu-Prep, 144
AccuNeb, 219–220
Accupril, 59, 66
Accuretic, 72, 73
Accutane Roche, 97
acebutolol, 82
acellular pertussis vaccine, 165, 166
acemannan, 157
Aceon, 59, 65
Acetadote, 231

acetaminophen, 2–3, 9–11, 153, 184, 227, 231
acetazolamide, 197
acetic acid, 133, 134
acetylcysteine, 231
acetylcysteine—inhaled, 222
acetylsalicylic acid, 2–4, 9–10, 80, 140
Acidophilus, 161
AcipHex, 142
acitretin, 101
Aclasta, 111–112
aclidinium, 222
Aclovate, 95
acrivastine, 130
Actemra, 228
ActHIB, 165
Acticin, 101
Acticlate, 56
Actidose-Aqua, 231–232
Actifed Cold & Allergy, 129
Actifed Cold & Sinus, 129
Actigall, 148
Actiq, 6–7
Activase, 90
Activase rt-PA, 90
activated charcoal, 231–232
Activella, 187
Actonel, 111

Actoplus Met, 113
Actoplus Met XR, 113
Actos, 119
Actron, 5
Acular, 199
Acular LS, 199
Acuvail, 199
acyclovir, 24–25, 37, 105, 184
acyclovir—topical, 102
Aczone, 32–33
Adacel, 163, 165
Adalat, 84
Adalat CC, 84
Adalat XL, 84
adalimumab, 225, 226
adapalene, 96, 97
Adcirca, 90
Adderall, 214
Adderall XR, 214
adefovir, 35
Adempas, 89
Adenocard, 68
adenosine, 68
ADH, 88
Adipex-P, 215
Adoxa, 56
Adrenalin, 88
Adriamycin, 191
Adrucil, 191
Advagraf, 167
Advair, 217, 220
Advair HFA, 217
Advicor®, 60, 77
Advil, 5
Aerius, 130

AeroBid, 221
AeroBid-M, 217, 221
Aerospan, 217, 221
Aesculus hippocastanum, 160
Afeditab CR, 84
Afinitor, 191
aflibercept, 200
Afluria, 164–166
Afrezza, 116
African plum tree, 161
Afrin, 135
Aggrastat, 81
Aggrenox, 80
Agrylin, 155
Airomir, 219–220
AK-Mycin, 194
AK-Pentolate, 199
AK Tracin, 194
Akarpine, 198
Akineton, 177
Akurza, 97
Akynzeo, 138, 229
ALA, 157
Alavert, 131
Alavert D-12, 129
Alaway, 193
Albalon, 193
albendazole, 33
Albenza, 33
albiglutide, 115
Albumarc, 91
albumin, 91, 155
Albuminar, 91

albuterol, 219–220
albuterol—inhaled, 220, 221
alcaftadine, 193
Alcaine, 200
alclometasone dipropionate, 95
Aldactazide, 72, 73
Aldactone, 66
Aldara, 102
aldesleukin, 191
Aldoril, 72, 73
alemtuzumab, 176, 191
alendronate, 111
Alertec, 215
Alesse, 184
Aleve, 5–6
alfuzosin, 39, 63, 233
Align, 161
Alimta, 191
Alinia, 34
alirocumab, 79
aliskiren, 73, 74
aliskirin, 73
alitretinoin, 103
Alka-Seltzer, 140
Alkeran, 191
All Clear, 193
Allegra, 131
Allegra-D 12-h, 129
Allegra-D 24-h, 129
Aller-Chlor, 131
Aller-Max, 131
Aller-Relief, 131
Allerdryl, 131
Allerfrim, 129

AllerNaze, 135
Alli, 148
Allium sativum, 159
allopurinol, 153, 228, 230
Alluna, 162
Almora, 122
almotriptan, 175
Alocril, 194
aloe vera, 157
alogliptin, 114, 115
Alomide, 194
Aloprim, 230
Alora, 186–187
alosetron, 146, 203
Aloxi, 138
alpha-galactosidase, 146
alpha-glucosidase inhibitors, 107, 113
alpha lipoic acid, 157
Alphagan, 199
Alphagan P, 199
alprazolam, 211
alprostadil, 234–235
Alrex, 196
Alsuma, 176
Altabax, 99
Altace, 59, 66
Altavera, 182, 184
alteplase, 90, 151
Alternagel, 140
Altoprev, 77
altretamine, 191
Alu-Cap, 140
Alu-Tab, 140
aluminum acetate, 133
aluminum chloride, 103
aluminum hydroxide, 2, 140

Alupent, 217, 220
Alvesco, 217, 221
alvimopan, 146
Alyacen 1/35, 182, 185
Alyacen 7/7/7, 183, 185
amantadine, 45
Amaryl, 118
Amatine, 88
AmBisome, 31
ambrisentan, 88–89
amcinonide, 95
Amerge, 175
Amethia, 183
Amethia Lo, 184
Amethyst, 183
Amicar, 155
Amidate, 13
amifostine, 191
Amigesic, 4
amikacin, 29
amiloride, 73, 86
aminocaproic acid, 155
aminoglycoside, 29
amiodarone, 63, 69, 78, 153
Amitiza, 145
amitriptyline, 201
AmLactin, 104
AmLactin AP, 104
amlexanox, 134
amlodipine, 73, 77–78, 84
Amnesteem, 97
amoxicillin, 15, 20, 22–23, 53, 141
amoxicillin-clavulanate, 18–19, 22–23, 53–54

amphetamine, 214
Amphojel, 140
amphotericin B, 29
amphotericin B deoxycholate, 31
amphotericin B lipid formulations, 31
ampicillin, 15, 20, 54
ampicillin-sulbactam, 18, 54
amprenavir, 153
Ampyra, 177
Amrix, 1
Amturnide, 72, 73
anabolic steroids, 110–111
Anacin, 3–4
Anafranil, 201
anagrelide, 63, 155
anakinra, 227
Analpram-HC, 103
Anaprox, 5–6
Anaspaz, 142–143
anastrozole, 191
Ancobon, 31
Andriol, 110–111
Androcur Depot, 191
Androderm, 110–111
AndroGel, 110–111
androgens, 110–111
Anectine, 14
Anexsia, 9
Angeliq, 187
Angiomax, 149
anhydrous glycerins, 133

anidulafungin, 30
Ansaid, 5
Antabuse, 212
antacids, 184
Antara, 75
antazoline, 193
Anthemis
  nobilis—
  Roman chamo-
  mile, 157
anthralin, 101
antipyrine, 133
Antivert, 132
Antizol, 232
Anzemet, 138
Aphthasol, 134
Apidra, 116, 117
apixaban, 149
Aplenzin,
  204–205
Aplisol, 167
Apo-Salvent,
  219–220
Apokyn, 178
apomorphine,
  178
apremilast, 230
aprepitant, 138,
  229
Apresazide,
  72, 73
Apresoline, 74
Apri, 182, 185
Apriso, 146
Aprodine, 129
Aptensio XR,
  215
Aptiom, 171
Aptivus, 45
AquaMephyton,
  126
Aquasol E, 127
AraC, 191
Aralen, 31–32
Aranelle, 183
Aranesp, 155
Arava, 228
Arcapta, 219
Aredia, 111

arformoterol, 219
argatroban, 149
Aricept, 169
Arimidex, 191
aripiprazole, 206,
  207
Aristocort, 95, 96
Aristospan, 113
Arixtra, 149–150
armodafinil, 214
Arnuity Ellipta,
  221
Aromasin, 191
Arranon, 191
arsenic, 231
arsenic trioxide,
  63, 191–192
Artane, 177
artemether, 32
Arthrotec, 4
articaine, 13
artichoke leaf
  extract, 157
artificial tears,
  200
Arzerra, 191
ASA, 4, 153
Asacol HD, 146
Asaphen, 3–4
ascorbic acid,
  124–125
Ascriptin, 2
asenapine, 206,
  208
Aslera, 158
Asmanex, 217
Asmanex HFA,
  221
Asmanex
  Twisthaler,
  221
asparaginase,
  192
aspirin, 3–4, 80,
  151
Astagraf XL, 167
Astelin, 135
Astepro, 135
astragalus, 157

Astragalus mem-
  branaceus, 157
Atacand, 67
Atacand HCT,
  72, 73
Atacand Plus,
  72, 73
Atarax, 131
Atasol, 11
Atasol 8, 10
Atasol 15, 10
Atasol 30, 10
atazanavir,
  42–43, 63,
  229
atazanavir–
  darunavir, 43
atazanavir–
  ritonavir,
  39, 43
atazanavir with
  or without
  ritonavir, 78
Atelvia, 111
atenolol, 73, 82
Atgam, 167
Ativan, 171
atomoxetine, 214
atorvastatin,
  60, 62, 64,
  73, 77
atovaquone,
  32, 34
Atralin, 97
Atripla, 38
AtroPen, 69
atropine, 14,
  69, 137, 142,
  231, 234
atropine—oph-
  thalmic, 199
Atrovent, 222
Atrovent HFA,
  217, 222
Atrovent Nasal
  Spray, 135
ATV, 42–43

Augmentin,
  53–54
Augmentin
  ES-600,
  53–54
Augmentin XR,
  53–54
Auralgan, 133
Auryxia, 123–124
Auvi-Q, 88
Avage, 97
Avalide, 72, 73
avanafil, 235
Avandamet, 113
Avandaryl,
  113–114
Avandia, 119
Avapro, 67
Avastin, 191
Avaxim, 165
Aveed, 110–111
Aveeno, 105
Avelox, 55
Aventyl, 202
Aviane, 181
Avinza, 8
Avodart, 233
Avonex, 177
Avycaz, 50
Axert, 175
Axid, 141
Axid AR, 141
Axiron, 110–111
Aygestin, 189
AZA, 228
azacitidine, 191
Azactam, 56
Azasan, 228
AzaSite, 194
azathioprine,
  154, 228
azelaic acid, 96
azelastine—nasal,
  135

azelastine—ophthalmic, 193
Azelex, 96
Azilect, 179
azilsartan, 67, 73
azithromycin, 15, 24, 26, 28, 51–52, 63, 154, 184
azithromycin—ophthalmic, 194
Azmacort, 221
Azo-Gesic, 234
Azo-Septic, 234
Azo-Standard, 234
Azopt, 197
Azor, 72, 73
Azourinary Pain Relief, 234
AZT, 42
aztreonam, 56
Azulfidine, 146, 229
Azulfidine EN-tabs, 146, 229
Azurette, 182, 185

B

B-D Glucose, 119
BabyBIG, 167
Bacid, 161
Bacillus of Calmette & Guerin, 191
bacitracin—ophthalmic, 194, 195
bacitracin—topical, 98–99
baclofen, 1
Bactrim, 55
Bactroban, 98–99
BAL, 231
balsalazide, 146
Balziva, 182, 185
banana bag, 123
Banophen, 131
Banzel, 174
baraclude, 35
barbiturates, 154
Baridium, 234
barium sulfate, 93
Basaljel, 140
basiliximab, 167
Bayer, 3–4
Baygam, 167
bazedoxifene, 188
BCG vaccine, 165, 191
BCNU, 191
Beano, 146
becaplermin, 104
beclomethasone, 184
beclomethasone HFA MDI, 218
beclomethasone—inhaled, 221
beclomethasone—nasal, 134
Beconase AQ, 134
bedaquiline, 63
belatacept, 167
Belsomra, 212
Belviq, 147
Benadryl, 131
Benadryl Allergy/Coldt, 129
Benadryl-D Allergy/Sinus Tablets, 129
benazepril, 59, 65, 73
bendamustine, 191
bendroflumethiazide, 73
Benicar, 67
Benicar HCT, 72, 73
Bentyl, 142
Bentylol, 142
Benylin, 132
Benzac, 96
Benzaclin, 96
Benzagel 10%, 96
Benzamycin, 96
benzathine penicillin, 28, 52
benzocaine, 135
benzocaine—otic, 133
benzodiazepines, 203, 231
benzoic acid, 233, 234
benzonatate, 132
benzoyl peroxide, 96–97, 184
benztropine mesylate, 177
benzyl alcohol, 100
bepotastine, 193
Bepreve, 193
besifloxacin, 194
Besivance, 194
beta-blockers, 231
Betagan, 197
Betaject, 112
Betaloc, 83
betamethasone, 101, 108, 112
betamethasone dipropionate, 95, 96
betamethasone valerate, 95
betamethasone—topical, 101, 103
Betapace, 72
Betapace AF, 72
Betaseron, 177
betaxolol, 82
betaxolol—ophthalmic, 197
bethanechol, 234
Bethkis, 29
Betimol, 197
Betoptic, 197
Betoptic S, 197
bevacizumab, 191
bexarotene, 192
Bexsero, 164, 166
Beyaz, 181
bezafibrate, 75
Bezalip SR, 75
Biaxin, 52
bicalutamide, 191
bicarbonate, 140, 142
Bicillin C-R, 52
Bicillin L-A, 52
Bicitra, 235
BiCNU, 191
BiDil, 91
Bifantis, 161
Bifidobacteria, 161
bile acid sequestrants, 60
bimatoprost, 198
Binosto, 111
BioGaia, 161
Bionect, 104
BioRab, 166
biotin, 125
biperiden, 177
Biphentin, 215

bisacodyl, 145, 184

bismuth subcitrate potassium, 141

bismuth subsalicylate, 137

bisoprolol, 73, 82

bisphosphonates, 111–112

bivalirudin, 149

Blenoxane–Canada only, 191

bleomycin, 191

Bleph-10, 195

Blephamide, 195

Blocadren, 83

Bloxiverz, 14

boceprevir, 78, 229

Bonine, 132

Boniva, 111

Boostrix, 163, 165

boric acid, 189

bortezomib, 192

bosentan, 39, 89, 154

Botox, 180

Botox Cosmetic, 180

botulinum toxin type B, 179

botulism immune globulin, 167

Breo Ellipta, 220

Brevibloc, 82

Brevicon, 182

Brevital, 13

brexpiprazole, 208

Briellyn, 182, 185

Brilinta, 80

brimonidine, 104, 198, 199

Brintellix, 203

brinzolamide, 197, 198

bromazepam, 210

Bromday, 199

bromfenac—ophthalmic, 199

Bromfenex, 129

bromocriptine, 127

brompheniramine, 129

Brovana, 219

buckeye, 160

budesonide, 146–147, 184, 218

budesonide DPI, 218

budesonide—inhaled, 221

budesonide—nasal, 134

Bufferin, 2

bumetanide, 85

Bumex, 85

Buminate, 91

Bunavail, 213

bupivacaine, 13

Buprenex, 6

buprenorphine, 1, 6, 213

Buproban, 204–205

bupropion, 147, 184, 204–205

Burinex, 85

burn plant, 157

Buscopan, 142

buspirone, 184, 212

busulfan, 191

Busulfex, 191

butalbital, 2–3, 9

butamben, 135

butenafine, 99

butorphanol, 1, 6

Butrans, 6

butterbur, 157

Bydureon, 115

Byetta, 115

Bystolic, 83

C

C. monogyna, 160

C. oxyacantha, 160

cabazitaxel, 191

cabergoline, 127

Caduet, 72, 73, 77

Caelyx, 191

Cafcit, 214

Cafergot, 176

Caffedrine, 214

caffeine, 2–3, 9, 10, 176, 214

calamine, 104

Calan, 85

Calan SR, 85

Calciferol, 125

Calcijex, 125

Calcimar, 127

calcipotriene, 101

calcipotriol, 101

calcitonin, 127

calcitriol, 125

calcium acetate, 120

calcium carbonate, 2, 120, 140, 141, 190

calcium channel blockers, 231

calcium chloride, 120, 231

calcium citrate, 120

calcium gluconate, 120

Caldolor, 5

CaloMist, 125

Calsan, 120

Caltine, 127

Caltrate, 120

Cambia, 4

Camellia sinensis, 160

Camila, 182, 184

Campath, 191

Campral, 212

Camptosar, 191

Camrese, 183

Camrese Lo, 184

canagliflozin, 107, 114, 118

canakinumab, 227

Canasa, 146

Cancidas, 30

candesartan, 67, 73

CanesOral, 29

Canesten, 99, 190

cangrelor, 80

Cankermelt, 160

capecitabine, 191

Capital with Codeine Suspension, 9

Capoten, 59, 65

Capozide, 72, 73

capsaicin, 104

captopril, 59, 65, 73

Carac, 98

Carafate, 143

carbachol, 198

carbamazepine, 35, 36, 41, 70, 81, 154, 170–171

carbamide peroxide, 133

Carbatrol, 170–171

carbidopa, 179
carbidopa-
    levodopa, 178
Carbocaine, 13
carboplatin, 191
carboprost, 189
Cardene, 84
Cardene SR, 84
Cardizem, 84, 85
Cardizem CD, 84
Cardizem LA,
    84, 85
Cardura, 68
Cardura XL, 68
Carimune, 167
cariprazine, 208
carisoprodol, 1,
    3, 9, 10
carmustine, 191
Carnitor, 123
carteolol—oph-
    thalmic, 197
Cartia XT, 84, 85
carvedilol, 81, 82
cascara, 145
Casodex, 191
caspofungin, 30
castor oil, 145
Cataflam, 4
Catapres, 67
Catapres-TTS, 67
Cathflo, 90
Caverject,
    234–235
Caverject
    Impulse,
    234–235
Cayston, 56
Caziant, 183
CCNU, 191
Ceclor, 48
Cedax, 50
CeeNu, 191
cefaclor, 48

cefadroxil, 48
cefazolin, 15, 48
cefdinir, 22–23,
    50
cefditoren, 50
Cefepime, 50
cefixime, 18, 50,
    153
cefixime-azithro-
    mycin, 28
cefoperazone, 153
cefotaxime, 18,
    26, 50
cefotetan, 27,
    153, 154
cefoxitin, 48
cefpodoxime, 18,
    22–23, 50
cefprozil, 48
ceftaroline, 51
ceftazidime, 50
ceftazidime-avi-
    bactam, 50
ceftibuten, 50
Ceftin, 48
ceftolozane-
    tazobactam, 50
ceftriaxone, 15,
    18, 22–24,
    26–28, 50
cefuroxime,
    22–23, 48
Celebrex, 3
celecoxib, 3, 4,
    153
Celestone, 112
Celestone
    Soluspan, 112
Celexa, 202
CellCept, 167
Celsentri, 38
Cena-K, 122,
    123
Centany, 98–99
cephalexin,
    15, 48
cephalosporins,
    22–23, 49–51,
    184

Cerebyx, 171
Certain Dri, 103
certolizumab,
    225, 226
Cerubidine, 191
Cervarix, 165
Cervidil, 188
C.E.S., 187
Cesamet, 139
Cetacaine, 135
cetirizine, 131
Cetraxal, 133
cetuximab, 191
cevimeline, 134
chamomile, 157
Champix, 213
Chantix, 213
CharcoAid,
    231–232
charcoal,
    231–232
Charcodote,
    231–232
chasteberry, 157
Chemet, 232
ChiRhoStim,
    148
chlamydia, 24
Chlor-Trimeton,
    131
chlorambucil,
    191
chloramphenicol,
    56, 153
chlordiazepoxide,
    210
chlordiazepox-
    ide–clinidium,
    147
Chlordrine SR,
    129
chlorhexidine glu-
    conate, 134
chlorodeoxy-
    adenosine, 191
chloroquine,
    31–32, 63
chlorothiazide,
    86

chlorpheniramine,
    129–132
chlorpromazine,
    63, 207
chlorthalidone,
    73, 86
chlorzoxazone, 1
cholecalciferol,
    126–127
cholesterol
    absorption
    inhibitor, 60
cholestyramine,
    60, 75, 154
choline magne-
    sium trisalicy-
    late, 4
chondroitin, 157
choriogonadotro-
    pin alfa, 188
Chrysanthemum
    parthenium,
    158
Ci-wu-jia, 159
Cialis, 235
ciclesonide—
    inhaled, 221
ciclesonide—
    nasal,
    134–135
ciclopirox, 99
cidofovir, 35
cilazapril, 65, 73
cilostazol, 91
Ciloxan, 194
cimetidine, 80,
    140, 153,
    184
Cimzia, 226
Cipralex, 202
Cipro, 54–55
Cipro HC Otic,
    133
Cipro XR, 54–55
Ciprodex Otic,
    133
ciprofloxacin,
    19–20, 24, 26,
    54–55, 229

ciprofloxacin—ophthalmic, 194
ciprofloxacin—otic, 133
cisapride, 63, 203
cisatracurium, 14
cisplatin, 191
citalopram, 63, 202
Citanest, 14
Citracal, 120
citrate, 140, 235
Citrucel, 143
cladribine, 191
Claforan, 50
Claravis, 97
Clarinex, 130
Clarinex-D 24-h, 129
Claripel, 104
clarithromycin, 15, 35, 52, 63, 70, 78, 81, 141, 154, 229, 233
Claritin, 131
Claritin-D 12-h, 129
Claritin-D 24-h, 129
Claritin Hives Relief, 131
Claritin RediTabs, 131
Clarus, 97
Clavulin, 53–54
Clear Eyes, 193
Clearasil, 96
Clearasil Cleanser, 97
clemastine, 131
Cleocin, 57, 190
Cleocin T, 97
clevidipine, 84
Cleviprex, 84
Climara, 186–187

Climara Pro, 187
Clindagel, 97
clindamycin, 15, 18–20, 22–24, 27, 32, 57, 184
clindamycin—topical, 96–98
clindamycin—vaginal, 190
Clindesse, 190
Clindoxyl, 97
Clinoril, 6
clobazam, 171
clobetasol, 96
clocortolone pivalate, 95
Cloderm, 95
clofarabine, 191
Clolar, 191
Clomid, 188
clomiphene citrate, 188
clomipramine, 201
Clonapam, 210
clonazepam, 210
clonidine, 67, 73, 81
clopidogrel, 80
clorazepate, 210–211
Clorpres, 72, 73
Clotrimaderm, 99, 190
clotrimazole, 24, 29, 184
clotrimazole—topical, 99, 103
clotrimazole—vaginal, 190
clozapine, 63, 206, 208
Clozaril, 208
coal tar, 104
Coartem, 32
COBI, 43

cobicistat, 39, 43, 44, 229
cobicistat-ata-zanavir, 40
cocaine, 63
codeine, 1, 6, 9–10, 130, 184
coenzyme Q10, 154, 158
Cogentin, 177
Colace, 145
Colazal, 146
colchicine, 229–230
Colcrys, 230
Cold-FX, 159
Cold-FX Extra, 159
colesevelam, 60, 75
Colestid, 75
Colestid Flavored, 75
colestipol, 60, 75, 154
colistin, 133
Colyte, 144
Combantrin, 34
Combigan, 198
Combipatch, 188
Combivent Inhalation Soln, 221
Combivent Respimat, 220
Combivir, 38
Combodart, 233
Combunox, 9
Commit, 213
Complera, 38–39
Comtan, 178
Comvax, 164, 165
Concerta, 215

concomitant amiodarone, 81
Condyline, 102
Condylox, 102
cone flower, 158
Congest, 187
conivaptan, 229
conjugated estrogens, 188
Conray, 94
Constella, 147
Contrave, 147
ConZip, 11
Copaxone, 177
Copegus, 36
CoQ-10, 158
Cordarone, 69
Cordran, 95
Coreg, 82
Coreg CR, 82
Corgard, 83
Corlanor, 91
Corlopam, 74
Cormax, 96
Correctol, 145
Cortaid, 95
Cortef, 112
Cortenema, 112
Corticaine, 95
corticosteroids, 108, 112–113
cortisone, 108, 112
Cortisporin, 103
Cortisporin Otic, 133
Cortisporin TC Otic, 133
Cortisporin—Ophthalmic, 195
Cortone, 112
Cortrosyn, 120

Corvert, 71
Corzide, 72, 73
Cosamin DS, 159
Cosentyx, 227
Cosmegen, 191
Cosopt, 198
cosyntropin, 120
Cotazym, 148
cotrimoxazole, 55
Coumadin, 153
Coversyl, 65
Cozaar, 67
Cranactin, 158
cranberry, 158
Crataegus laevigata, 160
Crataegutt, 160
creatine, 158
Creon, 148
Cresemba, 29
Crestor, 78
crizotinib, 229
crofelemer, 147
Crolom, 193
cromolyn, 184
cromolyn—inhaled, 222
cromolyn—nasal, 135
cromolyn—ophthalmic, 193
crotamiton, 100
Cryselle, 181, 182
Cubicin, 57
Culturelle, 161
Cutar, 104
Cutivate, 95
Cutter, 104
Cuvposa, 147
cyanide, 231
cyanide antidote kit, 231

cyanocobalamin, 125, 190
Cyanokit, 231, 232
Cyclafem 1/35, 182, 185
Cyclafem 7/7/7, 183, 185
Cyclen, 185
Cyclessa, 183
cyclobenzaprine, 1
Cyclocort, 95
Cyclogyl, 199
cyclopentolate, 199
cyclophosphamide, 191
Cycloset, 127
cyclosporine, 77–78, 92, 167, 229
cyclosporine—ophthalmic, 200
Cymbalta, 204
Cynara scolymus, 157
cyproheptadine, 131
cyproterone, 97, 191
Cystografin, 93
Cystospaz, 142–143
cytarabine, 191
cytarabine liposomal, 191
Cytomel, 124
Cytosar, 191
Cytotec, 143, 188
Cytovene, 35

D

dabigatran, 149
dacarbazine, 191
daclatasvir, 36

Dacogen, 191
dactinomycin, 191
Daklinza, 36
Dalacin, 190
Dalacin C, 57
Dalacin T, 97
dalbavancin, 51
dalfampridine, 177
dalfopristin, 57
Daliresp, 223
dalteparin, 150
Dalvance, 51
danazol, 77–78, 153
danshen, 153
Dantrium, 1–2
dantrolene, 1–2
dapagliflozin, 115, 118
dapsone, 32–33
Daptacel, 165
daptomycin, 57
darbepoetin, 155
darifenacin, 233
darunavir, 43, 44
darunavir-ritonavir, 229
dasabuvir, 39
dasatinib, 191
Dasetta 1/35, 182, 185
Dasetta 7/7/7, 183, 185
daunorubicin, 191
Daxas, 223
Daypro, 6
Daysee, 183
Daytrana, 215
DDAVP, 127
DDI, 41
DDrops, 126–127
Debacterol, 134
Debrox, 133
Decadron, 112
decitabine, 191
Deconamine, 129

Deconamine SR, 129
Deconsal I, 129
deet, 104
deferasirox, 155
deferoxamine, 231, 232
degarelix, 191
dehydroepiandrosterone, 158
Delatestryl, 110–111
Delsym, 132
Delzicol, 146
Demadex, 86
demeclocycline, 56
Demerol, 7
Denavir, 102
denileukin, 191
denosumab, 127
deoxycholic acid, 104
Depacon, 175
Depade, 212
Depakene, 175
Depakote, 175, 205–206
Depakote ER, 175, 205–206
Depo-Cyt, 191
Depo-Estradiol, 186
Depo-Medrol, 112
Depo-Provera, 189
Depo-SubQ Provera 104, 189
Depo-Testosterone, 110–111
DepoDur, 8
Deproic, 175
Dermaloc, 104
DermOtic, 133
Desferal, 232

desipramine, 184, 201
desirudin, 149
desloratadine, 129, 130
desmopressin, 127
Desogen, 182, 185
desogestrel, 182, 183, 185
desonide, 95
DesOwen, 95
desoximetasone, 95
Desquam, 96
desvenlafaxine, 204
Detrol, 234
Detrol LA, 234
Devil's claw, 158
Dex-4, 119
DexAlone, 132
dexamethasone, 81, 108, 112
dexamethasone—ophthalmic, 195–196
dexamethasone—otic, 133
Dexasone, 112
dexbrompheniramine, 129
dexchlorpheniramine, 131
Dexedrine, 214
DexFerrum, 121
Dexilant, 141
Dexiron, 121
dexlansoprazole, 141
dexmedetomidine, 13, 63
dexmethylphenidate, 214
DexPak, 112
dexrazoxane, 191
dextran, 91

dextroamphetamine, 214
dextromethorphan, 129, 130, 132, 179
dextrose, 119
D.H.E. 45, 176
DHEA, 158
DiaBeta, 118–119
Diamicron, 118
Diamicron MR, 118
Diamox, 197
Diamox Sequels, 197
Diane-35, 97
Diarr-Eze, 137
Diastat, 211
Diastat AcuDial, 211
diatrizoate, 93
Diazemuls, 211
diazepam, 211
dibucaine, 103
Dicetel, 148
Diclectin, 139
Diclegis, 139
diclofenac, 4
diclofenac—ophthalmic, 199
diclofenac—topical, 98
dicloxacillin, 53, 154
dicyclomine, 142
didanosine, 41
Didronel, 111
dienogest, 183, 186
difenoxin, 137
Differin, 94
Dificid, 52
diflorasone diacetate, 96
Diflucan, 29
diflunisal, 4

difluprednate, 196
dig immune Fab, 231
Digibind, 70
DigiFab, 70
Digitek, 69
digoxin, 69, 81, 92, 231
digoxin immune fab, 70
dihydrocodeine, 10
dihydroergotamine, 176
Dilacor XR, 84, 85
Dilantin, 174
Dilatrate-SR, 87
Dilaudid, 7
Diltia XT, 84, 85
diltiazem, 77–78, 84, 91, 92, 229
Diltiazem CD, 84
Diltzac, 84, 85
dimenhydrinate, 139
dimercaprol (BAL), 231
Dimetane-DX, 129
Dimetapp Cold & Allergy Elixir, 129
Dimetapp Decongestant Infant Drops, 133
Dimetapp DM Cold & Cough, 129
dimethyl fumarate, 177
dinoprostone, 188
Diocarpine, 198
Diogent, 194
Diovan, 67

Diovan HCT, 72, 73
Dipentum, 146
Diphen, 131
Diphenhist, 131
diphenhydramine, 129, 131, 134
diphenoxylate, 137
diphtheria, 163, 165
diphtheria tetanus, 166
diphtheria–tetanus toxoid, 165
Diprivan, 13
Diprolene, 96
Diprolene AF, 96
dipyridamole, 80, 89
Disalcid, 4
Diskets, 8
disopyramide, 63, 70, 81
disulfiram, 153, 212
Ditropan, 233
Ditropan XL, 233
Diuril, 86
divalproex, 175, 205–206
Divigel, 181
Dixarit, 67
dobutamine, 88
docetaxel, 191
docosanol, 102
Docu-Liquid, 145
Docu-Soft, 145
docusate, 145, 184
dofetilide, 63, 70
DOK, 145

dolasetron, 63, 138
Dolobid, 4
Dolophine, 8
Doloral, 8
Doloteffin, 158
dolutegravir, 39
Domeboro Otic, 133
domperidone, 139
Dona, 159
donepezil, 169, 170
dong quai, 153
DONNATAL, 142
dopamine, 88
Doribax, 48
doripenem, 48
dornase alfa, 222
Doryx, 56
dorzolamide, 197, 198
Dostinex, 127
Dovobet, 101
Dovonex, 101
doxazosin, 68
doxepin, 184, 201
doxepin—topical, 104
doxercalciferol, 125
Doxil, 191
doxorubicin lipo-somal, 191
doxorubicinnon-liposomal, 191
Doxycin, 56
doxycycline, 18–20, 24, 26–28, 32, 56
doxylamine, 10, 139, 184

DPP-4 inhibitors (gliptins), 107, 115
Dramamine, 139
Drisdol, 125
Dristan 12 Hr Nasal, 135
Drithocreme, 101
Drixoral Cold & Allergy, 129
dronabinol, 139
dronedarone, 39, 63, 70, 77, 78, 229
droperidol, 63, 139
drospirenone, 181, 182, 185, 187
Droxia, 156, 191
DRV, 43
Dry Eyes, 200
Drysol, 103
DT, 165
D2T5, 165
DTaP, 165
DTG, 39
DTIC-Dome, 191
Duac, 97
Duavee, 188
Duetact, 114
dulaglutide, 115
Dulcolax, 145
Dulera, 221
duloxetine, 204
Duodart, 233
DuoLube, 200
Duoneb, 221
DUOPA, 178
Duragesic, 6–7
Duratuss, 129
Duratuss HD©II, 130
Durela, 11
Durezol, 196
dutasteride, 233
Dutoprol, 72, 73
Duvoid, 234
Dyazide, 72, 73

Dymista, 135
Dyrenium, 86
Dysport, 179
Dytan, 131

E

E. angustifolia, 158
E. pallida, 158
E. purpurea, 158
Ebixa, 170
EC-Naprosyn, 5–6
echinacea, 158
Echinacin Madaus, 158
EchinaGuard, 158
echinocandins, 30–31
econazole, 99
Econopred Plus, 196–197
Ecotrin, 3–4
Ecoza, 99
ED Spaz, 142–143
Edarbi, 67
Edarbyclor, 72, 73
Edecrin, 85
Edex, 234–235
edoxaban, 149
EDTA, 231
Edurant, 41
EES, 52
efavirenz, 30, 38, 40, 42, 43, 44
Effer-K, 122
Effexor, 204
Effexor XR, 204
Effient, 80
Efidac/24, 133
efinaconazole, 99
eflornithine, 104
Efudex, 98
EFV, 40
EGb 761, 159

Elavil, 201
Eldepryl, 179
elderberry, 158
Eldopaque, 104
Eldoquin, 104
Eldoquin Forte, 104
Electropeg, 144
Elepsia XR, 173
Elestat, 193
Elestrin, 186
eletriptan, 175
Eleutherococcus senticosus, 159
Elidel, 102
Eligard, 191
Elimite, 101
Elinest, 182
Eliphos, 120
Eliquis, 149
Elitek, 192
elixir, 223
Elixophyllin, 223
Ellence, 191
Elocon, 95
Eloxatin, 191
Elspar, 192
Eltroxin, 124
elvitegravir, 39
Emadine, 193
Emcyt, 191
emedastine, 193
Emend, 138
Emetrol, 139
EMLA, 13
Emoquette, 182, 185
empagliflozin, 114, 118
Empirin, 3–4
Empirin with Codeine, 9
Emsam, 202
emtricitabine, 38, 39, 41
Emtriva, 41
Enablex, 233

enalapril, 59, 65, 73
enalaprilat, 65
Enbrel, 226
Endocet, 10
Endocodone, 8
Enduron, 87
Enemeez, 145
Enemol, 144
Engerix-B, 165
enoxaparin, 150, 151
Enpresse, 183, 185
Enskyce, 182, 185
entacapone, 178, 179
entecavir, 35
Entereg, 146
Entex PSE, 130
Entocort EC, 146–147
Entozyme, 148
Entresto, 74
Entrophen, 3–4
Entsol, 136
Entyvio, 148
Enulose, 143
Envarsus XR, 167
Epaned, 65
Epanova®, 60, 79
Epaxal, 165
ephedrine, 88
Epiduo, 97
Epiduo Forte, 97
Epifoam, 103
epinastine, 193
epinephrine, 13–14, 88
epinephrine racemic, 222
EpiPen, 88
EpiPen Jr, 88
EpiQuin Micro, 104
epirubicin, 191
Epitol, 170–171

Epival, 175, 205–206
Epivir, 41
Epivir-HBV, 41
eplerenone, 66
epoetin alfa, 155
Epogen, 155
epoprostenol, 89
Eprex, 155
eprosartan, 67, 73
eptifibatide, 80
Epzicom, 39
Equalactin, 143
Equetro, 170–171
Eraxis, 49
Erbitux, 191
ergocalciferol, 125
ergot alkaloids, 39
ergotamine, 176
eribulin, 63
erlotinib, 153, 191
Errin, 182, 184
Ertaczo, 100
ertapenem, 48
Ery-Sol, 97
Ery-Tab, 52
Eryc, 52
Erycette, 97
Eryderm, 97
Erygel, 97
EryPed, 52
Erythrocin IV, 52
erythromycin, 24, 26, 63, 77–78, 91, 154, 184
erythromycin base, 52
erythromycin base—topical, 96
erythromycin ethylsuccinate, 24, 26, 52

erythromycin lactobionate, 52
erythromycin—ophthalmic, 194
erythromycin—topical, 97
erythropoietin alpha, 155
Esbriet, 223
escitalopram, 63, 202
Esgic, 2
eslicarbazepine, 171
esmolol, 82
esomeprazole, 80, 141
Esoterica, 104
Estalis, 188
Estarylla, 182, 185
estazolam, 211
esterified estrogens, 186
Estrace, 187
estradiol, 186–188
estradiol acetate vaginal ring, 186
estradiol cypionate, 186
estradiol gel, 186
estradiol transdermal patch, 186–187
estradiol transdermal spray, 187
estradiol vaginal ring, 187
estradiol vaginal tab, 187
estradiol valerate, 186
Estradot, 186–187
estramustine, 191

Estring, 187
Estrogel, 186
estrogen vaginal cream, 187
estrogens conjugated, 187–188
Estrostep Fe, 182, 185
eszopiclone, 212
etanercept, 225, 226
ethacrynic acid, 85
ethambutol, 33
ethinyl estradiol, 97, 181–186
ethosuximide, 171
ethylene glycol, 231
ethynodiol, 182
Ethyol, 191
Etibi, 33
etidronate, 111
etodolac, 4, 5
etomidate, 13
etonogestrel vaginal ring, 186
Etopophos, 191
etoposide, 191
ETR, 40
etravirine, 38, 40, 80, 153
Euflex, 191
Euglucon, 118–119
Eulexin, 191
Eurax, 100
Euthyrox, 124
Evamist, 187
everolimus, 167, 191
EVG, 39

Evista, 189, 191
Evoclin, 97
evolocumab, 79
Evotaz, 43
Evoxac, 134
Evra, 186
Ex-Lax, 145
Exalgo, 7
Excedrin
    Migraine, 2
Exelon, 170
Exelon Patch,
    170
exemestane,
    191
exenatide, 115
Exforge, 72, 73
Exforge HCT,
    72, 73
Exjade, 155
Exsel, 105
extended-release
    dipyridamole,
    80
extended-release
    niacin, 60, 78
extended release
    nicotinic acid,
    60
Extina, 99–100
Eylea, 200
EZ-Char,
    231–232
ezetimibe, 60,
    77, 79
Ezetrol, 171
ezogabine, 171

F

Fabior, 97
Factive, 55
Fallback Solo,
    181, 186

Falmina, 181,
    184
famciclovir,
    24–25, 38,
    184
famotidine, 63,
    141, 154,
    184
Fampyra, 177
Famvir, 38
Fanapt, 208
Fareston, 191
Farxiga, 118
Faslodex, 191
fat emulsion, 123
FazaClo ODT, 208
febuxostat, 230
Feen-a-Mint, 145
felbamate, 63, 80
Feldene, 6
felodipine, 84
Femaprin, 157
Femara, 191
Femcon Fe, 182
Femizol-M, 190
Femring, 186
fenofibrate, 60,
    75, 78
fenofibric acid, 76
Fenoglide, 75
fenoldopam, 74
fentanyl, 1, 6–7
fentanyl trans-
    dermaldose, 7
Fentora, 6–7
fenugreek, 158
Feosol, 121
Fer-In-Sol, 121
Feraheme, 121
Fergon, 121
Ferodan, 121
Ferrex 150, 121
ferric carboxy-
    maltose, 120
ferric citrate,
    123–124
ferric gluconate
    complex,
    120–121

Ferrlecit,
    120–121
ferrous fumarate,
    184, 185
ferrous gluconate,
    121
ferrous sulfate,
    121
ferumoxsil, 93
ferumoxytol, 121
fesoterodine, 233
Fetzima, 204
feverfew, 158
Fexicam, 6
fexofenadine,
    129, 131
FFP, 231
Fiberall, 143
FiberCon, 143
fibrates, 60, 61,
    153
Fibricor, 76
fidaxomicin, 52
Fidelin, 158
15-methyl-pros-
    taglandin F2
    alpha, 189
filgrastim, 155
filgrastim-sndz,
    155
Finacea, 96
finasteride, 233
Finevin, 96
fingolimod, 63,
    177
Fioricet, 3
Fioricet with
    Codeine, 9
Fiorinal, 3
Fiorinal C-1/2, 9
Fiorinal C-1/4, 9
Fiorinal with
    Codeine, 9
Firmagon, 191
5-aminosalicylic
    acid, 146
5-Aspirin, 146
5-FU, 98, 191

FK 506, 167
Flagyl, 57
Flagyl ER, 57
Flamazine, 99
Flarex, 196
flavocoxid, 158
Flebogamma,
    167
flecainide, 63, 70
Flector, 4
Fleet, 143, 145
Fleet enema, 144
Fleet EZ-Prep,
    144
Fleet Mineral Oil
    Enema, 145
Fleet Pain Relief,
    103
Fleet Sof-Lax,
    145
Fletcher's
    Castoria, 145
Flexeril, 1
Flo-Pred, 113
Flolan, 89
Flomax, 233
Flonase, 135
Florastor, 161
Florinef, 112
Flovent Diskus,
    221
Flovent HFA,
    217, 221
Floxin Otic, 133
floxuridine, 191
Fluarix, 165–166
Flublok,
    165–166
Flucelvax,
    164–166
fluconazole, 24,
    29, 63, 80,
    153, 228,
    229
flucytosine, 31
Fludara, 191
fludarabine, 191
fludrocortisone,
    108, 112

FluLaval, 164–166
Flumadine, 45
flumazenil, 231, 232
FluMist, 166
flunarizine, 176
flunisolide HFA MDI, 218
flunisolide—inhaled, 221
flunisolide—nasal, 135
fluocinolone, 95, 105
fluocinolone—otic, 133
fluocinolone—topical, 105
fluocinonide, 96
Fluor-A-Day, 121
fluoride, 121
fluorometholone, 196
Fluoroplex, 98
fluoroquinolones, 153
fluorouracil, 153, 191
fluorouracil—topical, 98
fluoxetine, 80, 202–203, 208–209, 212
fluphenazine, 206, 207
flurandrenolide, 95
flurazepam, 211
flurbiprofen, 4, 5
flurbiprofen—ophthalmic, 199
flutamide, 191
fluticasone DPI, 218
fluticasone furoate, 221

fluticasone HFA MDI, 218
fluticasone propionate, 95
fluticasone—inhaled, 220, 221
fluticasone—nasal, 135
fluvastatin, 60, 62, 64, 77
fluvastatin XL, 62, 64
Fluviral, 165–166
Fluvirin, 165–166
fluvoxamine, 80, 153, 203
Fluzone, 165–166
Fluzone HD, 164
Fluzone ID, 164, 165
FML, 196
FML Forte, 196
FML-S Liquifilm, 195
Focalin, 214
Focalin XR, 214
folate, 125
folic acid, 125, 190
folinic acid, 192
Folotyn, 191
Folvite, 125
fomepizole, 231, 232
fondaparinux, 149–150
Foradil, 217, 219
Forfivo XL, 204–205
formoterol, 219, 221
Fortamet, 119
Fortaz, 50
Forteo, 128
Fortical, 127
Forxiga, 118

Fosamax, 111
Fosamax Plus D, 111
fosamprenavir, 43–44, 229
fosamprenavir-ritonavir, 39, 44, 229
fosaprepitant, 138
Fosavance, 111
foscarnet, 35, 63
Foscavir, 35
fosfomycin, 57
fosinopril, 59, 65, 73
fosphenytoin, 63, 153, 154, 171
Fosrenol, 124
FPV, 43–44
Fragmin, 150
Frisium, 171
Frova, 175
frovatriptan, 175
FSH, 188
FTC, 41
Fucidin, 98
Fucidin-H, 103
fucithalmic, 194
FUDR, 191
Fulyzaq, 147
fulvestrant, 191
Fulyzaq, 147
Furadantin, 57
furosemide, 85
fusidic acid—ophthalmic, 194
fusidic acid—topical, 98, 103
Fusilev, 192
Fycompa, 173

Gadavist, 93
gadobenate, 93
gadobutrol, 93
gadodiamide, 93
gadopentetate, 93
gadoteridol, 93
gadoversetamide, 93
galantamine, 169–170
Galexos, 36
Galzin, 123
Gamastan, 167
gamma hydroxy-butyrate, 180
Gammagard, 167
Gammaplex, 167
Gamunex, 167
ganciclovir, 35
ganciclovir—oph-thalmic, 195
ganirelix, 187
Garamycin, 194
Gardasil, 164, 165
garlic supple-ments, 159
Gas-X, 143
Gastrocrom, 222
Gastrografin, 93
GastroMARK, 93
gatifloxacin, 63
Gattex, 148
Gaviscon, 140
gefitinib, 191
Gelclair, 134
Gelnique, 233
gemcitabine, 153, 191
gemfibrozil, 60, 76–78, 153
gemifloxacin, 26, 55, 63

G

G115, 159
G-CSF, 155
gabapentin, 171
Gabitril, 174

Gemzar, 191
Gen-K, 123
Gengraf, 167
Genisoy, 162
Genoptic, 194
Genotropin, 128
Gentak, 194
gentamicin,
    27, 29
gentamicin—oph-
    thalmic, 194,
    196
gentamicin—topi-
    cal, 98
GenTeal, 200
Gentran, 91
Geodon, 210
Gerber Soothe
    Colic drops,
    161
GHB, 180
GI cocktail, 142
Gianvi, 181,
    185
Giazo, 146
Gildess Fe
    1.5/30, 182
Gildess Fe 1/20,
    181, 184
Gilenya, 177
ginger, 159
ginkgo, 153
ginkgo biloba,
    159
Ginkgold, 159
Ginkoba, 159
Ginsana, 159
ginseng—
    American,
    154, 159
ginseng—Asian,
    159

ginseng—
    Siberian, 159
glatiramer, 177
Glatopa, 177
Gleevec, 191
Gliadel, 191
gliclazide, 118
glimepiride,
    113–114, 118
glipizide, 115,
    118
GLP-1 agonists,
    107, 115–116
GlucaGen, 119
glucagon, 119,
    231
Glucobay, 113
GlucoNorm, 118
Glucophage, 119
Glucophage XR,
    119
glucosamine, 159
glucosamine-
    chondroitin,
    153
Glucotrol, 118
Glucotrol XL, 118
Glucovance, 118
Glumetza, 119
Glutose, 119
glyburide, 114,
    118–119
glycerin, 143
GlycoLax, 144
glycopeptides, 51
glycopyrrolate,
    14, 147
Glycyrrhiza
    glabra, 160
Glycyrrhiza ura-
    lensis, 160
Glynase PresTab,
    118–119
Glyquin, 104
Glyset, 113

GoLYTELY, 144
gonadotropins,
    188
gonorrhea, 24
Goody's Extra
    Strength
    Headache
    Powder, 3
goserelin, 191
Gralise, 171
gramicidin, 195
granisetron, 63,
    138
Granix, 155
Gravol, 139
green goddess,
    142
green tea, 160
Grifulvin V, 31
griseofulvin, 31,
    154, 183
guaifenesin, 129,
    130, 132
Guaifenex PSE,
    130
guanfacine, 68,
    214
Guiatuss, 132
GuiatussPE, 129
Gyne-Lotrimin,
    190

H

H-BIG, 167
Habitrol, 213
haemophilus B
    vaccine, 165
halcinonide, 96
Halcion, 212
Haldol, 207
HalfLytely, 144
Halfprin, 3–4
halobetasol pro-
    pionate, 96
halofantrine, 63
Halog, 96
haloperidol, 63,
    206, 207

Harpadol, 158
Harpagophytum
    procumbens,
    158
Harvoni, 36
Havrix, 165
hawthorn, 160
HCQ, 228
HCTZ, 63, 73, 86
Healthy Woman,
    162
HeartCare, 160
Heather, 182,
    184
Hecoria, 167
Hectorol, 125
Hemabate, 189
HepaGam B, 167
heparin, 65,
    150–153, 156,
    184, 231
hepatitis A
    vaccine, 163,
    165, 166
hepatitis B
    immune globu-
    lin, 167
hepatitis B
    vaccine, 163,
    165–166
Hepsera, 35
Heptovir, 41
Herceptin, 191
Hespan, 91
hetastarch, 91
Hexabrix, 94
Hexalen, 191
Hextend, 91
Hiberix, 165
histrelin, 191
Histussin D©II,
    130
Histussin HC©II,
    130
Hizentra, 167
Holkira Pak, 37
homatropine—
    ophthalmic,
    199

honey, 160
Horizant, 171
horse chestnut seed extract, 160
HP-Pac, 141
huang qi, 157
Humalog, 116, 117
Humalog Mix 50/50, 116, 117
Humalog Mix 75/25, 116, 117
human growth hormone, 128
human papillomavirus recombinant vaccine, 165
Humatrope, 128
Humibid DM, 130
Humira, 226
Humulin 70/30, 116, 117
Humulin N, 116, 117
Humulin R, 116, 117
hyaluronic acid, 104
Hycamtin, 191
Hycotuss©II, 130
hydralazine, 73, 74, 91, 184
hydraSense, 136
Hydrea, 156, 191
hydrochlorothiazide, 86
Hydrocil, 143
hydrocodone, 1, 9–11, 130, 132
hydrocortisone, 95, 103, 105, 108, 112, 134

hydrocortisone acetate, 95
hydrocortisone butyrate, 95
hydrocortisone valerate, 95
hydrocortisone—ophthalmic, 195
hydrocortisone—otic, 133
hydrocortisone—topical, 103, 105
Hydromorph Contin, 7
hydromorphone, 1, 7
hydroquinone, 104–105
hydroxocobalamin, 231, 232
hydroxychloroquine, 225, 228
hydroxychloroquine sulfate, 228
hydroxyprogesterone caproate, 190
hydroxypropyl cellulose, 200
hydroxyurea, 156, 191
hydroxyzine, 131
hyoscine, 142
hyoscyamine, 142–143, 233–234
Hyosol, 142–143
Hyospaz, 142–143
Hypaque, 93
HyperHep B, 167
Hypericum perforatum, 162
HyperRAB S/D, 167

HyperRHO S/D, 190
Hypocol, 161–162
Hypotears, 200
Hytone, 95
Hytuss, 132
Hyzaar, 72, 73

I

ibandronate, 111
ibritumomab, 191
Ibudone, 9
ibuprofen, 4, 5, 9, 10
ibutilide, 63, 71
icosapent ethyl, 79
Idamycin, 191
idarubicin, 191
Ifex, 191
ifosfamide, 153, 191
Ilaris, 227
Ilevro, 200
iloperidone, 63, 206, 208
iloprost, 89
Ilotycin, 194
imatinib, 153, 191, 229
imipenem-cilastatin, 48
imipramine, 201–202
imiquimod, 102
Imitrex, 176
Immucyst, 191
immune globulin—intramuscular, 167
immune globulin—intravenous, 167
immune globulin—subcutaneous, 167

Imodium, 137
Imodium AD, 137
Imodium Multi-Symptom Relief, 137
Imogam Rabies-HT, 167
Imovane, 212
Imovax Rabies, 166
Imuran, 228
Inapsine, 139
incobotulinumtoxin A, 180
Incruse Ellipta, 223
indacaterol, 219
indapamide, 86
Inderal, 83
Inderal LA, 83
Inderide, 72, 73
indinavir, 229
Indocin, 5
Indocin IV, 5
Indocin SR, 5
indomethacin, 4, 5
Infanrix, 165
InFeD, 121
Inflamase Forte, 196–197
infliximab, 227
influenza vaccine, 163
influenza vaccine—inactivated injection, 165–166
influenza vaccine—live intranasal, 166
Infufer, 121

ingenol, 98
INH, 33
Inhibace, 65
Inhibace Plus, 72, 73
Injectafer, 120
InnoPran XL, 83
Inspra, 66
Insta-Glucose, 119
insulin, 107, 116–118, 118
insulin aspart, 116
insulin aspart protamine, 116
insulin degludec/ aspart, 116
insulin detemir, 116
insulin glargine, 116
insulin glulisine, 116
insulin lispro, 116
insulin lispro protamine, 116
insulin—inhaled short-acting, 116
insulin—injectable combinations, 117
insulin—injectable intermediate, 117
insulin—injectable, long-acting, 117–118
insulin—injectable short-/rapid-acting, 117

Intal, 222
Integrilin, 80
Intelence, 40
interferon alfa-2b, 47, 191
interferon beta-1a, 177
interferon beta-1b, 177
interleukin-2, 191
Intestinex, 161
Intralipid, 123
intravaginal, 153
intravaginal butoconazole, 24
Intron-A, 47, 191
Introvale, 183, 185
Intuniv, 214
Intuniv XR, 68
Invanz, 48
Invega, 209
Invega Sustenna, 209
Invega Trinza, 209
Invirase, 44
Invokamet, 114
Invokana, 118
iodixanol, 93
iohexol, 93
iopamidol, 94
iopromide, 94
iothalamate, 94
ioversol, 94
ioxaglate, 94
ioxilan, 94
ipecac syrup, 232
IPOL, 166
ipratropium—inhaled, 220–222
ipratropium—nasal, 135
Iprivask, 149
Iquix, 197
irbesartan, 67, 73

Iressa, 191
iron, 231
iron dextran, 121
iron polysaccharide, 121
iron sucrose, 121
isavuconazole, 29, 229
isavuconazonium, 29
Isentress, 40
isocarboxazid, 202
isoniazid, 33, 153
isopropyl alcohol, 133
isoproterenol, 71
Isoptin SR, 85
Isopto Atropine, 199
Isopto Carbachol, 198
Isopto Carpine, 198
Isopto Homatropine, 199
Isordil, 87
isosorbide dinitrate, 87, 91
isosorbide mononitrate, 87
Isotamine, 33
isotretinoin, 97
Isovue, 94
isradipine, 63, 84
Istalol, 197
Istodax, 192
Isuprel, 71
itraconazole, 30, 35, 70, 77–78, 81, 90, 91, 153, 229, 233
ivabradine, 91
ivermectin, 27, 34

ivermectin—topical, 104
ixabepilone, 191
Ixempra, 191
Ixiaro, 166

J

Jalyn, 233
Jantoven, 153
Janumet, 114
Janumet XR, 114
Januvia, 115
Japanese encephalitis vaccine, 166
Jardiance, 118
Jencycla, 182, 184
Jentadueto, 114
Jevtana, 191
Jin Fu Kang, 157
Jolessa, 181
Jolivette, 182, 184
Jublia, 99
Junel 1.5/30, 182
Junel 1/20, 181
Junel 1.5/30 Fe, 182
Junel Fe 1/20, 181, 184

K

K+8, 123
K+10, 123
K-Dur 10, 123
K-Dur 20, 123
K-G Elixir, 122
K-Lor, 123
K-Lyte, 122
K-Lyte/Cl, 122
K-Lyte/Cl 50, 122
K-Lyte DS, 122
K-Norm, 123
K-Phos, 122

K-Tab, 123
K-vescent, 122
Kabikinase; 91
Kadian, 8
Kaletra, 44
Kaochlor 10%, 122
Kaochlor S-F, 122
Kaon, 122
Kaon-Cl 20%, 122
Kaopectate, 137
Kapvay, 67
Kariva, 182, 185
Kay Ciel, 122, 123
Kayexalate, 128
Kaylixir, 122
Kazano, 114
K+Care, 123
K+Care ET, 122
Kcentra, 156
Keflex, 48
Kelnor 1/35, 182
Kenalog, 95, 96, 113
Kengreal, 80
Kepivance, 191
Keppra, 173
Keppra XR, 173
Kerlone, 82
Ketalar, 13
ketamine, 13
Ketek, 58
ketoconazole, 35, 70, 77–78, 80, 81, 90, 91, 153, 229, 233
ketoconazole—topical, 99–100
Ketoderm, 99–100
ketoprofen, 4, 5
ketorolac, 4, 5
ketorolac—ophthalmic, 199

ketotifen, 222
ketotifen—ophthalmic, 193
Khedezla, 204
Kidrolase, 192
Kineret, 227
Kitabis Pak, 29
Kivexa, 39
Klaron, 97
Klean-Prep, 144
Klonopin, 210
Klonopin Wafer, 210
Klor-Con, 123
Klor-Con 8, 123
Klor-Con 25, 123
Klor-Con/EF, 122
Klor-Con M20, 123
Klor-Con M10 Klotrix, 123
Klorvess Effervescent, 122
Kolyum, 122
Kombiglyze XR, 114
Komboglyze, 114
Kondremul, 145
Konsyl, 143
Konsyl Fiber, 143
Korean red ginseng, 159
Kristalose, 143
Krystexxa, 230
Ku-Zyme, 148
Ku-Zyme HP, 148
Kurvelo, 182, 184
Kwai, 159
Kwellada-P, 101
Kybella, 104
Kyolic, 159

lacosamide, 172
Lacri-lube, 200
Lacrisert, 200
Lactaid, 147
lactase, 147
lactic acid, 104
lactulose, 143, 184
Lamictal, 172–173, 205
Lamictal CD, 172–173, 205
Lamictal ODT, 172–173, 205
Lamictal XR, 172–173, 205
Lamisil, 31, 100
Lamisil AT, 100
lamivudine, 35, 38, 39, 41
lamotrigine, 172–173, 205
Lanoxin, 69
lansoprazole, 6, 141–142
Lansoyl, 145
lanthanum carbonate, 124
Lantus, 116–118
Lantus SoloSTAR, 118
Lanvis, 191
lapatinib, 63, 191
Larin Fe 1.5/30, 182
Larin Fe 1/20, 181, 184
Lasix, 85
Lastacaft, 193
latanoprost, 198
Latisse, 198
Latuda, 208
Lax-A-Day, 144
Lazanda, 6–7
lead, 231
Lectopam, 210
ledipasvir, 36
Leena, 183

LEF, 228
leflunomide, 153, 225, 228
Legalon, 160
Lemtrada, 176
lenalidomide, 191
lepirudin, 153
Lescol, 77
Lescol XL, 77
Lessina, 181, 184
Letairis, 88–89
letrozole, 191
leucovorin, 192
Leukeran, 191
Leukine, 155
leuprolide, 63, 187, 191
Leustatin, 191
levalbuterol, 220
Levaquin, 55
Levbid, 142–143
Levemir, 116–118
Levemir FlexTouch, 118
levetiracetam, 173
Levitra, 235
Levo-Dromoran, 7
levobunolol, 197
levocabastine—nasal, 135
levocarnitine, 123
levocetirizine, 132
levodopa, 179
levofloxacin, 18–19, 24, 26, 55, 63

L

levofloxacin—
ophthalmic,
194
levoleucovorin,
192
levomilnacipran,
204
Levonest, 183,
185
levonorgestrel,
181–185, 187
levonorgestrel—
intrauterine,
186
levonorgestrel—
single dose,
186
Levophed, 88
Levora, 181,
182, 184
levorphanol, 1, 7
levothyroxine,
124, 153,
184
Levsin, 142–143
Lexapro, 202
Lexiva, 43–44
LH, 188
Lialda, 146
licorice, 160
Lidex, 96
lidocaine, 71
lidocaine—local
anesthetic, 13
lidocaine—oph-
thalmic, 200
lidocaine—
topical, 13,
104–105
lidocaine—vis-
cous, 134
Lidoderm,
104–105
Limbrel, 158

linaclotide, 147
linagliptin, 114,
115
lindane, 100
linezolid, 20, 57
Linzess, 147
Lioresal, 1
Lioresal D.S., 1
liothyronine, 124,
184
Lipidil EZ, 75
Lipidil Micro, 75
Lipidil Supra, 75
Lipitor, 77
Lipofen, 75, 76
lipoic acid, 157
Liposyn, 123
Liptruzet®, 60,
77
Liqui-Doss, 145
liraglutide, 116
lisdexamfe-
tamine,
214–215
lisinopril, 59,
65, 73
lisinopril HCTZ,
73
Lithane, 205
lithium, 63, 205
Lithobid, 205
Livalo, 78
Livostin, 135
LMX, 104–105
Lo Loestrin Fe,
181
Lo Media 1/20,
181
Lo Minastrin Fe,
181
Lo/Ovral, 181,
182
Locoid, 95
Lodalis, 75
lodoxamide, 194
Loestrin 1.5/30,
182
Loestrin-21 1/20,
181

Loestrin-24 Fe,
181
Loestrin Fe, 184
Loestrin Fe
1.5/30, 182
Loestrin Fe 1/20,
181
Logestrel, 182
lomitapide, 78
Lomotil, 137
lomustine/gleo-
stine, 191
Loperacap, 137
loperamide, 137,
184
Lopid, 76
lopinavir, 44
lopinavir-ritonavir,
39, 44, 229
lopinavir with
ritonavir, 78
Lopressor, 83
Lopressor HCT,
72, 73
Loprox, 99
Loprox TS, 99
loratadine, 129,
131
lorazepam, 211
lorcaserin, 147
Lorcet, 9
Lortab, 9
Loryna, 181,
185
Lorzone, 187
losartan, 67, 73
LoSeasonique,
181, 183,
184
Losec, 142
Lotemax, 196
Lotensin, 59, 65
Lotensin HCT,
72, 73
loteprednol, 196
Lotrel, 72
Lotriderm, 103
Lotrimin AF, 99,
100

Lotrimin Ultra,
99
Lotrisone, 103
Lotronex, 146
lovastatin, 39,
60, 62, 64,
77, 92
Lovaza®, 60, 79
Lovenox, 150
low molecular wt
heparins, 184
Low-Ogestrel,
181
loxapine, 206
Lozide, 86
LPV/R, 44
lubiprostone, 145
luliconazole, 100
lumefantrine, 32
Lumigan, 198
Luminal, 173
Lunesta, 212
Lupaneta Pack,
187
Lupron, 191
Lupron Depot,
191
Lupron Depot-
Ped, 191
lurasidone, 206,
208
Luride, 121
Lustra, 104
Lutera, 181
Luvox, 203
Luvox CR, 203
Luxiq, 95
Luzu, 100
Lybrel, 183
lymphocyte
immune globu-
lin, 167
Lyrica, 174
Lysodren, 192

M

M-Eslon, 8
M-M-R II, 166

M-Zole, 190
Maalox, 140
MabCampath, 191
macitentan, 89
Macrobid, 57
Macrodantin, 57
Macrodex, 91
macrolides, 51–52, 153
mafenide, 98
Mag-200, 122
Mag-Ox 400, 122
Magic Mouthwash, 134
Maglucate, 122
magnesium carbonate, 2, 140
magnesium chloride, 121
magnesium citrate, 144
magnesium gluconate, 122
magnesium hydroxide, 2, 140, 141, 144
magnesium oxide, 2, 122
magnesium sulfate, 122, 144
Magnevist, 93
Magtrate, 122
Makena, 190
Malarone, 32
malathion, 27, 101
maltodextrin, 134
mangafodipir, 93
manganate, 122
mannitol, 180
Mantoux, 167
maraviroc, 38
Marcaine, 13
Marinol, 139

Marlissa, 182, 184
Marplan, 202
Marvelon, 185
Matricaria recutita—German chamomile, 157
Matulane, 191
Matzim LA, 84, 85
Mavik, 59, 66
Maxair Autohaler, 217, 220
Maxalt, 176
Maxalt MLT, 176
Maxeran, 139
Maxiflor, 96
Maxilene, 104–105
Maximum Strength Pepcid AC, 141
Maxipime, 50
Maxitrol, 195–196
Maxivate, 96
Maxzide, 72, 73
MD-Gastroview, 93
measles, 166
mechlorethamine, 191
Meclicot, 132
meclizine, 132, 184
meclofenamate, 4, 5
Medihoney, 160
Medispaz, 142–143
Medivert, 132
Medrol, 112
medroxyprogesterone, 188, 189
medroxyprogesterone—injectable, 189

mefenamic acid, 5
mefloquine, 32
Megace, 189
Megace ES, 189
megestrol, 189
meglitinides, 107, 118
Melaleuca alternifolia, 162
Melaleuca oil, 162
Melanex, 104
melatonin, 160
meloxicam, 4, 5
melphalan, 191
memantine, 170
Menactra, 164, 166
Menest, 186
Meni-D, 132
meningococcal vaccine, 166
Menjugate, 166
Menomune-A/C/Y/W-135, 166
Menopur, 188
Menostar, 186–187
menotropinsx, 188
Mentax, 99
Mentha x piperita oil, 160
Menveo, 164, 166
meperidine, 1, 7, 184
Mephyton, 126
mepivacaine, 13
Mepron, 34
mercaptopurine, 154, 191
mercury, 231
meropenem, 20, 48
Merrem IV, 48
Mersyndol with Codeine, 10

mesalamine, 146, 154
Mesasal, 146
mesna, 191
Mesnex, 191
Mestinon, 177
Mestinon Timespan, 177
mestranol, 182
Metadate CD, 215
Metadate ER, 215
Metadol, 8
Metaglip, 115
Metamucil, 143
metaproterenol, 220
Metastron, 191
metaxalone, 2
metformin, 107, 113–115, 119
methadone, 1, 8, 63, 184
Methadose, 8
methanol, 231
methazolamide, 197
methemoglobin, 231
methenamine, 233–234
Methergine, 189
methimazole, 124, 154
methocarbamol, 2
methohexital, 13
methotrexate, 191, 225–228
methotrexate—rheumatology, 228
methyclothiazide, 87

methylaminolevu-
linate, 98
methylcellulose,
143
methyldopa, 68,
73, 184
methylene blue,
231–234
methylergonovine,
189
Methylin, 215
Methylin ER, 215
methylnaltrexone,
147
methylphenidate,
215
methylpred-
nisolone, 108,
112, 227
metipranolol, 197
metoclopramide,
139, 184
metolazone, 87
metoprolol, 83
metoprolol suc-
cinate, 73
metoprolol
tartrate, 73
Metozolv ODT,
139
MetroCream, 98
MetroGel, 98
MetroGel-Vaginal,
190
MetroLotion, 98
metronidazole,
21, 24,
26–28, 57,
141, 153,
184
metronidazole—
topical, 98
metronidazole—
vaginal, 190

Metvix, 98
Metvixia, 98
Mevacor, 77
mexiletine, 71
Mexitil, 71
Miacalcin, 127
micafungin, 31
Micardis, 67
Micardis HCT,
72, 73
Micardis Plus,
72, 73
Micatin, 100
miconazole, 24,
153, 190
miconazole—buc-
cal, 30
miconazole—
topical, 100,
105
Micozole, 190
MICRhoGAM,
190
Micro-K, 123
Micro-K 10, 123
Microgestin
1.5/30, 182
Microgestin 1/20,
181
Microgestin Fe
1.5/30, 182
Microgestin Fe
1/20, 181,
184
Micronor, 182,
184
Microzide, 86
Midamor, 86
midazolam, 13
midodrine, 88
Midol Teen
Formula, 11
miglitol, 113
Migranal, 176
MigreLief, 158
Milk of Magnesia,
144
milk thistle, 160
Millipred, 113

milnacipran, 180
milrinone, 88
Min-Ovral, 184
Minastrin 24 Fe,
181
mineral oil, 145
Minipress, 68
Minirin, 127
Minitran, 87
Minivelle,
186–187
Minizide, 72, 73
Minocin, 56
minocycline, 56,
225
Minoxidil for
Men, 105
minoxidil—topi-
cal, 105
Miostat, 198
mirabegron, 63,
205
MiraLax, 144
Mirapex, 178
Mirapex ER, 178
Mircette, 182,
185
Mirena, 186
mirtazapine, 63,
205
Mirvaso, 104
misoprostol, 4,
143
misoprostol—OB,
188
Mitigare, 230
mitomycin, 191
Mitomycin-C,
191
mitotane, 154,
192
mitoxantrone,
191
Mobic, 5
Mobicox, 5
modafinil, 215
Modecate, 207
Modicon, 182
Moduret, 72, 73

Moduretic, 72,
73
moexipril, 59,
63, 65, 73
molindone, 206
mometasone DPI,
218
mometasone
furoate, 95
mometasone—
inhaled, 221
mometasone—
nasal, 135
Monascus
purpureus,
161–162
Monazole, 190
Monistat, 190
Mono-Linyah,
182, 185
Monocor, 82
Monodox, 56
Monopril, 59
Monopril HCT,
72, 73
montelukast,
184, 222
Montmorency
cherry, 162
Monurol, 57
Morinda citrifolia,
160
morphine, 1, 7, 8
M.O.S., 8
Motofen, 137
Motrin, 5
Movantik, 147
MoviPrep, 144
Moxatag, 53
Moxeza, 194
moxifloxacin,
18–19, 26,
55, 63
moxifloxacin—
ophthalmic,
194
MS Contin, 8
MSIR, 8
MTX, 228

Mucaine, 140
Mucinex, 132
Mucinex-DM
    Extended-
    Release, 129
Mucomyst, 222,
    231
Multaq, 70
MultiHance, 93
multivitamins,
    125
mumps, 166
Mupirocin,
    98–99
Murine Ear, 133
Muse, 234–235
Mustargen, 191
Mutamycin, 191
MVC, 38
MVI, 125
Myambutol, 33
Mycamine, 31
Mycelex, 99
Mycelex 7, 190
Mycobutin, 33
Mycolog II, 103
mycophenolate
    mofetil, 167
Mycostatin, 100
Mydriacyl, 199
Myfortic, 167
Mylanta, 134,
    140
Mylanta
    Children's,
    120
Myleran, 191
Mylicon, 143
Myobloc, 179
Myocet, 191
Myorisan, 97
Myotonachol,
    234
Myrbetriq, 234
Mysoline, 174
Mytussin DM,
    129
Myzilra, 183,
    185

N

N-acetyl-5-
    methoxytrypta-
    mine, 160
N-acetylcysteine,
    231
NABI-HB, 167
nabilone, 139
nabumetone, 4, 5
nadolol, 73, 83
nafcillin, 53, 154
naftifine, 100
Naftin, 100
nalbuphine, 1, 6
Nalcrom, 222
naloxegol, 147
naloxone, 6, 11,
    213, 231
naltrexone, 147,
    212
Namenda, 170
Namenda XR,
    170
NAMZARIC, 170
naphazoline, 193
Naphcon, 193
Naphcon-A, 193
Naprelan, 5–6
Naprosyn, 5–6
naproxen, 4–6,
    176
naratriptan, 175
Narcan, 11
Nardi, 202
Nasacort AQ, 135
Nasacort HFA,
    135
NaSal, 136
NasalCrom, 135
Nasalide, 135
Nascobal, 125
Nasonex, 135
natalizumab, 177
Natazia, 183, 186
nateglinide, 118
Natesto,
    110–111

Natpara, 128
Natrecor, 92
Natroba, 101
Navelbine, 191
nebivolol, 83
Necon 1/35,
    182, 185
Necon 7/7/7,
    183, 185
nedocromil, 184
nedocromil—oph-
    thalmic, 194
nefazodone, 70,
    77–78, 81,
    229, 233
nelarabine, 191
nelfinavir, 41,
    229, 233
Neo-Fradin, 147
Neo-Synephrine,
    135
neomycin, 153
neomycin—
    ophthalmic,
    195–196
neomycin—oral,
    147
neomycin—otic,
    133
neomycin—topi-
    cal, 99, 103
NeoProfen, 5
Neoral, 167
Neosar, 191
Neosporin Cream,
    99
Neosporin
    Ointment, 99
Neosporin
    Ointment—
    Ophthalmic,
    195
Neosporin
    Solution—
    Ophthalmic,
    195
neostigmine, 14
nepafenac, 200
Nephro-Vite, 125

Nephrocap, 125
Nesina, 115
nesiritide, 92
NESP, 155
netupitant, 138,
    229
Neulasta, 155
Neumega, 155
Neupogen, 155
Neupro, 179
Neurontin, 171
Neutra-Phos,
    122
Nevanac, 200
nevirapine, 38,
    40–41, 44
Nexavar, 191
Nexium, 141
Next Choice One-
    Step, 186
niacin, 60,
    61, 77, 78,
    125–126
Niacor, 125–126
Niaspan®, 60,
    125–126
nicardipine,
    63, 84
NicoDerm CQ,
    213
Nicolar, 125–126
Nicorette,
    212–213
Nicorette DS,
    212–213
Nicorette Inhaler,
    213
nicotine gum,
    212–213
nicotine inhala-
    tion system,
    213
nicotine lozenge,
    213

nicotine nasal spray, 213
nicotine patches, 213
nicotinic acid, 60, 125–126
Nicotrol, 213
Nicotrol Inhaler, 213
Nicotrol NS, 213
Nidagel, 190
Nidazol, 57
nifedipine, 84, 184
Niferex, 121
Niferex-150, 121
Nikki, 181, 185
Nilandron, 191
nilotinib, 63, 191
nilutamide, 191
Nimbex, 14
nimodipine, 180
Nimotop, 180
nintedanib, 222
Nipent, 191
Niravam, 211
nisoldipine, 84
nitazoxanide, 34
Nitoman, 180
Nitro-BID, 87
Nitro-Dur, 87
nitrofurantoin, 57, 184
nitroglycerin intravenous infusion, 87
nitroglycerin ointment, 87
nitroglycerin spray, 87
nitroglycerin sublingual, 87

nitroglycerin sustained release, 87
nitroglycerin transdermal, 87
nitroglycerin—rectal, 148
Nitrolingual, 87
NitroMist, 87
Nitropress, 74
nitroprusside, 74
Nitrostat, 87
nizatidine, 141, 154, 184
Nizoral, 99–100
Nizoral AD, 99–100
n,n-diethyl-m-toluamide, 104
NoDoz, 214
noni, 160
Nor-Q.D., 182, 184
Nora BE, 182, 184
Norco, 10
Norcuron, 14
Nordette, 181, 182, 184
Norditropin, 128
Norditropin FlexPro, 128
Norditropin NordiFlex, 128
norelgestromin, 186
norepinephrine, 88
Norethin 1/35, 182
norethindrone, 181–185, 187
norethindrone acetate, 188, 189
Norflex, 2

Norgesic, 3
norgestimate, 185, 188
norgestrel, 182
Norinyl 1+35, 182, 185
Norinyl 1+50, 182
Noritate, 98
Norlutate, 189
Norpace, 70
Norpace CR, 70
Norpramin, 201
Nortrel 0.5/35, 182
Nortrel 1/35, 182, 185
Nortrel 7/7/7, 183, 185
nortriptyline, 202
Norvasc, 84
Norvir, 44
Nostrilla, 135
Novantrone, 191
Novasen, 3–4
Novasoy, 162
Novolin 70/30, 116, 117
Novolin N, 116, 117
Novolin R, 116, 117
NovoLog, 116, 117
NovoLog Mix 70/30, 116, 117
NovoRapid, 117
Noxafil, 30
NPH, 116
Nu-Iron 150, 121
Nubain, 6
Nucynta, 11
Nucynta ER, 11
Nuedexta, 179
NuLev, 142–143
Nulojix, 167
NuLYTELY, 144

Numby Stuff, 104–105
Nupercainal, 103
Nuprin, 5
Nutropin AQ, 128
Nutropin Depot, 128
Nuvaring, 186
Nuvessa, 190
Nuvigil, 214
NVP, 40–41
Nyaderm, 100
Nyamyc, 100
Nymalize, 180
nystatin, 31, 184
nystatin—topical, 100, 103
Nytol, 131

O

oatmeal, 105
Ocean, 136
Ocella, 182, 185
Octagam, 167
Octostim, 127
octreotide, 147
Octycine, 145
Ocufen, 199
Ocuflox, 194
Ocupress, 197
Oesclim, 186–187
ofatumumab, 191
Ofev, 222
Off, 104
Ofirmev, 11
ofloxacin, 24, 26, 55, 63
ofloxacin—ophthalmic, 194
ofloxacin—otic, 133
Ogestrel, 181, 182
olanzapine, 63, 203, 206, 208–209, 212

Oleptro, 205
Olestyr, 75
olmesartan, 67, 73
Olmetec, 67
olodaterol, 219
olopatadine, 193
olopatadine—nasal, 135
olopatadine—ophthalmic, 193
olsalazine, 146, 153
Olux, 96
Olysio, 36
ombitasvir, 37
ombitasvir-paritaprevir-ritonavir, 37
omega-3-acid ethyl esters, 79
omega-3-carboxylic acids, 79
omega3 fatty acids, 60
omeprazole, 80, 142, 153
Omnaris, 134–135
Omnicef, 50
Omnipaque, 93
Omniscan, 93
Omnitrope, 128
Omtryg, 79
onabotulinum toxin type A, 180
Onbrez Breezhaler, 219
Oncaspar, 192
Oncotice, 191
Oncovin, 191
ondansetron, 63, 138, 184
Onexton, 97
ONFI, 171

Onglyza, 115
Onmel, 30
Onsolis, 6–7
Ontak, 191
Onxol, 191
Opana, 8
Opana ER, 8
Ophthaine, 200
Ophthetic, 200
opiates, 231
opioids, 231
opium, 138
opium tincture, 138
oprelvekin, 155
Opsumit, 89
Opticrom, 193
OptiMARK, 93
Optipranolol, 197
Optiray, 94
Optivar, 193
Oracea, 56
Oracit, 235
OraDisc A, 134
Oramorph SR, 8
Orap, 207
Orapred, 113
Orapred ODT, 113
Oravig, 30
Orazinc, 123
Orbactiv, 51
orciprenaline, 220
Orencia, 227
Orenitram, 90
Oretic, 86
Orgalutran, 187
organophos-phates, 231
oritavancin, 51
orlistat, 128
orphenadrine, 2, 3
Orsythia, 181, 184
Ortho-Cept, 182, 185

Ortho-Cyclen, 182, 185
Ortho Evra, 186
Ortho-Novum 1/35, 182, 185
Ortho-Novum 7/7/7, 183, 185
Ortho Tri-Cyclen, 183, 185
Ortho Tri-Cyclen Lo, 183, 185
Orudis, 5
Orudis KT, 5
Oruvail, 5
Os-Cal, 120
oseltamivir, 45, 46
Oseni, 115
Osmitrol, 180
OsmoPrep, 144
ospemifene, 189
Osphena, 189
Osteoforte, 125
Otezla, 230
Otrexup, 228
Ovcon-35, 182, 185
Ovide, 101
Ovidrel, 188
Ovol, 143
oxacillin, 53
oxaliplatin, 191
oxaprozin, 4, 6
oxazepam, 211
oxcarbazepine, 173
Oxecta, 8
Oxeze Turbuhaler, 219
oxiconazole, 100
Oxilan, 94
Oxistat, 100
Oxizole, 100
Oxtellar XR, 173
oxybate, 180
Oxybutyn, 233
oxybutynin, 233

Oxycocet, 10
Oxycodan, 10
oxycodone, 1, 8–10, 184
OxyContin, 8
OxyFAST, 8
OxyIR, 8
oxymetazoline, 135
oxymorphone, 1, 8
OxyNEO, 8
oxytocin, 63, 188
Oxytrol, 233
Oyst-Cal, 120

P

Pacerone, 69
Pacis, 191
paclitaxel, 191
palifermin, 191
paliperidone, 63, 206, 209
palivizumab, 47
palonosetron, 138
pamabrom, 11
Pamelor, 202
pamidronate, 111
Panadol, 11
Panax ginseng, 159
Panax quinquefo-lius L., 159
pancreatin, 148
Pancreaze, 148
Pancrecarb, 148
pancrelipase, 148
panitumumab, 191
Panretin, 103
Pantoloc, 142

pantoprazole, 142
pantothenic acid, 125
paracetamol, 11
Parafon Forte DSC, 1
Paraplatin, 191
parathyroid hormone, 128
Parcopa, 178
paregoric, 138
paricalcitol, 126
Pariet, 142
paritaprevir, 44
Parlodel, 127
Parnate, 202
paromomycin, 34
paroxetine, 153, 203
Parvolex, 231
Pataday, 193
Patanase, 135
Patanol, 193
Paxil, 203
Paxil CR, 203
Pazeo, 193
pazopanib, 191
P.C.E., 52
PediaCare Infants' Decongestant Drops, 133
Pediapred, 113
Pediarix, 166
Pediatrix, 11
PedvaxHIB, 164, 165
Peg-Lyte, 144
pegaspargase, 192
Pegasys, 48
pegfilgrastim, 155

peginterferon, 43
peginterferon alfa-2A, 48
peginterferon alfa-2B, 48
PegIntron, 48
pegloticase, 230
pemetrexed, 191
penciclovir, 102
penicillin, 20, 52–54, 153, 184
penicillin G, 20, 28, 53
penicillin V, 53
Penlac, 99
Pennsaid, 98
pentamidine, 63
Pentasa, 146
pentazocine, 1, 6
Pentolair, 199
pentostatin, 191
pentoxifylline, 92, 153
Pepcid, 141
Pepcid AC, 141
Pepcid Complete, 141
peppermint oil, 160
Peptic Relief, 141
Pepto-Bismol, 137
peramivir, 45, 46
perampanel, 173
Percocet, 10
Percocet-demi-, 10
Percodan, 10
Percolone, 8
perflutren lipid microspheres, 63
Perforomist, 219
Pergonal, 188
Peri-Colace, 145
Periactin, 131
Peridex, 134

perindopril, 59, 65, 73
Periogard, 134
Perlane, 104
permethrin, 27, 101, 184
perphenazine, 206, 207
Persantine, 80
Petadolex, 157
Petasites hybridus, 157
pethidine, 7
petrolatum, 200
Pexeva, 203
PGE1, 143, 188
PGE2, 188
Pharmorubicin, 191
Phazyme, 143
Phenazo, 234
phenazopyridine, 234
Phenegran/ Dextromethorphan, 130
Phenegran VC, 130
Phenegran VC w/ codeine©V, 130
phenelzine, 202
Phenergan, 139
pheniramine, 193
phenobarbital, 35, 41, 70, 142, 173, 174
phentermine, 148, 215
phentolamine, 75
phenyl salicylate, 233–234
phenylephrine, 129, 130, 133
phenylephrine— intravenous, 88

phenylephrine— nasal, 135
phenylephrine— ophthalmic, 199
Phenytek, 174
phenytoin, 35, 41, 70, 81, 153, 154, 174
Philith, 182, 185
Phoslax, 144
PhosLo, 120
Phoslyra, 120
phosphorated carbohydrates, 139
phosphorus, 122
Photofrin, 192
Phrenilin, 3
Phyto soya, 162
phytonadione, 126
Picato, 98
pilocarpine, 134
pilocarpine—ophthalmic, 198
pimecrolimus, 102
pimozide, 39, 63, 203, 206, 207
Pimtrea, 182, 185
Pin-X, 34
pinaverium, 148
pindolol, 83
Pinworm, 34
pioglitazone, 113–115, 119
piperacillin-tazobactam, 54
pirbuterol, 220
pirfenidone, 223
Pirmella 1/35, 182, 185
Pirmella 7/7/7, 185
piroxicam, 4, 6

pitavastatin, 62, 64, 78
Pitocin, 188
Plan B One-Step, 181, 186
Plaquenil, 228
Plasbumin, 91
plasma protein fraction, 91
Plasmanate, 91
Plasmatein, 91
Platinol-AQ, 191
Plavix, 80
Plendil, 84
Pletal, 91
Pliaglis, 105
Pneumo 23, 166
pneumococcal 13-valent conjugate vaccine, 163, 166
pneumococcal 23-valent vaccine, 163, 166
Pneumovax, 166
Pneumovax 23, 163
Podocon-25, 102
Podofilm, 102
podofilox, 102
Podofin, 102
podophyllin, 102
Polaramine, 131
polio vaccine, 166
Polocaine, 13
polycarbophil, 143
Polycitra, 235
Polycitra-K, 235
Polycitra-LC, 235
polyethylene glycol, 144
polyethylene glycol with electrolytes, 144

polymyxin—ophthalmic, 195–196
polymyxin—otic, 133
polymyxin—topical, 99, 103
Polyphenon E, 160
Polysporin, 99
Polysporin—Ophthalmic, 195
Polytar, 104
polythiazide, 73
Polytopic, 99
Polytrim—Ophthalmic, 195
Ponstan, 5
Ponstel, 5
Pontocaine, 200
porfimer, 192
Portia, 181, 182, 184
posaconazole, 30, 77, 78, 229
Posanol, 30
Potasalan, 122
potassium, 123
potassium sulfate, 144
potentiates warfarin, 222
Potiga, 171
Power-Dophilus, 161
PPD, 167
Pradaxa, 149
Pralatrexate, 191
pralidoxime, 231, 232
Praluent, 79
pramipexole, 178
pramlintide, 107, 119
Pramosone, 103, 105
Pramox HC, 105

pramoxine, 103
pramoxine—topical, 103, 105
Prandimet, 115
Prandin, 118
Prasterone, 158
prasugrel, 80
Pravachol, 78
pravastatin, 60, 62, 64, 78, 154
praziquantel, 34
prazosin, 68, 73
Precedex, 13
Precose, 113
Pred Forte, 196–197
Pred G, 196
Pred Mild, 196–197
prednisolone, 108, 113
prednisolone—ophthalmic, 195–197
prednisone, 108, 113, 184
Prednisone Intensol, 113
Prefest, 188
pregabalin, 174
Prelone, 113
Premarin, 187
Premesis-RX, 190
Premphase, 188
PremPlus, 188
Prempro, 188
Prepidil, 188
Prepopik, 144
Pressyn AR, 88
Prestalia, 72, 73
Pretz, 136
Prevacid, 141–142
Prevacid NapraPAC, 5–6
Prevalite, 75

Previfem, 182, 185
Prevnar 13, 163, 166
PrevPac, 141
Prezcobix, 44
Prezista, 43
Priftin, 33
prilocaine, 14
prilocaine—topical, 13
Prilosec, 142
Primadophilus, 161
primaquine, 32
primaxin, 48
Primella 7/7/7, 183
primidone, 154, 174
Primsol, 58
Prinivil, 59, 65
Prinzide, 72, 73
Priorix, 166
Pristiq, 204
Privigen, 167
Pro-Banthine, 143
ProAir HFA, 217, 219–220
ProAir RespiClick, 219–220
probenecid, 230
probiotics, 161
procainamide, 63, 71
procaine penicillin, 52–53
procarbazine, 191
Procardia, 84
Procardia XL, 84
ProCentra, 214

prochlorperazine, 139
Procrit, 155
Proctofoam HC, 103
ProctoFoam NS, 103
Prodium, 234
progesterone micronized, 189
Prograf, 167
proguanil, 32
ProHance, 93
Prolensa, 199
Proleukin, 191
Prolia, 127
Proloprim, 58
Promensil, 161
promethazine, 63, 130, 139
Prometrium, 189
propafenone, 71, 153
propantheline, 143
proparacaine, 200
Propecia, 233
propofol, 13
propoxyphene, 153
propranolol, 73, 83, 222
Propyl Thyracil, 124
propylene glycol, 134
propylthiouracil, 124, 154
ProQuad, 166
Proscar, 233
Prosed/DS, 233
ProSom, 211

prostaglandin E1, 234–235
Prostin E2, 188
Prostin VR, 234–235
Prostin VR Pediatric, 234–235
protamine, 156, 231
protease inhibitors, 183
Protenate, 91
prothrombin complex concentrate, 156
Protonix, 142
Protopam, 232
Protopic, 102
protriptyline, 202
Protropin, 128
Proventil HFA, 217, 219–220
Provera, 189
Provigil, 215
Prozac, 202–203
Prozac Weekly, 202–203
Prudoxin, 104
Prunus cerasus, 162
pseudoephedrine, 129, 130, 132, 133
pseudoephedrine chlorpheniramine, 129
pseudoephedrinedesloratadine, 129
Psorcon, 96
psyllium, 143, 184
PTU, 124
Pulmicort, 217
Pulmicort Flexhaler, 221
Pulmicort Respules, 221

Pulmicort Turbuhaler, 221
Pulmozyme, 222
Purinethol, 191
pygeum africanum, 161
Pylera, 141
pyrantel, 34
pyrazinamide, 33
pyrethrins, 101
Pyriate, 234
Pyridium, 234
pyridostigmine, 177
pyridoxine, 125, 126, 139, 190
PZA, 33

Q

Qnasl, 134
Qsymia, 148
Quadramet, 191
Qualaquin, 32
Quartette, 183
Quasense, 181, 183, 185
Qudexy XR, 174–175
Quelicin, 14
Questran, 75
Questran Light, 75
quetiapine, 63, 206, 209
Quick-Pep, 214
Quillivant XR, 215
quinapril, 59, 66, 73
quinidine, 63, 71, 153, 179
quinine, 32, 153
quinolones, 54–55
quinupristin, 57
Quixin, 194

Qutenza, 104
QVAR, 217, 221

R

RabAvert, 166
rabeprazole, 142
rabies immune globulin human, 167
rabies vaccine, 166
Rabies Vaccine Adsorbed, 166
RAL, 40
Ralivia, 11
raloxifene, 154, 189, 191
raltegravir, 38, 40
ramelteon, 212
ramipril, 59, 66
Ranexa, 92
ranitidine, 141, 154, 184
ranolazine, 63, 78, 92, 229
Rapaflo, 233
Rapamune, 167
Rapivab, 45, 46
rasagiline, 179
rasburicase, 192
Rasilez, 74
Rasilez HCT, 72, 73
Rasuvo, 228
raxibacumab, 20
Rayos, 113
Razadyne, 169–170
Razadyne ER, 169–170
R&C, 101
Re-Azo, 234
Reactine, 131
Rebetol, 36
Rebif, 177
Reclast, 111–112

Silenor, 201
...odosin, 233
...adene, 99
... sulfadia-
... mari-
99
60
38

...00
...ni, 211
RestoroLAX, 144
Restylane, 104
... M, 200
...esh Tears, 200
Regitine, 75
Reglan, 139
Regonol, 177
Regranex, 104
Rejuva-A, 97
Relafen, 5
Relenza, 45, 46
ReliOn Novolin 70/30, 117
ReliOn Novolin N, 117
Relistor, 147
Relpax, 175
Remeron, 205
Remeron SolTab, 205
Remicade, 227
Reminyl, 169–170
Remodulin, 90
Remular-S, 1
Renagel, 124
Renedil, 84
Reno-60, 93
Reno-DIP, 93
RenoCal, 93
Renografin, 93
Renova, 97
Renvela, 124
ReoPro, 79
repaglinide, 115, 118
Repatha, 79
Repel, 104

Rifadin, 33
Rifamate, 33
rifampin, 33, 35, 36, 39, 70, 81, 90, 154, 183
rifapentine, 33, 39, 154
Rifater, 33
rifaximin, 57
rilpivirine, 38–39, 41
Rilutek, 180
riluzole, 180
rimantadine, 45
rimexolone, 197
riociguat, 89
Riomet, 119
risedronate, 111
Risperdal, 210
Risperdal Consta, 210
Risperdal M-Tab, 210
risperidone, 63, 206, 210
Ritalin, 215
Ritalin LA, 215
Ritalin SR, 215
ritonavir, 37, 38, 39, 42, 43, 44, 70, 154, 229, 233
Rituxan, 191, 227
rituximab, 191, 227
rivaroxaban, 150
rivastigmine, 170
Rivotril, 210
rizatriptan, 176
Robaxin, 2
Robaxin-750, 2
Robinul, 147
Robinul Forte, 147
Robitussin, 132
Robitussin AC ©V, 130

retapamulin, 99
Retavase, 90, 151
Retin-A, 97
Retin-A Micro, 97
Retisol-A, 97
Retrovir, 42
Revatio, 89
ReVia, 212
Revlimid, 191
Revonto, 1–2
Rexulti, 208
Reyataz, 42–43
Rezira, 132
Rheomacrodex, 91
Rheumatrex, 228
Rhinalar, 135
Rhinocort Allergy Spray, 134
Rhinocort Aqua, 134
RHO immune globulin, 190
RhoGAM, 190
Rhophylac, 190
Rhotral, 82
Ribasphere, 36
ribavirin, 43, 154
ribavirin—oral, 36
riboflavin, 125, 126
RID, 101
rifabutin, 33, 154, 183

Robitussin CF, 129
Robitussin Cough, 132
Robitussin DAC ©V, 130
Robitussin DM, 129
Robitussin PE, 129
Rocaltrol, 125
Rocephin, 50
rocuronium, 14
Rofact, 33
roflumilast, 223
Rogaine, 105
Rogaine Extra Strength, 105
Rogitine, 75
Rolaids, 140
Romazicon, 232
romidepsin, 192
Rondec DM Oral Drops, 130
Rondec DM Syrup, 130
Rondec Oral Drops, 130
Rondec Syrup, 130
ropinirole, 178–179
Rosasol, 98
rosiglitazone, 113–114, 119
rosuvastatin, 60, 62, 64, 78
Rotarix, 164, 166
RotaTeq, 166
Rotateq, 164
rotavirus vaccine, 166
rotigotine, 179

Rowasa, 146
Roxanol, 8
Roxicet, 10
Roxicodone, 8
Rozerem, 212
RPT, 33
RPV, 41
RSV immune
 globulin, 167
RTV, 44
rubella vaccine,
 166
Rubex, 191
Rubini, 158
Rufen, 5
rufinamide, 174
Rum-K, 122
Ryanodex, 1–2
Rybix ODT, 11
Rylosol, 72
Rynatan, 130
Rynatan-P
 Pediatric, 130
Rytary, 178
Rythmol, 71
Rythmol SR, 71
rythromycin,
 229
Ryzodeg 70/30,
 116, 117
Ryzolt, 11

S

S-2, 222
S-adenosyl-
 methionine
 (SAM-e), 162
Saccharomyces
 boulardii, 161
sacubitril, 74
Safyral, 182
Saizen, 128
Salagen, 134
Salazopyrin
 EN-tabs, 146,
 229
salbutamol,
 219–220
Salflex, 4
Salicin, 162
Salicis cortex,
 162
salicylic acid, 97
saline nasal
 spray, 136
salmeterol, 39,
 219, 220
Salofalk, 146
salsalate, 4
samarium 153,
 191
Sambucol, 158
Sambucus nigra,
 158
Sanctura, 234
Sanctura XR, 234
Sancuso, 138
Sandimmune,
 167
Sandostatin,
 147
Sandostatin LAR,
 147
Sans-Acne, 97
Saphris, 208
saquinavir, 44,
 63
saquinavir-ritona-
 vir, 229
Sarafem,
 202–203
sargramostim,
 155
Savaysa, 149
Savella, 180
saxagliptin, 114,
 115
Saxenda, 116
Scopace, 140
scopolamine,
 140, 142
SeaMist, 136
Seasonale, 181,
 183, 185
Seasonique, 181,
 183
Sebivo, 35
SecreFlo, 148
secretin, 148
Sectral, 82
secukinumab,
 227
Sedapap, 3
selegiline, 179
selegiline—trans-
 dermal, 202
selenium sulfide,
 105
Selsun, 105
Selzentry, 38
Semprex-D, 130
senna, 145
sennosides, 145
Senokot, 145
Senokot-S, 145
SenokotXTRA,
 145
Sensorcaine, 13
Septacaine, 13
Septra, 55
Serevent Diskus,
 217, 219
Serophene, 188
Seroquel, 209
Seroquel XR, 209
Serostim, 128
Serostim LQ, 128
sertaconazole,
 100
sertraline, 203
sevelamer, 124
sevoflurane, 63
SGLT2 inhibitors,
 118
short-acting
 inhaled beta-2
 agonists, 184
Silace, 145
Siladryl, 131
sildenafil, 39, 89,
 235
S_
si_.
 zi_
Silybu_
 anum_
Silymarin,
Simbrinza,
Simcor, 78
simeprevir, 36,
 39, 78
simethicone,
 137, 140,
 143, 184
Simponi,
 226–227
Simponi Aria,
 226–227
Simulect, 167
simvastatin, 39,
 60, 62, 64,
 78–79, 92
sinecatechins,
 102
Sinemet, 178
Sinemet CR,
 178
Singulair, 222
sirolimus, 92,
 167
sitagliptin, 114,
 115
Sitavig, 37
Sivextro, 58
6-MP, 191
Skelaxin, 2
Sklice, 104
Slo-Niacin®, 60,
 125–126
Slow-Fe, 121
Slow-K, 123
Slow-Mag, 121
SMV, 36
sodium bicarbon-
 ate, 72, 231
sodium phos-
 phate, 144,
 234

sodium picosulfate, 144
sodium polystyrene sulfonate, 128
sodium sulfate, 144
sodium valproate, 175
SOF, 35–36
sofosbuvir, 35–36
Solaquin, 104
Solaraze, 98
Solia, 181
solifenacin, 233–234
Solodyn, 56
Soltamox, 189
Solu-Cortef, 112
Solu-Medrol, 112
Solugel, 96
Soma, 1
Soma Compound, 3
Soma Compound with Codeine, 10
somatropin, 128
Sominex, 131
Sonata, 212
Soolantra, 104
sorafenib, 191
sorbitol, 144
Soriatane, 101
Sorilux, 101
sotalol, 63, 72
Sotret, 97
Sotylize, 72
sour cherry, 162
Sovaldi, 35–36
soy, 162
Spacol, 142–143
Spasdel, 142–143
Spectracef, 50
spinosad, 101
Spiriva, 217, 223
Spiriva HandiHaler, 223

Spiriva Respimat, 223
spironolactone, 66, 73
Sporanox, 30
Sprintec, 182, 185
Sprycel, 191
SQV, 44
Sronyx, 181
St. John's wort, 39, 70, 162
Stadol, 6
Stadol NS, 6
Stalevo, 179
starch, 103
Starlix, 118
Statex, 8
statins, 60, 64, 153
Stavzor, 175, 205–206
Staxyn, 235
Stay Awake, 214
Stelara, 101–102
Stemetil, 139
Stendra, 235
Stieprox shampoo, 99
Stieva-A, 97
Stimate, 127
Strattera, 214
Streptase, 91
streptokinase, 91
streptomycin, 29
streptozocin, 191
Striant, 110–111
Stribild, 39, 205
Stridex Pads, 97
Striverdi Respimat, 219
Stromectol, 34
strontium-89, 191

succimer, 231, 232
succinylcholine, 14
Suclear, 144
sucralfate, 134, 143
sucroferric oxyhydroxide, 124
Sudafed, 133
Sudafed 12 Hour, 133
Sudafed PE, 133
Sular, 84
Sulcrate, 143
Sulf-10, 195
Sulfacet-R, 97
sulfacetamide—ophthalmic, 195, 196
sulfacetamide—topical, 97
Sulfamylon, 98
sulfasalazine, 225
sulfasalazine—gastroenterology, 146
sulfasalazine—rheumatology, 229
Sulfatrim Pediatric, 55
sulfinpyrazone, 153
sulfonamides, 55, 153
sulfonated phenolics, 134
sulfonylureas, 107, 118–119
sulfur, 97
sulfuric acid, 134
sulindac, 9, 153
sumatriptan, 176
Sumavel, 176
sunitinib, 63, 191
sunscreen, 105

succimer, 231, 232

265
Index

Supeudol, 8
Supprelin LA, 191
Suprax, 50
Suprenza, 215
Suprep, 144
Supro, 162
Surpass, 120
Sustiva, 40
Sutent, 191
suvorexant, 212
Swim-Ear, 133
Syeda, 182, 185
Symax, 142–143
Symbicort, 221
Symbicort Turbuhaler, 221
Symbyax, 212
Symlin, 119
SymlinPen, 119
Synacthen, 120
Synagis, 47
Synalar, 95
Synalgos-DC, 10
Synera, 105
synercid, 57
Synthroid, 124
Systane, 200

T

T3, 124
T4, 124
T-Phyl, 223
Tabloid, 191
Taclonex, 101
tacrolimus, 63, 92, 167
tacrolimus—topical, 102
Tactuo, 97
tadalafil, 39, 89, 90, 235

tafluprost, 198
Tagamet, 140
Tagamet HB, 140
Talwin NX, 6
Tamiflu, 45, 46
Tamofen, 189
Tamone, 189
tamoxifen, 63, 153, 189
tamsulosin, 233
Tanacetum parthenium L., 158
Tanafed, 130
Tanzeum, 115
Tapazole, 124
tapentadol, 11
Tarceva, 191
Targretin, 192
Tarka, 72, 73
Tarsum, 104
Tart cherry, 162
Tasigna, 191
Tavist-1, 131
Tavist ND, 131
Taxol, 191
Taxotere, 191
tazarotene, 97
Tazicef, 50
Tazocin, 54
Tazorac, 97
Taztia XT, 84, 85
tbo-filgrastim, 155
TCAs, 153, 231
Td, 165
Tdap, 163, 165
TDF, 42
tea tree oil, 162
Tears Naturale, 200
Tebrazid, 33
Tecfidera, 177
technivie, 37

Tecta, 142
tedizolid, 58
teduglutide, 148
Teflaro, 51
Tegretol, 170–171
Tegretol XR, 170–171
Tegrin, 104
Tekamlo, 72, 73
Tekturna, 74
Tekturna HCT, 72, 73
telavancin, 51
telbivudine, 35
telithromycin, 58, 63, 77–78, 81, 229
telmisartan, 67, 73
Telzir, 43–44
temazepam, 211
Temodal, 191
Temodar, 191
Temovate, 96
temozolomide, 191
Tempra, 11
temsirolimus, 191
tenecteplase, 91, 151
Tenex, 68
teniposide, 191
tenofovir, 38–39, 41, 42
Tenoretic, 72, 73
Tenormin, 82
Terazol, 190
terazosin, 68
terbinafine, 31
terbinafine—topical, 100
terconazole, 24, 190
teriparatide, 128
Tersi, 105
Teslascan, 93
Tessalon, 132

Tessalon Perles, 132
Testim, 110–111
Testopel, 110–111
testosterone, 110–111
Testro AQ, 110–111
tetanus, 163, 165
tetanus toxoid, 166
tetrabenazine, 180
tetracaine, 135
tetracaine—ophthalmic, 200
tetracaine—topical, 105
tetracyclines, 32, 56, 141
Teveten, 67
Teveten HCT, 72, 73
thalidomide, 191
Thalomid, 191
Theo-24, 223
Theo-Dur, 223
Theolair, 223
theophylline, 89, 184, 203, 222, 223
TheraCys, 191
thiamine, 125, 126
thiazide, 62
thiazolidinediones, 107, 119
thioctic acid, 157
thioguanine, 191
Thioplex, 191
thioridazine, 63, 203, 206, 207
thiotepa, 191
thiothixene, 206, 207
Thisilyn, 160

thonzonium, 133
3TC, 41
tiagabine, 174
Tiazac, 84
ticagrelor, 80
Tice BCG, 191
ticlopidine, 80, 81
Tigan, 140
tigecycline, 58, 153
Tikosyn, 70
Tilia Fe-28, 185
timolol, 83
timolol—ophthalmic, 197, 198
Timoptic, 197
Timoptic Ocudose, 197
Timoptic XE, 197
Tinactin, 100
Tindamax, 34
tinidazole, 26–28, 34
tioconazole, 24
tiotropium, 223
tipranavir, 45, 153
tipranavir-ritonavir, 38, 39, 229
tirofiban, 81
Tirosint, 124
Tivicay, 39
tizanidine, 2, 63, 203
TMP-SMX, 55
TNKase, 151
Tobi, 29
Tobradex, 196
Tobradex ST, 196
tobramycin, 29
tobramycin—ophthalmic, 194, 196
Tobrex, 194
tocilizumab, 228
tocopherol, 127
Toctino, 103

tofacitinib, 228
Tofranil, 201–202
Tofranil PM, 201–202
Tolectin, 6
tolmetin, 4, 6
tolnaftate, 100
Toloxin, 69
tolterodine, 63, 234
Topamax, 174–175, 205
Topicort, 95
topiramate, 148, 174–175, 205
Toposar, 191
topotecan, 191
Toprol-XL, 83
Toradol, 5
toremifene, 191
Torisel, 191
torsemide, 86
Totect, 191
Toujeo, 116
Toujeo SoloSTAR, 118
Toujeo Tresiba, 117–118
Toviaz, 233
TPA, 90
tPA, 90
TPV, 45
Tracleer, 89
Tradjenta, 115
Trajenta, 115
Tramacet, 3
tramadol, 3, 11, 153
Trandate, 82
trandolapril, 59, 66, 73
Transderm-Nitro, 87
Transderm-Scop, 140
Transderm-V, 140
transdermal fentanyl, 7

Tranxene, 210–211
tranylcypromine, 202
trastuzumab, 191
Travatan Z, 198
travoprost, 198
trazodone, 205
Treanda, 191
Trefoil, 161
Trelstar Depot, 191
treprostinil sodium—injectable, 90
treprostinil—inhaled solution, 90
Tresiba, 116
Tresiba FlexTouch, 118
tretinoin, 98, 105, 192
tretinoin—topical, 97
Trexall, 192
Treximet, 176
Tri-Cyclen, 185
Tri-Estarylla, 183, 185
Tri-K, 122
Tri-Legest, 182
Tri-Legest Fe, 182, 185
Tri-Linyah, 183, 185
Tri-Luma, 105
Tri-Nasal, 135
Tri-Norinyi, 183
Tri-Previfem, 183, 185
Tri-Sprintec, 183, 185
triamcinolone, 95, 96, 108, 113
triamcinolone—inhaled, 221

triamcinolone—nasal, 135
triamcinolone—topical, 103
Triaminic Cold & Allergy, 129
Triaminic Oral Infant Drops, 133
triamterene, 73, 86
Trianal, 3
Trianal C-1/2, 9
Trianal C-1/4, 9
Triazide, 72
triazide, 73
triazolam, 39, 212
Tribenzor, 72, 73
TriCor, 75
Tridesilon, 95
Tridural, 11
Triesence, 113
trifluoperazine, 206, 207
trifluridine, 195
Trifolium pratense, 161
Triglide, 75
Trigonelle foenum-graecum, 158
trihexyphenidyl, 177
Trileptal, 173
TriLipix, 76
Trilisate, 4
TriLyte, 144
trimethobenzamide, 140, 184
trimethoprim, 58
trimethoprim-sulfamethoxazole, 26, 55
trimethoprim—ophthalmic, 195
Trinipatch, 87
Trinovin, 161

Trintellix, 203
Triostat, 124
Tripacel, 165
triprolidine, 129
triptorelin, 191
Trisenox, 191–192
Triumeq, 39
Trivora, 181
Trivora-28, 183, 185
Trizivir, 39
Trokendi XR, 174–175
Tropicacyl, 199
tropicamide, 199
Trosec, 234
trospium, 234
Trulicity, 115
Trumenba, 166
Trumendat, 164
Trusopt, 197
Truvada, 39
tryptophan, 203
tuberculin PPD, 167
Tubersol, 167
Tucks, 103
Tucks Hemorrhoidal Ointment, 103
Tucks Suppositories, 103
Tudorza Pressair, 222
Tums, 120
Turdoza Genuair, 222
Tussionex©II, 130
Twin-K, 122
Twinrix, 163, 164, 166

292 Tab, 9
2-PAM, 232
Twynsta, 72, 73
Tybost, 43
Tygacil, 58
Tykerb, 191
Tylenol, 11
Tylenol #1, 10
Tylenol #2, 10
Tylenol #3, 10
Tylenol #4, 10
Tylenol with
    Codeine, 10
Tylox, 10
Typherix, 167
Typhim Vi, 167
typhoid vaccine—
    inactivated
    injection, 167
typhoid vaccine—
    live oral, 167
Tysabri, 177
Tyvaso, 90
Tyzeka, 35

U

ubiquinone, 158
Uceris, 146–147
Ulesfia, 100
Uloric, 230
Ultracet, 3
Ultram, 11
Ultram ER, 11
Ultraquin, 104
Ultrathon, 104
Ultravate, 96
Ultravist, 94
Ultresa, 148
umeclidinium,
    223
Unasyn, 54
Uni-retic, 72
Uniphyl, 223

Uniretic, 73
Unisom
    Nighttime
    Sleep Aid, 139
Unithroid, 124
Univasc, 59, 65
Urecholine, 234
Uricalm, 234
Urised, 234
Uristat, 234
Urocit-K, 235
Urodol, 234
Urogesic, 234
Urolene Blue,
    232
Uromax, 233
Uromitexan, 191
UroXatral, 233
URSO, 148
URSO Forte, 148
ursodiol, 148
ustekinumab,
    101–102
UTA, 234
UTI Relief, 234
Utira-C, 234

V

Vaccinium macro-
    carpon, 158
Vagifem, 187
valacyclovir,
    24–25, 38,
    184
Valcyte, 35
valerian, 162
Valeriana offici-
    nali, 162
Valium, 211
valproate, 153,
    172
valproic acid,
    175, 205–206
valrubicin, 191
valsartan, 67,
    73, 74
Valstar, 191

Valtaxin, 191
Valtrex, 38
Valtropin, 128
Vancocin, 51
vancomycin,
    21–22, 51
Vandazole, 190
vandetanib, 63
Vaniqa, 104
Vantas, 191
Vaponefrin, 222
Vaqta, 165
vardenafil, 63,
    89, 235
varenicline, 213
varicella vaccine,
    166, 167
Varilrix, 167
Varivax, 167
Vascepa®, 60, 79
Vascoray, 94
Vaseretic, 72, 73
Vasocidin, 196
Vasocon-A, 193
vasopressin, 88
Vasostrict, 88
Vasotec, 59, 65
Vaxigrip,
    165–166
VCR, 191
Vectibix, 191
vecuronium, 14
vedolizumab,
    148
Velban, 191
Velcade, 192
Veletri, 89
Velivet, 183
Velphoro, 124
Veltin, 98
Venastat, 160
venlafaxine, 63,
    204
Venofer, 121
Ventavis, 89
Ventolin HFA,
    217, 219–220
VePesid, 191
Veramyst, 135

verapamil, 73,
    77–78, 85,
    92, 229
Veregen, 102
Verelan, 85
Verelan PM, 85
Versacloz, 208
Versed, 13
Versel, 105
Vesanoid, 192
VESIcare,
    233–234
vetch, 157
Vexol, 197
Vfend, 30
Viactiv, 120
Viagra, 235
Vibativ, 51
Vibramycin, 56
Vicks 44 Cough,
    132
Vicks Sinex, 135
Vicks Sinex 12
    Hr, 135
Vicodin, 10
Vicoprofen, 10
Victoza, 116
Vidaza, 191
Videx, 41
Videx EC, 41
Viekira Pak, 37
Vigamox, 194
Viibryd, 205
vilanterol, 220
vilazodone, 205
Vimpat, 172
vinblastine, 191
Vincasar, 191
vincristine, 191
vinorelbine, 191
Viokace, 148
Viorele, 182, 185
Viramune, 40–41
Viramune XR,
    40–41
Viread, 42
Viroptic, 195
Visicol, 144
Visipaque, 93

Vistaril, 131
vitamin A, 126, 153
Vitamin A Acid Cream, 97
vitamin B1, 126
vitamin B2, 126
vitamin B3, 125–126
vitamin B6, 126
vitamin B12, 126
vitamin C, 124, 125, 154
vitamin D2, 125
vitamin D3, 126–127
vitamin E, 127, 153
vitamin K, 126, 231
Vitekta, 39
Vitex agnus castus fruit extract, 157
Vivactil, 202
Vivaglobulin, 167
Vivarin, 214
Vivelle Dot, 186–187
Vivitrol, 212
Vivotif Berna, 167
VLB, 191
VM-26, 191
Vogelxo, 110–111
Volibris, 88–89
Voltaren, 4, 98, 199
Voltaren Ophtha, 199
Voltaren Rapide, 4
Voltaren XR, 4
Voluven, 91
vorapaxar, 81
voriconazole, 30, 70, 77, 78, 80, 81, 153, 229

vorinostat, 153, 192
vortioxetine, 203
Vosol HC, 134
VoSpire ER, 219–220
Votrient, 191
VP-16, 191
Vraylar, 208
VSL#3, 161
Vumon, 191
Vusion, 105
Vyfemla, 182, 185
Vyloma, 102
Vytorin®, 60, 79
Vyvanse, 214–215

W

warfarin, 153, 154, 203, 231
Wartec, 102
Welchol, 75
Wellbutrin, 204–205
Wellbutrin SR, 204–205
Wellbutrin XL, 204–205
Wera, 182
Westcort, 95
white petrolatum, 105
willow bark extract, 162
Winpred, 113
WinRho SDF, 190
witch hazel, 103
Women's Rogaine, 105

X

Xalatan, 198
Xanax, 211
Xanax XR, 211

Xarelto, 150
Xatral, 233
Xeljanz, 228
Xeloda, 191
Xenazine, 180
Xenical, 148
Xeomin, 180
Xerese, 105
Xifaxan, 57
Xigduo XR, 115
Xodol, 11
Xolegel, 99–100
Xopenex, 220
Xopenex Concentrate, 220
Xopenex HFA, 217, 220
Xuezhikang, 161–162
Xulane, 186
Xylocaine, 13, 71, 104–105, 134
Xylocard, 71
Xyrem, 180
Xyzal, 132

Y

Yasmin, 182, 185
Yaz, 181, 185
yellow fever vaccine, 167
YF-Vax, 167
Yocon, 235
yohimbine, 235
Yohimex, 235

Z

Zaditen, 222
Zaditor, 193
zafirlukast, 153, 222
zaleplon, 212
Zanaflex, 2
zanamivir, 45, 46

269
Index

Zanosar, 191
Zantac, 141
Zantac 75, 141
Zantac 150, 141
Zantac EFFERdose, 141
Zarah, 182, 185
Zarontin, 171
Zarxio, 155
ZDV, 42
ZeaSorb AF, 100
Zebeta, 82
Zecuity, 176
Zegerid, 142
Zelapar, 179
Zeldox, 210
Zemplar, 126
Zemuron, 14
Zenatane, 97
Zenchent, 185
Zenhale, 221
Zenpep, 148
Zenzedi, 214
Zerbaxa, 50
Zestoretic, 72, 73
Zestril, 59, 65
Zetia, 79
Zetonna, 134–135
Zevalin, 191
Zhibituo, 161–162
Ziac, 72, 73
Ziagen, 41
Ziana, 98
zidovudine, 38, 39, 42
zileuton, 153, 222
Zinacef, 48
zinc acetate, 123
zinc oxide, 105
zinc sulfate, 123

Zincate, 123
Zinecard, 191
Zingiber offici-
nale, 159
Zingo, 104–105
Zioptan, 198
ziprasidone, 63,
206, 210
Zipsor, 4
Zirgan, 195
Zithranol, 101
Zithromax, 51–52

Zmax, 51–52
Zocor, 78
Zofran, 138
Zoladex, 191
zoledronic acid,
111–112
Zolinza, 192
zolmitriptan, 176
Zoloft, 203
Zomacton, 128
Zometa, 111–112
Zomig, 176
Zomig ZMT, 176
Zonalon, 104
Zonatuss, 132
Zonegran, 175
Zontivity, 81

zopiclone, 212
Zorbtive, 128
Zorcaine, 13
Zorprin, 3–4
Zortress, 167
Zorvolex, 4
Zostavax, 167
zoster vaccine—
live, 167
Zostrix, 104
Zostrix-HP, 104
Zosyn, 54
Zovia 1/35E,
182
Zovia 1/50E, 182
Zovirax, 37, 102
Zubsolv, 213

Zuplenz, 138
Zutripro, 132
Zyban, 204–205
Zyclara, 102
Zyflo CR, 222
Zylet, 196
Zyloprim, 230
Zyprexa,
208–209
Zyprexa Relprevv,
208–209
Zyprexa Zydis,
208–209
Zyrtec, 131
Zytram XL, 11
Zyvox, 57
Zyvoxam, 57

APPENDIX

ADULT EMERGENCY DRUGS (selected)

ALLERGY	diphenhydramine (*Benadryl*): 25 to 50 mg IV/IM/PO. epinephrine: 0.1 to 0.5 mg IM/SC (×1:1000 solution), may repeat after 20 minutes. methylprednisolone (*Solu-Medrol*): 125 mg IV/IM.
HYPERTENSION	esmolol (*Brevibloc*): 500 mcg/kg IV over 1 minute, then titrate 50 to 200 mcg/kg/min. fenoldopam (*Corlopam*): Start 0.1 mcg/kg/min, titrate up to 1.6 mcg/kg/min. labetalol: Start 20 mg slow IV, then 40 to 80 mg IV q10 min prn up to 300 mg total cumulative dose. nitroglycerin: Start 10 to 20 mcg/min IV infusion, then titrate prn up to 100 mcg/min. nitroprusside (*Nitropress*): Start 0.3 mcg/kg/min IV infusion, then titrate prn up to 10 mcg/kg/min.
DYSRHYTHMIAS / ARREST	adenosine (*Adenocard*): PSVT (not A-fib): 6 mg rapid IV and flush, preferably through a central line or proximal IV. If no response after 1-2 minutes, then 12 mg. A third dose of 12mg may be given prn. amiodarone: V-fib or pulseless V-tach: 300 mg IV/IO; may repeat 150 mg just once. Life-threatening ventricular arrhythmia: Load 150 mg IV over 10 min, then 1 mg/min × 6 h, then 0.5 mg/min × 18 h. atropine: 0.5 to 1 mg IV, repeat q 3-5 minutes prn to maximum of 3 mg. diltiazem (*Cardizem*): Rapid A-fib: bolus 0.25 mg/kg or 20 mg IV over 2 min. May repeat 0.35 mg/kg or 25 mg 15 min after 1st dose. Infusion 5-15 mg/h. epinephrine: 1 mg IV/IO q 3-5 minutes for cardiac arrest [1:10,000 solution]. lidocaine (Xylocaine): Load 1 mg/kg IV, then 0.5 mg/kg q 8-10 min prn to max 3 mg/kg. Maintenance 2 g in 250 mL D5W (8 mg/mL) at 1 to 4 mg/min drip (7-30 mL/h).
PRESSORS	dobutamine: 2 to 20 mcg/kg/min. 70 kg: 5 mcg/kg/min with 1 mg/mL concentration (e.g. 250 mg in 250 mL D5W) = 21 mL/h. dopamine: Start at 5 mcg/kg/min, increase prn by 5 to 10 mcg/kg/min increments at 10 min intervals, max 50 mcg/kg/min. 70 kg: 5 mcg/kg/min with 1600 mcg/mL concentration (e.g. 400 mg in 250 mL D5W) = 13 mL/h. Doses in mcg/kg/min: 2–4 = (traditional renal dose, apparently ineffective) dopaminergic receptors; 5–10= (cardiac dose) dopaminergic and beta1 receptors; >10 = dopaminergic, beta1, and alpha1 receptors. norepinephrine (*Levophed*): 4 mg in 500 mL D5W (8 mcg/mL), start 8 to 12 mcg/min (1 to 1.5 mL/h), usual dose once BP is stabilized 2 to 4 mcg/min. 22.5 mL/h = 3 mcg/min. phenylephrine: 20 mg in 250 mL D5W (80 mcg/mL), start 100 to 180 mcg/min (75 to 135 mL/h), usual dose once BP is stabilized 40 to 60 mcg/min (30 to 45 mL/h).
INTUBATION	etomidate (*Amidate*): 0.3 mg/kg IV. methohexital (*Brevital*): 1 to 1.5 mg/kg IV. propofol (*Diprivan*): 2.0 to 2.5 mg/kg IV. rocuronium (*Zemuron*): 0.6 to 1.2 mg/kg IV. succinylcholine (*Anectine, Quelicin*): 0.6 to 1.1 mg/kg IV. Peds (<5 yo): 2 mg/kg IV. thiopental: 3 to 5 mg/kg IV.
SEIZURES	diazepam (*Valium*): 5 to 10 mg IV, or 0.2 to 0.5 mg/kg rectal gel up to 20 mg PR. fosphenytoin (*Cerebyx*): Load 15 to 20 mg "phenytoin equivalents" (PE)/ kg IV, no faster than 100 to 150 mg PE/min. lorazepam (Ativan): Status epilepticus: 4 mg IV over 2 min, may repeat in 10-15 min. Anxiolytic/sedation: 0.04 to 0.05 mg IV/IM; usual dose 2 mg, max 4 mg. phenobarbital: Status epilepticus: 15 to 20 mg/kg IV load; may give additional 5 mg/kg doses q 15-30 mins to max total dose of 30 mg/kg. phenytoin (*Dilantin*): 15 to 20 mg/kg up to 1000mg IV no faster than 50 mg/min.

CARDIAC DYSRHYTHMIA PROTOCOLS (for adults and adolescents)

Chest compressions ~100/min. Ventilations 8-10/min if intubated; otherwise 30:2 compression/ventilation ratio. Drugs that can be administered down ET tube (use 2–2.5 × usual dose): epinephrine, atropine, lidocaine, naloxone, vasopressin*.

V-Fib, Pulseless V-Tach

Airway, oxygen, CPR until defibrillator ready
Defibrillate 360 J (old monophasic), 120–200 J (biphasic), or with AED
Resume CPR × 2 min (5 cycles)
Repeat defibrillation if no response
Vasopressor during CPR:
- Epinephrine 1 mg IV/IO q 3–5 minutes, or
- Vasopressin* 40 units IV to replace 1st or 2nd dose of epinephrine
Rhythm/pulse check every ~2 minutes
  Consider antiarrhythmic during CPR:
- Amiodarone 300 mg IV/IO; may repeat 150 mg just once
- Lidocaine 1.0–1.5 mg/kg IV/IO, then repeat 0.5–0.75 mg/kg to max 3 doses or 3 mg/kg
- Magnesium sulfate 1–2 g IV/IO if suspect torsades de pointes

Asystole or Pulseless Electrical Activity (PEA)

Airway, oxygen, CPR
Vasopressor (when IV/IO access):
- Epinephrine 1 mg IV/IO q 3–5 min, or
- Vasopressin* 40 units IV/IO to replace 1st or 2nd dose of epinephrine
Consider atropine 1 mg IV/IO for asystole or slow PEA. Repeat q 3–5 min up to 3 doses.
Rhythm/pulse check every ~2 minutes
Consider 6 H's: hypovolemia, hypoxia, H+acidosis, hyper/ hypokalemia, hypoglycemia, hypothermia
Consider 5 T's: Toxins, tamponade-cardiac, tension pneumothorax, thrombosis (coronary or pulmonary), trauma

Bradycardia, <60 bpm and Inadequate Perfusion

Airway, oxygen, IV
Prepare for transcutaneous pacing; don't delay if advanced heart block
Consider atropine 0.5 mg IV; may repeat q 3–5 min to max 3 mg
Consider epinephrine (2–10 mcg/min) or dopamine(2–10 mcg/kg/min)
Prepare for transvenous pacing

Tachycardia with Pulses

Airway, oxygen, IV
If unstable and heart rate >150 bpm, then synchronized cardioversion
If stable narrow-QRS (<120 ms):
- Regular: Attempt vagal maneuvers, If no success, adenosine 6 mg IV, then 12 mg prn (may repeat q 1),
- Irregular: Control rate with diltiazem or beta blocker (caution in CHF or severe obstructive disease).
If stable wide-QRS (>120 ms):
- Regular and suspect V-tach: Amiodarone 150 mg IV over 10 min; repeat prn to max 2.2 g/24 h. Prepare for elective synchronized cardioversion.
- Regular and suspect SVT with aberrancy: adenosine as per narrow-QRS above.
- Irregular and A-fib: Control rate with diltiazem or beta blocker (caution in CHF/ severe obstructive pulmonary disease).
- Irregular and A-fib with pre-excitation (WPW): Avoid AV nodal blocking agents; consider amiodarone 150 mg IV over 10 min,
- Irregular and torsades de pointes: magnesium 1–2 g IV load over 5–60 min, then infusion.

bpm=beats per minute; CPR=cardiopulmonary resuscitation; ET=endotracheal; IO=intraosseous; J=Joules; ms=milliseconds; WPW=Wolff-Parkinson-White. Sources: Circulation 2005; 112, suppl IV; *NEJM 2008;359:21–30 (demonstrated no benefit over epinephrine and worse long-term neurological outcomes).

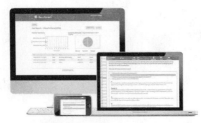
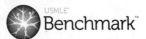